Blood and St

Blood and Steel

*Ryan White, the AIDS Crisis
and Deindustrialization
in Kokomo, Indiana*

RUTH D. REICHARD

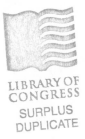
McFarland & Company, Inc., Publishers
Jefferson, North Carolina

ISBN (print) 978-1-4766-8489-5
ISBN (ebook) 978-1-4766-4264-2

LIBRARY OF CONGRESS AND BRITISH LIBRARY
CATALOGUING DATA ARE AVAILABLE

Library of Congress Control Number 2021017863

Cover image: Ryan White talking to reporters on February 21, 1986;
aerial view of Continental Steel Corporation, ca. 1950
(courtesy Howard County Historical Society, Kokomo, Indiana).

Printed in the United States of America

*McFarland & Company, Inc., Publishers
Box 611, Jefferson, North Carolina 28640
www.mcfarlandpub.com*

Writing these words during a new and frightening outbreak of a contagious disease, I am acutely aware of the emotional toll that sickness and death takes on both individuals and communities. To all who have endured, may we vow that the lives lost not have been in vain. We can learn from history, both recent and past, and change for the better.

This book is dedicated to anyone who has ever lost a job due to mismanagement, globalization, or the whims of our nation's unique type of capitalism. May the fact that you are not alone offer you some comfort.

This book is also dedicated to anyone who has ever faced prejudice and discrimination. To those who ever doubted whether they had enough courage to face another day, take heart from the example of Ryan White, his mother Jeanne, and his sister Andrea.

May Ryan's memory be a blessing.

Acknowledgments

I offer my profound thanks to Eric Sandweiss, who has been a patient and steadfast source of intellectual and academic support throughout this project. His insight and wisdom have made me a better writer, a better thinker, and a better scholar, and knowing him has also made me a better person. My sincere thanks also go to Michael McGerr, whose generous comments and critical inquiry were so helpful in conceptualizing this project. I also thank Colin Johnson, James Madison, Krista Maglen, Khalil Gibran Muhammad, and Nancy Robertson for pointing me in the right direction within their respective fields of expertise, and for their encouragement and collegiality.

I would also like to thank the dedicated and professional associates and staff of the Howard County Historical Society in Kokomo, Indiana, for their invaluable archival assistance with this project, particularly the then–Executive Director Dave Broman, Curator Stewart Lauterbach, Indiana University Emeritus Professor Allen Safianow, and Bonnie Van Kley. Thanks also to Doria Lynch, the historian at the United States District Court for the Southern District of Indiana, for her archival assistance. I am very grateful to the wonderful staff of the Children's Museum of Indianapolis for granting me unfettered access to their Ryan White Collection and for their warm hospitality and logistical support; in particular, Janna Bennett, Jennifer Nofze, Jennifer Pace-Robinson, and Louis Cavallari were especially helpful.

Very special thanks go to Jeanne White Ginder and Christopher Mac-Neil for allowing me to interview them about times past that were, in some respects, still very painful to recall even decades afterward. They were so generous with their time, and unfailingly gracious about recounting events that left an indelible mark on their lives for the historical record, even though I was a complete stranger to them both.

Finally, my deepest thanks go to my friends, for their good cheer, support, and inspiration, and to my family—especially Jean and Julia—for their love.

Table of Contents

Preface

In December 1984, 13-year-old Ryan White lay in a bed at Riley Children's Hospital in Indianapolis recovering from pneumocystis pneumonia. He had just learned the reason for his severe illness, along with the fevers, increasing weakness, and other health issues he had been battling the past several months: he had AIDS. In 1984, AIDS was not the chronic, treatable condition it is today—it was lethal. The primary question facing many AIDS patients in the 1980s was when, not if, they would die. Ryan, too, realized that he would die, but he could have had no inkling of what the next five-and-one-half years of his life would bring. He would be shunned—left alone and isolated by his community, unable to attend school, even ignored in church. But he would also become an international celebrity, receive thousands of cards and letters from around the world, appear in a made-for-TV movie about his life, and find himself a sought-after speaker, all before graduating from high school. His endurance in the face of these unexpected sources of pressure required that he defy not only his weak body but also the social norms that governed the behavior of the sick generally, as well as the more particular anxieties of an urban community seized by economic uncertainty.

By the time that HIV and AIDS first appeared in the West in the late 1970s, routine vaccinations had made many diseases of the past (including smallpox, polio, and diphtheria) unthinkable to boys Ryan's age. A purified water system ensured that cholera and typhoid fever were also consigned to history, and advances in immunology, virology, and bacteriology enabled swifter responses to new strains of influenza. But the appearance in the United States in 1979 of symptoms eventually associated with HIV and AIDS puzzled medical scientists and frightened everyone. During those early years, a leadership vacuum combined with a popular discourse of misinformation and prejudice to result in discrimination against the sick. For those infected with HIV and ill with AIDS, even the simple act of traveling from private to public space transgressed social and spatial

1

boundaries that had been erected centuries earlier, but in many ways sub-merged during subsequent years of steadily improved public health condi-tions. The case of Ryan White in Kokomo, Indiana, was one of a handful to spark nationwide debate over whether children infected with HIV should be allowed to attend public school. Ryan missed a year of school because of Western School Corporation's refusal to allow him to attend. According to his mother, Jeanne White Ginder, "It was really bad. People were really cruel, people said that he had to be gay, that he had to have done some-thing bad or wrong, or he wouldn't have had it. It was God's punishment, we heard the 'God's punishment' a lot. That somehow, some way he had done something he shouldn't have or he wouldn't have gotten AIDS."[1]

The question of whether Ryan White should be allowed to attend school divided his community. Kokomo residents fell into three camps: a passionately outspoken minority who feared that one undersized teenager could contaminate an entire school by his mere presence; a much quieter minority who believed strongly that the youth should be allowed to attend classes; and a very silent majority whose beliefs, prejudices, fears, and incli-nations went virtually unrecorded. Members of the latter group refused publicly to choose a side, although their silence effectively aided and abet-ted Ryan's opposition. Instead of defining themselves and staking out their positions, they left it to others on either extreme to assert that "most peo-ple" agreed with them. As they did so, media and popular perception con-structed an increasingly coherent image of Kokomo as an intolerant place populated by ignorant, mean-spirited folks. A proud, mid–American city of innovators and solid blue-collar values, Kokomo watched as outsiders defined it as a narrow and prejudiced place.

As emotions over Ryan White reached a boiling point in Kokomo, executives at the city's third-largest employer, Continental Steel, ordered the gates to its massive campus padlocked. After years of financial strug-gles, company officials had decided to file for bankruptcy, and any hope of restructuring the firm's debt (always a long shot) had recently vanished: the once-mighty steel mill would have to liquidate its assets. More than one thousand steelworkers would lose their jobs, their paychecks, and most of their pensions. The mill's closure came as the forces of global competi-tion, a declining American auto industry, and a weakening in the power of U.S. labor unions rendered Kokomo's working class especially vulnerable. Continental Steel had been a bulwark of the city's identity and economy for nearly a century; generations of families had worked in its mills and offices for secure pay with good benefits. The company was a solid citizen, its executives serving on local boards and its employees donating to the United Way. But a corporate takeover in the late 1960s, followed by poor management of its new parent company, slowly but inexorably robbed

Continental of its capital and contributed to its dire financial straits in the mid–1980s.

Like Ryan White's illness, Continental Steel's decline divided Kokomo; both labor and management engaged in finger pointing. Were the company's money troubles due to lackluster productivity and lazy workers, or foreign competition and cheap imported steel? Did Continental's debt arise from inept management with no real connection to the city, or a risky equipment upgrade worth millions of dollars? Newly jobless workers, who a few years earlier had agreed to make concessions resulting in lower wages, found themselves blamed for the company's woes and vilified for seeking government "handouts." Although Ryan White's opponents, armed with outrage and fear of a dreaded disease, could raise thousands of dollars for their cause in one weekend, ex-steelworkers had trouble making ends meet. Some gathered by their shuttered company just to pray.

And while fear of contamination forced Ryan and his family to endure ostracism in Kokomo's churches, schools, grocery stores, and restaurants, Continental Steel's closure revealed another, very real sort of contamination: the site was a toxic mess. Environmental inspections conducted shortly after the mill's closure uncovered evidence that the steel operation had been fouling the air, soil, and water on the city's west side for decades. Kokomo *was* contaminated, but not by the sick teenager, and it would take decades to remediate that damage, just as it would take decades to restore the city's image from the beating it took in the international media.

The story of Ryan White, Continental Steel, and the city of Kokomo, Indiana, is at its root a story of sickness and work in a midsized American city in the late twentieth century. Through the person of Ryan White, a frightening new illness connected itself to the sickness of a place, and the decline of one body paralleled the deindustrialization that threatened to unravel a whole town—like many Midwestern towns—during the 1980s. In Kokomo, the elements of blood and steel combined in a toxic mix of disease, stigma, decline, division, and mistrust—each marking the other in high relief. Ryan White, who had lived with a chronic blood disease his entire life, survived and even flourished after he learned of his AIDS diagnosis partly because of his steadfast refusal to take "no" for an answer. Those who opposed his public presence showed their mettle, as well, by resorting to lawsuits to keep him out of school and away from their children. But many of the same people who stigmatized Ryan and his family found themselves stigmatized by the nation's reaction to media accounts of Ryan's ill treatment. And as Ryan's immune system slowly broke down, so did a mainstay of his city's manufacturing economy—a site whose continued well-being in earlier decades had long contributed to the city's collective resistance to crisis. The two narratives—one of blood and the other of steel—joined one another in a larger tale of fear, disaster, division, and—ultimately—resilience.

AIDS in the 1980s spread far beyond cities such as New York, San Francisco, and Los Angeles. It affected men, women, and children in towns and cities across America—in places without gay enclaves, without chapters of ACTUP, and without gay pride marches: places where, in the words of Harry Britt, "they are not gay, because they are invisible." In short, AIDS happened in places like Kokomo, and Ryan White's very visible story helps bring to light the stories of the countless others whose stigmatization drove them underground. Likewise, deindustrialization spread beyond places like Detroit and Cleveland; many who lost their jobs in the 1970s and 1980s lived in cities, like Kokomo, that had become even more singularly dependent upon manufacturing. Continental Steel's story is a tragic example of the human costs of global economic change and the toll that dishonest corporate dealings took on local economies.[2]

Yet more than two decades after their demise, it may be easier to see Continental Steel's legacy as something more than a record of contamination and loss, just as it is clear that Ryan White deserves to be remembered as something more than a life cut too short. By exploring the intersection of blood and steel in Kokomo, Indiana, we can hope to better understand the powerful convergence of deindustrialization and of the AIDS pandemic as Americans experienced these phenomena in the 1980s. Americans' reaction to AIDS—and to people with AIDS—should not be considered in isolation from the larger social and economic context of events that formed the backdrop to AIDS' appearance, including in particular the economic uncertainty that affected so many American communities scarred by deindustrialization during those years. Interpreting AIDS in America during the 1980s requires a focus wider than the by-now familiar concern that historians and social critics have shown toward homophobia, puritanical attitudes toward sex, or the rise of the religious right—although these factors certainly played a part in Americans' collective response to the disease. Studies of deindustrialization, in turn, fail to include the manner in which the rise of AIDS and the increased visibility of gay Americans accompanied a decreasing faith in the ability of science, medicine, business, and technology to handle crises. In fact, by the 1980s, both the spread of HIV/AIDS and the widening reach of deindustrialization owed their prominence to the pivotal forces of globalization, capital, and commodification.

Choosing to focus on Ryan White, Continental Steel, and the city of Kokomo, Indiana, as subjects in the same story both augments and shifts existing scholarly conversations on AIDS and deindustrialization. The literature on—and from—the early years of the AIDS pandemic traverses the gamut from personal memoirs to contemporary chronicles, and from scientific and medical accounts to political, social, sexual, and cultural renderings. The memoirs of such diverse figures as Sean Strub, Shawn Decker, Jay Hoyle, Elton John, Kate Scannell, Cleve Jones, and C. Everett Koop all recount the frightening debut of the AIDS virus in the 1980s.[3] Decker, Koop, and Hoyle credit Ryan White with blazing a trail for students with AIDS, while John writes of the profound personal impact of his relationship with Ryan (and with Jeanne and Andrea, Ryan's mother and sister), a legacy that remains influential. Journalist Randy Shilts' riveting account of the beginning of the pandemic, *And the Band Played On*, is still vital reading, even with thirty years' hindsight, for its immediacy and urgency; *The Plague Years*, a collection of David Black's essays for *Rolling Stone*, offers a taste in real time of Western culture's response to the crisis, and it is not flattering.[4] Another contemporaneous account, David L. Kirp et al.'s *Learning by Heart: AIDS and Schoolchildren in America's Communities*, unsparingly documents the struggles of pupils like Ryan White in communities large and small.[5]

The works of physician Mirko D. Grmek in 1990, and of microbiologist Jacques Pepin twenty years later, both explore the virus's provenance, strive to identify the earliest human cases, and place the disease in its epidemiological context in light of available scientific knowledge.[6] Medical historians Charles Rosenberg and Allan Brandt, who wrote in the pandemic's early years, placed AIDS in historical, social, and biological perspective and injected often fearful contemporary discourse with much-needed reason; Victoria Harden's work, written from the vantage of the twenty-first century, built on that foundation.[7] An important subset of these historical accounts looked specifically at the relationship between the human immunodeficiency virus (HIV), hemophilia, and the blood products industry, and recounted the disastrous consequences for people dependent on those products; these works include Susan Resnik's *Blood Saga: Hemophilia, AIDS, and the Survival of a Community*, Douglas Starr's *Blood: An Epic History of Medicine and Commerce*, and Stephen Pemberton's *The Bleeding Disease: Hemophilia and the Unintended Consequences of Medical Progress*.[8] Finally, *Blood Feuds: AIDS, Blood, and the Politics of Medical Disaster*, edited by Eric A. Feldman and Ronald Bayer, contributed a very detailed global history of HIV, the blood supply, and policy decisions to the historical record.[9]

Of course, many scholars working outside the disciplinary boundary of medical history have also written on AIDS. Early collections of essays, produced in the 1980s, explored policy implications for health care, individual liberty, education, and community cohesion. *AIDS: Public Policy Dimensions*, edited by John Griggs and published in 1987, is a prime example of such work. *AIDS: The Burdens of History*, edited by Elizabeth Fee and Daniel M. Fox and published in 1988, sought to place the new disease in historical perspective. Its essays showed that a society's response to a fatal outbreak had much to teach observers about not just the law, gender, history, or popular culture, but also about human nature. The year 1990 brought *Culture and AIDS*, edited by Douglas A. Feldman, which broadened the scope of the discussion to include Rwanda, Haiti, and London, as well as women and heterosexual men. As the emergence of pharmacologic treatments for HIV lengthened the lifespans of the infected, Fee and Fox reprised their editorial roles in 1992 for *AIDS: The Making of a Chronic Disease*, which looked outward from the North American continent toward Japan, Africa, and the United Kingdom, while also delving into questions of law, public policy, the ethics of clinical trials, and discrimination. And more recently, Phil Tiemeyer, in his 2013 work *Plane Queer: Labor, Sexuality, and AIDS in the History of Male Flight Attendants*, tied the virus's spread to large U.S. metropolitan areas to the deregulation of the airlines and the development of the "hub and spoke" route system in the 1980s, while Richard McKay zoomed in on the need for a scapegoat in his 2017 *Patient Zero and the Making of the AIDS Epidemic*.[10]

Other historical writers have taken a more specialized approach to AIDS, choosing to narrow in on politics and activism. Cathy J. Cohen's *The Boundaries of Blackness: AIDS and the Breakdown of Black Politics* focused on AIDS' impact on African Americans in particular; Jennifer Brier's *Infectious Ideas: U.S. Political Responses to the AIDS Crisis* critically examined federal and local AIDS policy, AIDS activism, and international AIDS relief from the beginning of the pandemic in the early 1980s through the early 2000s. Michael P. Brown's *RePlacing Citizenship: AIDS Activism and Radical Democracy* employed an ethnographic approach to argue that individual responses to AIDS in Vancouver re-ordered the relationships between people and their government. Deborah B. Gould, a sociologist, wrote on the rise, division, and fall of AIDS activism in *Moving Politics: Emotion and ACTUP's Fight Against AIDS*, and Steven Epstein's *Impure Science: AIDS, Activism, and the Politics of Knowledge*, revealed a grassroots activism that challenged not only formal political power, but also the scientific knowledge surrounding AIDS itself.[11]

Finally, scholars have written about AIDS in the context of sexuality, the body, gender, and discourse and rhetoric. Cindy Patton looked critically at the discourse surrounding AIDS in its early years in her 1990 *Inventing AIDS*, while Lee Edelman's 2004 work, *No Future: Queer Theory and the Death Drive*, discussed the social construct of the "innocent child" trope and heteronormativity. In *AIDS and the Body Politic: Biomedicine and Sexual Difference*, Catherine Waldby examined the rhetoric of AIDS in the early 1990s as it related to the body, to medicine, and to sex, in order to expose the normative messages contained therein. All of these works on AIDS—whether they parse the social and cultural meanings behind public policy, chronicle important events, highlight the individual's struggle against a judgmental community, or explore the power relations embedded in a community's response to the disease—do justice to the complexity of many dimensions of the pandemic. But telling Ryan White's story, with an eye toward understanding how AIDS and deindustrialization together laid bare the tensions of late twentieth-century urban life, brings together narratives of stigma, individualism, deviance, economic decline, and insecurity in a way that the others do not.[12]

As they have the AIDS epidemic, historians and other observers of recent American life have written a great deal on late twentieth-century urban decline and deindustrialization. Robert A. Beauregard's *Voices of Decline: The Postwar Fate of U.S. Cities* traces the evolution of a consensus depiction of a general postwar downward trajectory, fueled partly by cities' unhealthy economic dependence on the federal government and partly by Americans' longstanding general ambivalence toward cities. The history of deindustrialization in America is largely woven from narrative strands that combine general studies of such phenomena as capital flight and the weakening power of unions with stories of individual communities and people affected by external economic forces. Depending on their focus, the authors of those studies identify the origins of deindustrialization at different moments. Thomas J. Sugrue, in *The Origins of the Urban Crisis: Race and Inequality in Postwar Detroit*, put the beginning of deindustrialization in the 1950s, while Jefferson Cowie, in *Capital Moves: RCA's Seventy-Year Quest for Cheap Labor*, traced its roots to labor unrest in Camden, New Jersey, in the 1930s. Geographer David Harvey, in *A Brief History of Neoliberalism*, contended that deindustrialization had been well underway by the time of the Nixon administration; however, most discussions of deindustrialization identify the 1970s and 1980s as its chronological epicenter.[13]

Barry Bluestone and Bennett Harrison's 1982 work, *The Deindustrialization of America: Plant Closings, Community Abandonment, and the Dismantling of Basic Industry*, first popularized the term "deindustrialization," which they defined as "a widespread, systematic disinvestment in the nation's basic productive capacity." Their leftist interpretation cited international competition, weakened unions, and a shift in American capital to overseas investments and conglomeration as the chief drivers of the phenomenon. Such shifts, which Bluestone and Harrison traced to the 1970s, were well underway by the time Continental Steel went bankrupt in 1986. Like Bluestone and Harrison, Steven Dandaneau's 1996 case study of Flint, Michigan, blamed the structure of capitalism itself for deindustrialization. His avowedly Marxist *A Town Abandoned: Flint, Michigan, Confronts*

Deindustrialization focused on what Dandaneau described as the "destructive and corrosive" impact a flawed economic system could have on a community.[14]

In a turn away from an economic systems analysis, historians such as Nelson Lichtenstein, in his *State of the Union: A Century of American Labor*, and Steve Babson, in *The Unfinished Struggle: Turning Points in American Labor, 1877–Present*, cited a decline in the power of American labor unions as a contributor to the tenuous state in which American workers found themselves in the 1980s. Both works characterized unions' influence as fluctuating throughout the twentieth century; Babson, writing in the late 1990s, marked the Reagan administration's defeat of the PATCO union during the air traffic controllers' strike as an important turning point. Thanks to increasing dissension over issues of race and gender since the mid–1960s, labor was already vulnerable in the early 1980s. That weakening unity, coupled with a new aggressiveness on the part of employers (as evidenced by the tactic of hiring "permanent replacements") during that decade, spelled doom for laborers. Never again would they enjoy the job security and benefits that enabled so many to prosper.[15]

Other works on deindustrialization and labor have focused on the tragic stories of communities and individuals. Steven High's evocative titles, *Industrial Sunset: The Making of North America's Rust Belt, 1969–1984* and *Corporate Wasteland: The Landscape and Memory of Deindustrialization*, are representative of this genre. High's 2003 *Industrial Sunset*, which compared plant closings and relocations in the United States and Canada, identified contributing factors that were all too familiar to the workers of Continental Steel: "technological change, declining product demand, poor management, bankruptcy, new environmental regulations, consolidation, disinvestment, high labour costs, and the advancing age of facilities." *Corporate Wasteland*, a 2007 collaboration between High and photographer David W. Lewis, combined oral histories and historical essays with stunning photographs of ruins to drive home the human toll of deindustrialization. In *Steeltown U.S.A.: Work and Memory in Youngstown*, Sherry Lee Linkon and John Russo portrayed the fragmentation of a community wrought by deindustrialization, while the work of Dale Maharidge and Michael S. Williamson—*Journey to Nowhere: The Saga of the New Underclass*—traveled beyond the rust belt to chronicle the stories of individuals dealing with the fallout from deindustrialization.[16]

These works, laudable for their exploration of capitalism's effects on communities and individuals, nevertheless give short shrift to the effects of other contemporaneous phenomena on the people and places on which they focus. The appearance of AIDS, in particular, revealed the unsettling doubts about the adequacy of science, medicine, and government to protect the common good, while the prejudices associated with the disease's sexual means of transmission posed vexing social questions of how to curb its spread as well as what to do with its "innocent victims," such as Ryan White, who contracted it by other means. As surely as plant closings and relocations split communities, so did the emergence of HIV/AIDS. Yet even later considerations of deindustrialization, such as Cowie and Heathcott's *Beyond the Ruins* and Ruth Milkman's *Farewell to the Factory*, though they extended beyond tales of job loss, nostalgia, victimization, and the "capitalist vs. community" binary, continued to focus on labor and economic systems at the cost of considering such pressing questions.[17]

Two books on deindustrialization and globalization, however, moved the discussion closer to Kokomo: Richard Longworth's 2008 *Caught in the Middle: America's Heartland in the Age of Globalism* posited that "what happens to America happens first to the Midwest." Longworth's hometown of Boone, Iowa, with its Friday night summertime band concerts, is "pure community and holds real value." "If we lose it," Longworth warned, "we lose something important to the American soul." Such statements beg the question of what, precisely, is the value of "pure community" to "the heartland" and, by extension, to America. In his 1993 *Cities of the Heartland: The Rise and Fall of the Industrial Midwest*, Jon C. Teaford endeavored to prove why the Midwest was a region distinct from the rest of America. As much as shared waterways, railroads, natural resources, and fertile soil, Teaford maintained, geography influenced the development of a particular mindset, a "common heartland consciousness" that stemmed from residents' "realization that for better or worse they were in the interior of the continent, removed from either coast and one giant step from access to the world beyond the seas." The heartland consciousness waxed and waned over time; in the late nineteenth and early twentieth centuries, the Midwest could proudly claim to be the "Land of Lincoln," the locus of the nation's political virtue, and the "All-American" norm. Later, however, the region's residents developed feelings of inferiority, as Midwestern cities assumed the role of "cultural colonies" of the Eastern coastal cities. Teaford tells us that this feeling of detachment from the nation's cultural and economic centers only worsened in the 1970s, as the industrial belt transformed into the rust belt and the notion of a "bicoastal" America acquired greater economic and cultural currency. By Teaford's formulation, both isolation and imitation marked the heartland consciousness during the time that the fates of Ryan White and Continental Steel intersected in Kokomo.[18]

Ultimately, the story of blood and steel in Kokomo during the 1980s relates the struggle between community and individual interests in a nation that valued both. What happened to the Whites exposed the idea of a heartland community, as Longworth has described it, as illusory. Arguably,

Kokomo came together as a community during this crisis, not to help a teen with a fatal disease but to oppose his agency, to thwart his assertion of his right to attend school, and to deny him his right to join them in the public sphere—surely not the type of community Longworth envisioned. This story adds complexity both to Longworth's communal ideal and to Teaford's idea of a heartland consciousness by reminding readers that communities—wherever they are—have fault lines. Both Ryan White's resistance to his community's will and Continental Steel's long and tortuous separation from the working lives of more than a thousand Kokomo workers caused breaks along the seams of class. As Robert and Helen Lynd had discovered in their *Middletown* study of nearby Muncie, Indiana, some fifty years earlier, two classes dominated the twentieth-century heartland city: the business class and the working class. Continental Steel's demise exposed ruptures between the two, as each blamed the other for the mill's downfall. Against that troubled backdrop, Ryan White and his family very publicly left the confines of their working-class status: they flew abroad, attended lavish fundraisers on the coasts, and consorted with celebrities.[19]

Other fault lines—less directly tied to class—also appeared. Ryan's insistence that he be allowed to mix with his healthy peers at public school challenged deeply embedded social mores that governed the behavior of sick people. The media's attention to this story—to the actions of one person and his family, and to their effect upon his community—inscribed these tensions into the national narrative for several years. As Thomas Bender and Robert Bellah et al. wrote at roughly the same historical moment, Americans had long sought community. If the boundaries of neighborhood, town, or census tract failed, in themselves, to provide that sense of common interest, then individuals sought out other networks of the like-minded. Shunned by the people of his original geographic community, Ryan White turned both to a new "home"—the small town of Cicero, Indiana—and to an extended network of supportive outsiders.[20]

The clash between individual agency and community harmony underlies the tale of AIDS and deindustrialization—of blood and steel—as it is related in this book. The first chapter, "Steel, Blood and Ryan White, 1896–1980: Capital and Commodification," lays the groundwork for later chapters by tracing the history of Continental Steel in Kokomo, providing a background on hemophilia, and introducing the reader to Ryan White, his family, and his city. The forces of capital, commodification, and globalization appear throughout this chapter, affect the destinies of both steel and blood, and proceed along parallel tracks of promise and despair. Businesses were eager to invest in the city of Kokomo, as its seemingly abundant supply of natural gas provided a constant source of power. However, misuse of that commodity spelled its ruin, just as mismanagement, capital flight, and global competition would eventually combine to doom Continental Steel. Wonderful scientific discoveries led to both the capitalization and the commodification, in the United States, of blood products, as well as to the promise of normality for people with hemophilia, at the same time those very products infected them with serious illnesses. Globalization enhanced the ability of the AIDS virus to travel and spread efficiently, while the symbolic commodification of hemophilia promised to endow its patients with political clout. The processes described initially in Chapter 1 played out to destructive ends through the rest of this story.

"Russian Roulette, 1980–1984," the second chapter, chronicles the early years of the AIDS pandemic. The title, of course, refers to risk: the risks involved in gay sex during those early years, when the transmissibility of the AIDS virus was unclear; the risk of infection that Ryan White took every time he used Factor VIII for his hemophilia; and the risks that the managers and laborers at Continental Steel took during those years when they gambled on the company's future and agreed to concessions so the firm could reorganize and stay afloat. Gambling is also an apt metaphor for the risks faced by the National Hemophilia Foundation, the blood industry, and government scientists, as they struggled to understand the extent to which a new disease originated in patients' blood, and as they wrestled with the political, economic, and public health implications of restricting blood donors and regulating blood products. Representatives of those interests took calculated risks in the early 1980s, and their willingness to prioritize the profitable, stable status quo over patient safety would not be exposed until a decade later. And, not surprisingly, the world steel economy seemed to be a game of chance to those laborers and managers caught up in the woes of Continental Steel. This chapter demonstrates the risks undertaken by steelworkers who agreed to forego raises and benefits in the hopes of a big payout down the line.

Chapter 3, "'Somewhere, there's going to be that first student with AIDS wanting to go to school': 1985 and the Question of Public Knowledge," relates the beginnings of the conflict between Ryan White and his family and the communities of Kokomo and Russiaville. We learn that the self-image of Kokomo as a forward-thinking "City of Firsts" did not envision a "first" involving a child with AIDS wishing to attend public school. Jeanne White begins to understand that her hometown was not the welcoming place she thought it was, and that her neighbors and co-workers might abandon her instead of help her. The Whites' decision to disclose Ryan's condition was exceptional—most families in their position went underground, hid their diagnoses, and stayed silent. The events of this chapter center around the conflict between what is rightfully public knowledge, what information should be private, and on both the quantity and quality of the information imparted to the public. Many media organs chose to publish hysterical and speculative pieces on the AIDS crisis; what factual information they did share within an article was often obscured by a manipulative cover story designed for shock value. It is little wonder, then, that many people with hemophilia, AIDS, and HIV did not discuss their health—they kept their status a secret. Similarly, managers at Continental Steel were faced with a decision about how much to share about their company's health, or lack thereof, in 1985. Questions remained about how much the board knew—and when—as shareholders, steelworkers, and the public all wanted to believe the optimistic corporate pronouncements of an improving financial trajectory.

Chapter 4, "Four Months in a Blast Furnace: December 1985–March 1986," relates how the two main elements of this story—Ryan White and Continental Steel—converged in the same eventful week in late February 1986, to drive wedges into the community. Ryan's opponents came together and found their voice, but their message was not received warmly outside of Howard County. And, after a period of uncertainty, the legal die was finally cast for Continental's workers when officials decided to liquidate the company's assets. Incredibly, the gates to the plant were locked the very same week that Ryan White's return to school brought throngs of reporters to Kokomo. Both locally and nationally, AIDS and deindustrialization divided people into factions: healthy vs. unhealthy, straight vs. gay, employed vs. unemployed, and labor vs. management. Once-stable identities and once-secure positions of power began to shift during these months in response to the seismic forces of job loss and incurable disease.

The conflict, division, and stigmatization that started in early 1986 deepen in Chapter 5, "'He's the good guy, and I'm the bad guy': February 1986–May 1987." The nurturing civic image promoted by Kokomo radio station WWKI's "WE CARE" campaign belied the worsening experiences of both the White family and the displaced workers of Continental Steel in 1986 and 1987. The binary nature of the quotation in the chapter's title—good and bad—conveys a sense of the sharpness of the disagreements that divided the city. Citizens of Kokomo were either for the steelworkers, or against them. They either stood with the "Concerned Parents" who sued to keep Ryan White out of school, or they kept quiet—there was no middle ground in either conflict. Beyond Kokomo's city limits, national media constructed an equally stark narrative, pitching Ryan White as the good guy and Kokomo's citizens, collectively, as the bad guy.

In Chapter 6, "'I am ashamed to admit that I even live here!': Stigma and Transformation, 1987–1990," the town of Cicero, Indiana, emerges to supply the media with their "good guy," the attractive community that accepted Ryan and his family. The Whites' new neighbors welcomed them, and Ryan's fellow high school students included him as one of the crowd. Learning to drive and working part-time at a skateboard shop, he enjoyed the feeling of being a normal teenager, even as his peers and their families in his former home found themselves demonized in the popular media. Just as Ryan's life was transformed by the move, Americans' attitudes toward people with AIDS also began to undergo a slow transformation, as HIV-positive citizens began to beat back against relentless stigmatization. Ryan's old hometown felt the sting of national opprobrium, as a television movie of Ryan's story portrayed Kokomo as a regressive, mean-spirited place while depicting Cicero as a paragon of tolerance and enlightenment. The shame compounded in Kokomo, meanwhile, as the city learned the true extent of the environmental contamination left behind by Continental Steel.

Finally, Chapter 7, "Blood, Steel and Ryan White: Erasure and Visibility, 1990–2020," completes the stories of hemophilia, HIV/AIDS, and Continental Steel that were introduced in Chapter 1. Out of medical, social, economic, and environmental catastrophe has emerged hope, a measure of justice, remediation, and resilience. The impact of Ryan White's life and death has extended beyond his home to the nation. Jeanne White, embracing her identity as "Ryan's mom," finds herself leaving her job at Kokomo's Delco plant, lobbying in the halls of Congress, speaking at events all over the country, and, most importantly, working with the Children's Museum of Indianapolis to create an exhibition, *The Power of Children*. That exhibition, which ties Ryan's story to those of Anne Frank, Ruby Bridges, and, soon, Malala Yousafzai, uses the children's courageous actions to teach museumgoers that one person can make a difference in the world. The narrative of Ryan White's AIDS experience has been made visible for thousands to witness. The element of blood, as it relates to HIV/AIDS, likewise equates with visibility in this chapter. People with hemophilia emerge in the public arena as powerful agents who agitate for reform and restitution. Back in Ryan's old community of Kokomo, Indiana, however, residents find the events of the 1980s do not lend themselves to a simple story line. The element of steel in Kokomo—as in so many communities that experienced factory closures, job loss, and abandonment—becomes associated with erasure. Here, where chimneys once spewed smoke into the sky and waste heaps piled high next to busy neighborhoods, now sit flat, quiet, grassy expanses of land.

I close with two brief notes on sources. First, how I used a particular work determined whether I treated it as a primary source—in the sense that it served as an artifact—as opposed to a secondary source. Therefore, non-scholarly pieces written contemporaneously with the events that inspired them, such as David Black's work for *Rolling Stone*, or accounts that described a subject's thoughts and feelings about the events of the

1980s, such as Shawn Decker's memoirs or Jay Hoyle's remembrance of his son in *Mark*, qualified as primary sources for me as I conducted research, and are listed as such in the Bibliography. Second, the reader will observe that I quote from Ryan White's memoir (*Ryan White: My Own Story*, co-written with Ann Marie Cunningham and published posthumously in 1992) and Jeanne White's memoir (*Weeding Out the Tears: A Mother's Story of Love, Loss, and Renewal*, co-written with Susan Dworkin and published in 1997). Again, I treated them as primary sources that provided special insight into the events as the Whites experienced them. I established a factual timeline of events based on newspaper accounts and other independent documentary evidence (such as government records) and noted the very few times when the record I pieced together appeared to differ from the accounts in the Whites' memoirs. I was able to interview Jeanne White in person and ask her questions to help me clarify matters, so that I could portray the events recounted herein as accurately and faithfully as possible.

1

Steel, Blood
and Ryan White,
1896–1980

Capital and Commodification

Steel, blood, capital, and commodification would all prove fateful to the stories of Ryan White, Continental Steel, and the city of Kokomo in the 1980s. Although the city of Gary has historically been Indiana's best-known steel producer, Kokomo was also home to significant metals industries. It was there that Elwood Haynes invented several alloys in the early twentieth century, including a type of stainless steel in 1911. This chapter recounts the origins of the city's oldest steel company, Continental Steel, Kokomo's largest employer for many years. We also witness the beginning of its end, as a combination of market forces, industrial conglomerates, and one man's criminal misdeeds brought a bastion of the city's economy to its knees. Unfortunately for Continental Steel, just when it was at the height of its potential—stable, profitable, and well-maintained—it became attractive to a conglomerate whose leader plundered its capital and drained its liquid assets. Continental might have survived that attack if not for the fact that it, along with the entire United States steel industry, also faced a volatile global market with strong international competition, often funded by American banks. As Ryan White entered adolescence, Continental, a mainstay of Kokomo industry for more than eight decades, faced the prospect of locking its doors forever.[1]

As for blood, had Ryan not had severe hemophilia and needed regular, frequent treatments with a clotting factor, he most likely would not have contracted HIV. In the years just prior to his birth in 1971, rapid advancements in the treatment of hemophilia had enabled patients, for the first time in history, to enjoy life spans approaching those of the general population. Researchers had scored a victory against a ravaging and painful

15

disease, but the sophisticated science that empowered people like Ryan to administer the lifesaving blood products at home, as often as necessary, also carried a terrible risk. The treatments Ryan and his fellow hemophilia patients came to rely upon were, like steel, also subject to market forces. After World War II, an entire industry concerned with blood services and blood products arose. Just as conglomerates swallowed steel mills in order to increase profits, so too did pharmaceuticals and medical laboratories expand into the blood sector in the pursuit of profits. When researchers' discoveries fostered the production of portable, do-it-yourself injectable treatments for severe hemophilia, the blood industry charged as much as the market would bear for those treatments and exported their products worldwide. In the United States, thanks to labor unions' ability to negotiate "Cadillac" health insurance plans for automotive workers such as Ryan's mother, working-class families like the Whites could afford these wonder drugs. The patients got amazing treatments, and the blood industry got a golden ticket. But the expansion of scientific knowledge, the organization of families with hemophilia and growing visibility of the disease, and the promise of capital returns to large corporations all carried some drawbacks—chiefly the fact that the product carried incurable viruses.

This chapter explains how two vital commodities—steel and blood—when mixed with the forces and processes of capital, globalization (especially after the Second World War), and commodification, would become so integral to understanding the events of the 1980s in Kokomo.

Steel

In 1911, returning to Indiana after lengthy stays in Europe and New York City, Hoosier author Booth Tarkington remarked on the many changes to his "native soil." The always-keen observer noted that the "flat lands were bleaker than they had been aforetime; the ground was dark and fertile, but great stretches of forest were gone, leaving only clumps of woodland here and there." The farms' "old bosky 'snake fences' had disappeared, replaced by unamiable wire." Those wire fences, while suggesting to Tarkington a less friendly rural life than he had known, were the material embodiment of the prosperous, innovative, industrial economy of the north-central Indiana city of Kokomo.[2]

The Kokomo Fence Machine Company was founded in 1896 with an investment of $6,000 by John E. Frederick, J.H. Strofe, and Harry Ward. Earlier decades had seen important innovations in agriculture, such as the reaper, which enabled farmers in Indiana and elsewhere to expand production to unprecedented levels. As a nostalgic Tarkington would later observe, those farmers had begun to replace their traditional, split-rail wooden fences with fences made from wire, and Frederick, Strofe, and Ward had devised a portable machine that customers could use in the field. Farmers attached horizontal wires to a line of fence posts, and then used the machine to "weave" stays together. Although the process was slow and the results crude, there was a great demand for the fence weaving machine—so much so that after just three years, the Kokomo Fence Machine Company expanded, consolidated with other firms, and became the Kokomo Nail & Wire Company. As its name indicated, the new company produced wire and nails, as well as staples, in addition to the portable hand weaving fence machine. Kokomo Nail & Wire did not manufacture its own steel—instead, it produced the goods from steel rods it bought from other steel companies. By 1900, the company's stock had doubled in value, and a year later, it reorganized once again; capitalized at $1,000,000, its new name was the Kokomo Steel & Wire Company. In 1904, even in the wake of the collapse of Indiana's gas boom, Kokomo Steel & Wire was a $2,000,000 business.[3]

Although the city had been incorporated in 1854, the discovery of natural gas in the area in 1886 served as the real beginning of Kokomo's industrial path. Indiana historian James Glass notes that makers of glass, paper, and other materials flocked to Kokomo, lured by cheap and ample supplies of gas to power their ventures. Local businesses formed the Kokomo Improvement Company, which promised manufacturers cash subsidies and help with land acquisition in addition to affordable energy. The incentives worked: by the mid–1890s, Kokomo was the state's foremost "Gas Belt" city, outranking Marion, Muncie, and Anderson. The city's imposing city hall, built in 1893 despite the national economic depression, reflected its new prosperity.[4]

It was during these boom years that Kokomo began to associate its success with innovation. The commodification of natural gas attracted capital to the growing urban hub. Inventors like Elwood Haynes, who produced one of the first gasoline-powered automobiles there in 1894; D.C. Spraker, who invented the pneumatic rubber tire, also in 1894; and William "Billy" Johnson, developer of the first aluminum casting in 1895, all contributed to Kokomo's new nickname, "The City of Firsts." Haynes would go on to develop significant advances in the field of metallurgy— his high-performance alloys served as the foundation for a business that still thrives today (and is still headquartered in Kokomo), Haynes International.[5]

Although state geologist S.S. Gorby warned of a looming problem as early as 1889, cities and manufacturers splurged on natural gas. Glass quotes Gorby's report that "an average of 100 million cubic feet of gas were being wasted *each day* through wells and flambeaux" alone. (Cities and gas companies would regularly show off their abundant supplies of natural gas, and provide a scenic attraction to boot, by allowing the fires from the wells—"flambeaux"—to burn continuously throughout the day and night.) The state recorded declines in gas pressure throughout the 1890s; in response, the General Assembly passed conservation legislation and banned flambeaux in 1891. Indiana natural gas supervisor E.T.J. Jordan recommended selling gas under a metered system instead of using flat rates or simply providing it free to industrial concerns. Both producers and consumers largely ignored the official warnings, however, and gas pressure fell from its earlier peak of 325 pounds per cubic inch to below 100 pounds in 1901. Despite the reduction in its cheap energy supply, Kokomo Steel & Wire stayed put. In fact, the company expanded in 1901 by building a rod mill, which enabled it to produce its own steel rods (albeit from billets bought elsewhere) at a capacity of 250 tons a day.[6]

Two years later, in 1903, Kokomo Steel & Wire developed a machine that fabricated woven wire fencing in its own plant. The machine bundled the fencing in rods, which the company shipped to farmers in nearly every state. In 1914, the company decided at last to supply its own steel and built two 75-ton open-hearth furnaces that produced ingots, as well as a 34-inch blooming mill, which rolled the ingots into billets, or slabs, of steel. The mill then transformed the billets into wire rods. Kokomo Steel & Wire became a major supplier of steel during the Great War, shipping 30,000 tons of steel abroad before building its third open-hearth furnace in 1917. A 1918 *Kokomo Daily Tribune* article noted the firm's expansion and praised architects' conversion of a former machine plant into a "beautiful and artistic" workspace for its office and clerical staff, and described "a wealth of room, plenty of light and ventilation." After the war, the company supplied much of Europe with wire, nails, and fences to aid in the rebuilding effort, even as it continued to maintain its more traditional agricultural customer base.[7]

In 1927, Kokomo Steel & Wire merged with a Canton, Ohio, firm, Superior Sheet Steel, and an Indianapolis concern, Chapman Price Steel. The new entity, which now offered customers sheet steel in addition to its existing wire products, was called the Continental Steel Corporation. The Kokomo plant added two more open-hearth furnaces, a 19-inch continuous sheet bar and billet mill, and a separate sheet mill in the interwar years. As Continental added capacity and diversified its output, it also steadily expanded its customer base to include residential and industrial customers along with its agricultural buyers. The coming of the Second World War meant more defense-related production (barbed wire, nails, and sheet steel), and the company saw further expansions at the Kokomo plant after World War II. As the war had left German and Japanese steel manufacturers reeling, American companies such as Continental enjoyed a clear path to profit in the 1940s and 1950s while the defeated nations rebuilt their heavy industries. During these years, global competition was of little concern to the leaders of the U.S. steel powerhouses. Indeed, some manufacturers arguably became overconfident and failed to innovate—they kept their open-hearth furnace technology while their European and Japanese competitors incorporated the new, much faster basic oxygen steelmaking process into their rebuilt plants.[8]

Continental sold off its Superior Sheet Steel properties in 1946 and Chapman Price a year later, leaving the Kokomo location as its major producer. The company embarked on a program of continuous improvements over the following decades, including the addition of a $7.5 million continuous rod mill in 1953; a welded fabric department in 1955; a nail mill and warehouse in 1958; new shipping facilities in 1963; two new 150-ton electric furnaces to replace its five open-hearth furnaces in 1965; and a wire galvanizing unit in 1967. All of these modifications enabled Continental to increase its production of steel assembly to 455,000 tons annually by 1970. Continental products—nails, wire, fences, rods, and sheets—had helped rebuild European infrastructure twice, strengthened the domestic agricultural economy, and solidified Kokomo's place as an industrial heavyweight.[9]

In the late 1940s and early 1950s—"boom years" for Kokomo's manufacturing economy—jobs were plentiful at factories such as Delco, Haynes Stellite, and Pittsburgh Plate Glass, among others. Continental Steel, though, was Kokomo's largest employer at mid-century. Generations of residents had grown up counting on jobs at Continental after they finished high school or finding temporary work over the summers to help pay for college. The firm was also a good corporate citizen. Steve Daily, a former Continental employee who would go on to become the mayor of Kokomo in the 1980s, recalled that in the post–World War II years, newly hired workers typically signed three pieces of paper: an authorization for the company to take money out of their paychecks for hard hats, safety glasses, and steel-toed boots; a union dues card; and a card authorizing automatic payroll deductions for United Way contributions. Company executives regularly filled posts at the local Chamber of Commerce and served on boards of charitable and community organizations. Continental would continue to be one of the city's largest employers well into the 1980s, when only General Motors' Delco operation and Chrysler's transmission plant outranked it. Profitable, well-managed, and equipped with a stable workforce, it was also, by the late 1960s, an attractive target for a takeover. That—along with the reentry of Germany and Japan into world steel markets—was the beginning of its demise.[10]

The steel industry as a whole experienced a unique shift in the late 1960s, and Continental was destined to become a part of the trend. Four "intra-industry" mergers between nine steel companies, and ten "inter-industry" mergers involving ten steel companies and other firms— often conglomerates—occurred between 1968 and 1971. These seismic changes happened rapidly: the ten inter-industry mergers took place in 1968 and 1969 alone. By 1970, conglomerates owned more than 20 percent of the United States' primary metals manufacturers. These mergers, especially those involving conglomerates, had two major ramifications for the domestic steel industry. First, the steel unions saw their bargaining position during strikes weaken significantly, because large, diverse conglomerates could always shut down their steel divisions and still accrue profits from their other businesses instead of negotiating with the unions. Second, conglomerates bought solvent firms like Continental Steel, drained them of their assets for the sake of being able to show a short-run profit on paper, and then watched the venerable manufacturers dissolve. As the arrival of cheaper products from the United Kingdom, Europe, and Japan caused prices for steel to falter, the conglomerates' vampire-like behavior could not have come at a worse time.[11]

The conglomerate that ultimately bought Continental Steel was the New York–based Penn-Dixie Industries. Penn-Dixie Industries had begun as Penn-Dixie Cement, which it remained until 1967, when 32-year-old Jerome Castle bought it and expanded it into ventures such as construction, aggregates, chemicals, leasing, and steel. Castle, born Jerome Kesselman, had started his career as a broker in the mid–1950s. He was once suspended from trading for a month by the National Association of Securities Dealers because of questionable practices; after that incident, he changed his last name to Castle and went to work for another brokerage firm. A friend of Castle's persuaded the Axe-Houghton mutual funds to invest heavily in Penn-Dixie Cement stock, and Castle himself then persuaded Axe-Houghton's outside directors to back him against the cement company's existing management staff. When several of Castle's brokerage customers chipped in more capital, he took over the company. The board of directors of the newly constituted Penn-Dixie Industries included Castle himself as its chair, Castle's first wife, and four of Castle's longtime associates, including one who had helped Castle finance the initial takeover. These board members, Castle insiders all, regularly approved lavish compensation packages for their chairman (including $761,000 in cash and stock in 1975), placing him among the top five earners in *Forbes* magazine's list of highly paid American executives during the 1970s.[12]

Castle's generous pay, and the formation of the conglomerate through the purchase of other companies, came at the expense of Penn-Dixie's profits. The firm earned millions less in the mid–1970s than it had in 1967, when Castle bought the cement company, and its stock price lost half its value in that short time. "Virtually debt-free," according to *Forbes*, at the time of Castle's takeover, by the second quarter of 1976, Penn-Dixie was "more than $55 million in debt, with $33 million in unfunded pension liability" and $20 million owed to banks.[13]

Under Castle's direction, Penn-Dixie purchased Continental Steel in 1969 for an inflated price, which it paid primarily with Penn-Dixie's pension funds—essentially borrowed money. Due in large part to that purchase, Penn-Dixie's banks "came close to shutting [Castle] down; only the sale of Penn-Dixie's prize cement plant bailed the company out," according to *Forbes*. After that near miss with his creditors, Castle attempted to acquire the Continental hourly workers' pension fund in order to access liquid capital. However, the steelworkers in Kokomo went on strike and returned to work only after Castle backed away. Despite those dramatic events, in April 1973, Continental Steel shareholders approved plans for a merger with Penn-Dixie.[14]

The Securities and Exchange Commission began an investigation of Castle in 1977, and a federal grand jury indicted him and two others on fraud and conspiracy charges in October 1978. In the summer of 1979, Castle's first trial ended in a mistrial when the jury was unable to reach a unanimous verdict. The second trial began on August 20, 1979; nine days later, a federal jury convicted Castle of conspiracy, mail fraud, and wire fraud. In October, a judge sentenced him to 15 months in prison and a $12,000 fine; he also faced numerous civil suits.[15]

All of this occurred against a backdrop of steel shortages and global recession during the early to mid–1970s, and a worldwide oversupply of steel afterward, which lasted into the early 1980s. As American laborers coped with these fluctuations, steelmakers' debt increased amidst a shortage of capital, all while U.S. banks loaned hundreds of millions of dollars to foreign steel companies in the 1970s. For example, Citibank, Chase Manhattan, Bank of America, and other household names increased their loans to the six largest Japanese firms by 270 percent in just two years. These market forces, combined with a general pattern of disinvestment on the part of many American steel companies and slow but steady deindustrialization among the U.S. manufacturers, spurred a wave of plant closings and bankruptcy reorganizations between 1978 and 1982, resulting in the loss of more than 150,000 steel industry jobs during the same period. Among the casualties was Penn-Dixie Steel in Kokomo.[16]

Continental's parent company had not invested in improvements to the plant, despite the company's 70-year history of steadily upgrading its facilities and expanding its manufacturing capability. The steel operation had remained reasonably profitable into the mid–1970s despite Castle's dubious stewardship, but Penn-Dixie milked the steel plant for some $35 million without making the capital improvements needed to keep it competitive. Penn-Dixie dropped sheet steel from its product line in 1970. To make matters worse, during the global shortage in 1973–1974, the New York headquarters diverted supplies of the Kokomo plant's steel away from established customers and toward Castle's associates. One friend alone received 20 percent of the plant's 240,000 tons of total production during this period. According to *Inc.* magazine, "when the steel shortage turned to a glut by late 1975, this mistreatment of old customers devastated the Kokomo mill. Orders fell by more than 30 percent, and for the first time in its history, the company went into the red." Customers began to leave while cheaper imports further eroded the dominance of the American steel industry as a whole; in 1978, for example, imports filled nearly one-fifth—18.1 percent— of the U.S. appetite for steel. A casualty of disinvestment, mismanagement, and a cutthroat global environment, Penn-Dixie Steel filed for Chapter 11 bankruptcy reorganization on April 7, 1980.[17]

Blood

Although Hoosiers embraced innovation and modernity in industry and business, their mindset was very different when it came to innovations in policy and government—especially on those occasions when public health and public policy intersected. It had not always been so. The Indiana State Board of Health, established in 1881, lay relatively quiescent until a committed reformer, Dr. John N. Hurty, took its helm in 1896. During Hurty's 26-year tenure, the Board of Health tackled such public health problems as the food-, water-, and milk-borne diseases of typhoid and tuberculosis, which eventually led to better sanitation infrastructure around the state.[18]

Hurty's leadership also ushered in an unprecedented level of attention to children's health, which continued when Dr. Ada E. Schweitzer headed up the all-female Division of Infant and Child Hygiene—a department that became especially active during the 1920s. Fortunately for Schweitzer, in 1921 Congress passed the Sheppard-Towner Act, which allotted both direct and matching funds to state governments for education on maternal and infant health; in 1923, the Indiana General Assembly enacted legislation in order to qualify for the funds. The funds enabled Schweitzer to grow her staff, sponsor conferences on child health, organize lectures around the state on the importance of proper nutrition, advocate for pre- and post-natal care, develop literature and films, and achieve measurable improvements in infant mortality, children's weight gain, and infant diarrhea rates. Unfortunately for Schweitzer, however, the receipt of federal dollars with strings attached proved an intensely controversial notion in a state and nation infused with paranoia toward the political Left in the wake of the 1917 Russian Revolution. Both the American Medical Association and the Indiana State Medical Association (ISMA) had actively fought the Sheppard-Towner Act, which conservatives viewed as "an unwarranted, even radical, interference of government in individual and private concerns." Closer to home, the ISMA vocally criticized Schweitzer for failing to "provide a sufficiently large role for organized medicine," and charged that the "publicly-supported work interfered with the private practice of physicians in Indiana." In fact, the battle against the Division of Infant and Child Hygiene was part of a larger war waged by doctors' associations during the Red Scare against "state" or "socialized" medicine in the interwar years. The ISMA even opposed using the Indiana state laboratory for Wasserman tests for syphilis during the early 1930s and argued that the government engaged in unfair competition with private practitioners.[19]

Decades later, the legacy of mistrust and resentment of centralized government—whether it be the federal government in Washington, D.C., or the one located in the state capital, Indianapolis—would prove to be an important force in the story of the contaminated blood that entered the body of one Kokomo boy. Time and again in the 1980s, the people of Kokomo and its neighboring town of Russiaville both ignored and opposed the recommendations of the Indiana State Department of Health, the Board of Special Education Appeals, or even the Centers for Disease Control or National Institutes of Health, just because of their source.

The earliest historical references to bleeding disorders, and probably hemophilia, occurred as long ago as the second century CE, in rabbinical rulings exempting third-born sons from circumcision if two older male siblings had died from the procedure. During the eighteenth and nineteenth centuries, medical writers variously described "bleeders" and a "bleeding disease"; the term "hemophilia" first appeared in 1828. People with hemophilia (the vast majority of them male) have a genetic anomaly on the X chromosome that prevents their blood from clotting in a timely fashion. The disease, which is a "sex-linked recessive disorder," is usually transmitted from a mother to her son. According to Susan Resnik:

> this defective gene restricts the production of one of two essential clotting factors, known as Factor VIII and Factor IX. Lack of Factor VIII (also known as anti-hemophilic factor or AHF) results in what is called hemophilia A or "classical hemophilia"; lack of Factor IX (or plasmathromboplastin component) causes hemophilia B, also known as "Christmas disease," after a British family that had this form of the disease.

Depending on how much active clotting factor is present in a patient's blood, hemophilia is classified in one of three levels of severity: mild, moderate, and severe. People with mild hemophilia have the greatest amount of active clotting factor—between 5 and 50 percent of normal; for them, dental procedures, surgery, or trauma can trigger excessive bleeding, but they will not experience spontaneous bleeds into their joints and muscles. People with moderate hemophilia have clotting activity between 1 and 5 percent of the normal range; they will endure excessive bleeding for minor injuries, but, like those with the mild form, do not usually encounter spontaneous bleeding. People with severe hemophilia—unfortunately, the majority—have a clotting factor of less than 1 percent of normal. They suffer from spontaneous bleeding into their joints and muscles, which causes extreme pain as well as crippling orthopedic problems. Surgery and dental work can become life-threatening events.[20]

People with hemophilia endured brief, isolated, and painful lives until well into the twentieth century, when even a simple dental procedure—pulling a tooth—could mean death. Before the Second World War, most boys with the disease died between the ages of 12 and 19. Resnik quotes one of the few survivors of that era to live to an old age, Ben Lederman, who wrote in the early 1980s of his parents' fear that he would bleed to death when he was circumcised, and his subsequent avoidance of surgery for the next 60 years. For contemporary readers, Lederman described the various treatments he had endured in the 1930s: vitamins, brewer's yeast, cod liver oil, and "*fasting* for 48 hours was naturally the final prescription for getting a good clot…. [Even] a subcutaneous injection of cottonmouth moccasin venom was given … some of us are still hissing." As late as the end of the 1940s, people with hemophilia had a life expectancy of less than 30 years. Treatment consisted of icing joints where internal bleeding occurred and painful, time-consuming, expensive transfusions of whole blood. Whole-blood transfusions persisted as the primary means of treatment (for those who could afford them) into the 1950s. The suffering of people with hemophilia was often compounded by the financial strain on their families of lengthy hospital stays without health insurance.[21]

Nevertheless, the years immediately around World War II did bring developments that offered some hope: the nation's first blood bank was established at Chicago's Cook County Hospital in 1937. In 1941, scientists discovered how to separate plasma from whole blood in a process called fractionation, which led researchers to discover the problem with hemophilia patients' blood was in their plasma, not their platelets. (Eventually, physicians would transfuse people with hemophilia with only plasma.) In 1947, hospital-based and community blood centers formed an organization, the American Association of Blood Banks, as a counterweight to the American Red Cross's influence on policies and supply. And, in 1948, the National Institute of Health merged with other entities to become the National Institutes of Health, part of the U.S. Public Health Service. The NIH would become a significant source of funding for research involving hemophilia. Perhaps most importantly, that same year, Robert Lee Henry, a New York attorney and father of a son with hemophilia, established the Hemophilia Foundation, the precursor to the National Hemophilia Foundation (NHF). This development arguably marks the beginning of the symbolic commodification of hemophilia. Historian Keith Wailoo discusses the concept of the commodification of a disease in his examination of sickle cell anemia and the city of Memphis, Tennessee, *Dying in the City of the Blues: Sickle Cell Anemia and the Politics of Race and Health*. In the 1950s in particular, Wailoo writes, "[n]ew and tragic maladies, far from being civic blemishes or social burdens, were now positive centerpieces of social, political and economic relations." In essence, the commodification of a disease entails social, political, and economic processes that implicate both identity and power. In the United States, *who* gets sick matters. Society writ large responds differently to the suffering of those with power than it does to the suffering of those who, for whatever reason—race, class, sex, or sexuality—are powerless. What is important, Wailoo maintains in both *Dying in the City of the Blues* and his later *Pain: A Political History*, is to leverage the sympathy of liberal society to one's advantage. By establishing the foundation, Henry helped to legitimize hemophilia patients as people who deserved both society's notice and the drug companies' attention. A foundation affords one a seat at the table when blood banks and pharmaceuticals meet with government regulators; it enables one to raise funds from sympathetic donors; and it educates the public about both the sufferers and the symptoms of the disease. The creation of a foundation associated with a disease, with a board, a logo, an office, and a staff, enables the creation of an identity for its patients—a person with hemophilia—and in turn facilitates political power. The expansion of the federal role in alleviating suffering and providing access to medical care (chiefly via Social Security Disability Insurance, Medicare, and Medicaid) in the Eisenhower, Kennedy, and Johnson administrations—as well as the growth of private health insurance as an employee benefit—rendered these postwar scientific and medical developments in hemophilia treatment more accessible to patients. By founding a national organization, Henry did more than create a support group and fundraising vehicle—he harnessed the political power of an organized group of citizens (and consumers of current and future treatments) and applied that force to both commercial and governmental concerns. The trajectory of hemophilia's symbolic commodification reached its zenith in the early 1980s, when the NHF became the most powerful lobbying and advocacy group for people with hemophilia.[22]

Another important postwar development in the treatment of hemophilia involved the establishment of what Resnik refers to as the "blood services industry," with its "resources for collecting, storing, and transfusing blood." By 1956, the American blood industry had vastly increased the nation's capacity: blood service providers (blood banks and plasma manufacturers) had collected more than 5.1 million units of blood that year alone, and physicians transfused more than 4.5 million units. In 1952, Baxter Laboratories, already a successful biomedical company in its own right, acquired Hyland Laboratories of Glendale, California. Hyland was the first U.S. company to make plasma commercially available; Baxter's acquisition of Hyland was another indicator that, with the help of technology, blood was on its way to becoming a bona fide commodity in the U.S., subject to the supply-and-demand rules of the global marketplace and offering the potential for large profits. While the entry of blood into the for-profit sector was in keeping with the United States' overall system of capital markets, blood's literal commodification would prove to be a fateful development in later decades.[23]

The market for blood products grew apace with the scientific, medical, and technological advances that occurred after World War II. Since voluntary donations could never supply enough blood for the demand, blood service providers began in the early 1960s to purchase blood and plasma commercially, often from society's most vulnerable and destitute—and least healthy—members. This development was consistent with capitalism, but in direct contrast to the practices of other countries. Resnik points out that other countries did not commodify blood services and blood products during the postwar years; instead, governments classified blood services and blood products as a public good and subjected them to stricter monitoring and regulation.[24]

In the U.S., however, little government oversight attended these early years of capitalized blood. Compensated donations from denizens of urban skid rows and prisoners compromised the safety of blood products as early as the 1960s and 1970s, mainly due to a greater risk of hepatitis arising from donors' unprotected sex with multiple partners and intravenous drug use involving the sharing of needles. One 1970 estimate put the number of people sickened by blood products at 30,000 annually. The promise of payment for one's blood, and especially for one's plasma, motivated prospective donors to hide their medical histories. Plasma donation was particularly lucrative: plasmapheresis (the process by which the blood banks extracted blood from the donor, harvested the plasma, and then returned the red blood cells to the donor) was more time-consuming and, in the early decades, more painful than blood donation. Yet the American appetite for blood products was insatiable. In addition to medical innovations like open-heart surgery and organ transplantation, scientific and technical advances with respect to hemophilia also helped create the high demand for blood during the 1960s and 1970s. The capitalization of blood and the commodification of blood products, the scientific discoveries outlined below, the circulation of the blood products in international markets, and the hands-off regulatory posture of American governments, all contributed mightily to the global medical catastrophe of HIV.[25]

In the 1960s, the NIH routinely funded coagulation research, including the first clinical trials of treatments with Factor VIII in people with hemophilia. The first big advance of the decade came in 1965, when Dr. Judith Graham Pool, a Stanford coagulation researcher, published a paper describing her breakthrough discovery: cryoprecipitate. In her lab, Pool had noticed that Factor VIII stayed frozen at the bottom of a container of otherwise thawed plasma. Resnik writes:

> [n]ews of Pool's discovery was disseminated through National Hemophilia Foundation channels. […] [W]ord spread quickly that "the outlook for treatment improved almost overnight." Cryoprecipitate was adopted widely for routine treatment of hemophilia, marking an end to risky high-volume blood transfusions. It could be easily stored in hospitals and blood banks from single units of blood, refrozen, and stored for up to a year. It was described as safe, inexpensive, and effective.

There were two types of cryoprecipitate: single-donor, which resulted in smaller amounts, and pooled Factor, produced by using several bags of fresh-frozen plasma and then pooling it. A patient might need a larger amount of Factor for major surgery, tooth extractions, etc., and thus the pooled Factor enabled the blood industry to meet this demand at a relatively lower cost.[26]

A second major development occurred in 1966, when researchers led by Dr. Kenneth M. Brinkhous at the University of North Carolina and Dr. Edward Shanbrom of Hyland Laboratories in California developed a concentrate of Factor VIII. In order to develop the concentrate, labs pooled thousands of units of plasma in order to net large amounts of cryoprecipitate, then "treated [the cryoprecipitate] with chemicals, filtered it, and centrifuged it—all to produce a white crystalline powder of pure, highly concentrated Factor VIII…. Carried in a vial the size of a salt shaker, the concentrate had one hundred times the clotting power of raw plasma—so concentrated that the patient could inject it with a syringe if he wanted, instead of a blood bag." Concentrated Factor was more stable and more easily stored, since it no longer needed to be frozen like cryoprecipitate. The concentrate also helped with the treatment of orthopedic issues, because patients could administer the Factor more often and thus control, or even head off, painful and disabling bleeds in the joints. This development was not only transformative medically, but also socially—for men with hemophilia, the promise of a "normal" life (or at least a life that appeared normal) suddenly seemed attainable. Stephen Pemberton has written about the power that the quest for normalcy exerted over those involved in both the medical and social response to hemophilia. The lure of relegating hemophilia to the rank of a manageable condition (instead of a debilitating one) shaped consumers' response to this new product, just as it would shape the response of the NHF to the HIV/AIDS crisis two decades later.[27]

The FDA granted a license to Hyland Laboratories to produce a Factor VIII concentrate commercially in 1968, and so it became widely available to consumers as an injection. Factor VIII concentrate was extremely expensive—the treatment could cost a person with severe hemophilia tens of thousands of dollars a year—and it carried a huge risk of viral hepatitis infection, since the fractionators used plasma purchased from down-and-out donors in hepatitis "hot zones." The blood companies assumed that any attempt to sterilize the concentrate with heat would destroy the clotting factor, so the large pools of plasma purchased in this manner were extremely vulnerable to infection—just one infected donor could render an entire pool contaminated.[28]

By 1970, people with hemophilia could use the new Factor VIII concentrate to treat "even significant bleeding episodes effectively on an outpatient basis." Ironically, the very circumstance that rendered the new Factor VIII product so effective—the concentrated power of up to 10,000 donors' clotting factor in a single dose—was also what made it so dangerous. Diseases like malaria, hepatitis, and syphilis ran rampant in the nation's blood supply. In a parallel development that would compound the disaster that was HIV for people with hemophilia, by 1970 the blood industry had effectively secured legal immunity from liability for transfusion-related disease transmission in state after state. The blood industry had presented a stark calculus to elected officials: if biomedical companies had to worry about lawsuits every time a blood recipient contracted hepatitis, they could not stay in business. The "blood shield" laws, as they were known, reflected a legislative decision to value a sustainable business climate over the health of individual citizens. With the systematic adoption of these statutes, lawmakers throughout the nation chose to protect corporate interests and prioritize commerce over individual bodily integrity, and there would be an enormous outcry and pushback against the blood shield laws in the 1990s. Federal regulators, though, were not without recourse. The Food and Drug Administration, aware of the hepatitis risk with blood transfusions (one

New York Times story referred to it as "transfusion roulette" in 1970), could and did promulgate rules designed to make the blood safer. Scientists had begun working on a test to detect hepatitis B in 1964, and the FDA mandated the testing of donated blood for the disease in the 1970s. However, by 1975, even the best test was only 40 percent accurate. In 1978, the FDA hit on a new strategy: it required the blood banks and plasma centers to affix labels to blood bags indicating whether the donor of the product was paid or was a volunteer. Once the rules disclosing the provenance of the blood took effect in May of 1978, hospitals quickly ceased buying blood labeled "paid," and rates of infection with hepatitis B plummeted. Unfortunately, none of these safety measures helped people with hemophilia relying on the new Factor VIII concentrate; there was no alternative means of producing concentrate other than pooling thousands of units of donors' plasma. Blood-borne infection with hepatitis was the price that people with hemophilia paid for the convenience of using freeze-dried Factor VIII at home, and even with that risk, most opted to do so. That product was so precious because it enabled people with hemophilia finally to lead "normal" lives in the 1970s, for the first time in history.[29]

School-aged people with hemophilia—especially those living in urban areas with access to a treatment center or with a chapter of the NHF—could now attend classes on a regular basis, participate in sports, and attend summer camp. Adults could maintain careers, get married, and have children, while enjoying life spans that were previously unthinkable. In fact, between 1968 and 1979, health officials noted a drastic 67 percent decline in deaths occurring in people with hemophilia aged 0–19 years who had a Factor VIII deficiency, thanks to the availability of the concentrate. The example of just one state, Massachusetts, is striking: whereas in 1972 about half of all people with hemophilia were unemployable (and the average age of patients was only 11 years, due to their shorter life spans), by 1986, the average age of people with hemophilia had climbed to 24 years, and their unemployment rate was only three percent—lower than the rate for healthy people.[30]

By 1980, hemophilia was viewed as a manageable chronic condition with a cost-effective model for service delivery instead of a death sentence. An estimated 14,467 people with hemophilia with Factor VIII and IX deficiencies lived in the United States in 1980. Many of them had hepatitis B from using blood products. Although by this time the blood banks screened donors for hepatitis A and B, hepatitis C (then known as "non A non B hepatitis") was already present in the blood supply, and it could not yet be detected in tests. Another lethal virus was also present in the nation's blood supply in 1980—it did not yet have a name, but thanks to an efficient combination of science and commerce, it would ultimately infect and kill thousands of people with hemophilia around the world, including Ryan White.[31]

Ryan White

Jeanne Hale simply did not believe she was smart enough to go to college, so she applied for a job assembling car radios at one of Kokomo's largest employers, the Delco Electronics Corporation, right after finishing high school. After working a short summer job at Kroger, Jeanne started at Delco in the fall of 1965. Delco Electronics had been a fixture in Kokomo since 1936, when the company began its life as the Delco Radio Division, employing more than 400 people in a building once owned by the Haynes Automotive Company, and later by the Crosley Radio firm.[32]

Although Jeanne's first job at Delco had the typical drawbacks of working on an assembly line—monotony, the pressure to make quotas, fatigue, and rigid time discipline—it also provided financial security and enabled her to meet new friends. It was at Delco that Jeanne reconnected with her former neighbor and schoolmate, Wayne White. Wayne's parents, Mildred and Hubert White, had moved to Kokomo from Tennessee when he was young. Hubert worked at Continental Steel, but Wayne did not follow in his father's footsteps. After high school, he served in the Army in Germany and then returned to Kokomo and began working at Delco. Jeanne and Wayne started dating and were married in 1968; she continued working at Delco until she delivered their son, Ryan, in 1971.[33]

Jeanne, the oldest child in her family of two daughters and one son, was born and raised in Kokomo. Her parents, Gloria and Tom Hale, were also born and raised in Kokomo. Tom's parents, Mabel and Fred Hale, were Kokomo natives, too, while Gloria's parents had emigrated from Germany, where they had been farmers, before the Great Depression. Tom Hale had left high school to work at Kokomo's original Kroger store at age 16, when his father died. He would work for Kroger for the rest of his life, rising to become the head produce manager at the city's largest Kroger store. Tom and Gloria met and married when both were barely 20 years old, but by the mid–1950s, they were able to move their young and growing family to a modest suburban house in the Bon Air subdivision on Fischer Street, on the city's north side. Raised in a happy, loving, and stable family, Jeanne would go on to attend Kokomo High School and graduate in 1965.[34]

Jeanne was a fan of the actor Ryan O'Neal: she had watched him in the 1960s television soap opera *Peyton Place* and his role in the 1970 film *Love Story* affected her so much that she decided that if she ever had a boy, she would name him Ryan. When Ryan was born on December 6, 1971, two medical emergencies immediately confronted Jeanne and Wayne: first, Jeanne hemorrhaged so badly that she almost died. The second, of course, became apparent when Jeanne's obstetrician, Dr. Fred Swartz, circumcised the infant. Ryan could not stop bleeding—his blood would not clot at all. Swartz called in Ryan's pediatrician, Dr. Donald Fields, who was also unable to stop the bleeding. Fields was concerned about hemophilia, so the two doctors sent Ryan, Jeanne, and the Hales to Indianapolis to see Dr. Laurence Bates, a hematologist, in order to handle the immediate crisis. Soon thereafter, Fields referred the Whites to hematologists at Indianapolis's Riley Hospital for Children, where they began treatments with Factor VIII. Once that regimen began, Fields could take over giving the medicine locally, in Kokomo; for a long time, he mixed the Factor VIII powder with a liquid and injected the potent compound into Ryan's veins approximately twice a week in order to prevent bleeds. Eventually, Fields taught Jeanne how to administer the injections to Ryan at home, and mother and son began their routine.[35]

In the early 1970s, freeze-dried Factor VIII for home use was expensive: Jeanne White recalled the price as $350 a shot. Fortunately, Delco offered its workers an excellent benefits package, including health insurance. Wayne White continued to work at Delco, and Jeanne returned to her job once her maternity leave ended. Ryan thrived—he was the poster boy for the Howard County Hemophilia Society's 1973 fund drive, and a smiling picture of him graced the *Kokomo Tribune* that March.[36]

Her doctors had advised Jeanne not to get pregnant again due to the complications she suffered with Ryan's delivery; nevertheless, she did become pregnant again in 1973. As Jeanne had feared, the news made Wayne "furious"—she deliberately told him about her pregnancy at work, because she dreaded his response. Ryan's younger sister, Andrea, was born on October 15, 1973, without complications on the part of mother or child. In her memoir, Jeanne never used the term "domestic violence" to describe her relationship with Wayne White. However, her description of Wayne's reaction to the news of her pregnancy, and her efforts to make that disclosure in a public place where, presumably, he would be too inhibited to fully express his anger, suggest that their relationship was not a healthy one. According to Jeanne's memoir, Wayne began to drink after Ryan was born, and alcohol made him mean. Although he never hit her when he was sober, when drinking, she wrote that he "occasionally gave me a swat, and I couldn't stand for that. One night he shoved me so that I fell between these two stools. He stood there laughing while I floundered and flopped, trying to get up. When I finally regained my footing, I punched him in the stomach. He staggered back, hurt." Jeanne reported that Wayne never hit her again after that episode, but another incident, when Ryan was five, would mark the beginning of the end of their troubled marriage.[37]

Wayne and a "drinking buddy" took their sons on a fishing trip in which there was apparently little angling and much drinking. Wayne drove home under the influence, ran over someone's fence, and fled home only to drive into the wall of the garage, with Ryan in the car the entire time. After an argument during which Wayne harangued Jeanne about her weight, she went on a crash diet and became extremely ill. While she was hospitalized in Indianapolis with sarcoidosis, an infection of the lymph nodes in her lungs, a drunken Wayne verbally abused her, and she vowed that she would divorce him. After the Whites divorced in 1978, Wayne was largely absent from his children's lives. He and Jeanne did not stay in touch.[38]

The year 1980 found Jeanne, Ryan, and Andrea White living with Jeanne's second husband, Steve Ford, in a house on two acres of land on Route 213 in Windfall, Indiana. Windfall is in Tipton County, directly to the south of Howard County, where Kokomo is the county seat. Although Windfall is in a different county, Jeanne and Steve, who also worked at Delco, had only a twenty-minute drive to work. (The town got its name because of the many tornadoes that landed there.) Ryan was nine years old, and Andrea was seven and just beginning to take roller-skating lessons and to compete in that sport.[39]

As the forces of capital and global commerce shaped the commodities of steel and blood worldwide, their fates were just beginning to intersect in Indiana in 1980. Penn-Dixie Steel was still open and operating, but its future was uncertain. Ryan White, growing up near the city where the mill stood, had a serious, chronic disease—he did occasionally get "bleeds" in his joints—but regular doses of Factor VIII allowed him to go to school and enjoy childhood activities such as riding his bicycle. Ryan's treatment—a white powder that he and his mother mixed with liquid and injected into his veins—must have seemed both very convenient and very far removed from the actual blood of others. But the traits that distinguished the concentrate from the pure transfusions that people with hemophilia received in earlier decades would ultimately work to disastrous effect.

2

Russian Roulette, 1980–1984

Gambling was an apt metaphor for the early 1980s, and not just for families with Factor-dependent hemophilia patients like the Whites. The blood industry, federal health officials, the NHF, and consumers of blood products all played Russian roulette in the years between 1980 and 1984. At meetings to decide whether to impose restrictions on blood and plasma donors, the NHF, the blood companies, and their federal counterparts played a game of chance: just how communicable was the new disease, and what were the odds that a newly discovered and so-far incurable condition, believed to be transmissible via blood, would sicken consumers of blood products? If the likelihood was appreciable, did that mean every single patient would get sick? If the answer was "not everyone," then how many? What would it cost the blood services industry to restrict donations, and would that cost outweigh the benefit to patients? Would the cost be the same in the United States and in other countries to which the blood industry exported its products? This calculus of science and commerce presented itself in a very real way to all of the players along the line, from the producers to the consumers, repeatedly during these years. And, while the stakes (life vs. death) were not exactly the same for the U.S. steel industry, the vagaries of the global economy, combined with corporate disinvestment and capital flight, dealt a losing hand to steelworkers during those same years. This chapter recounts events that occurred in Kokomo, but which echoed nationally as well, as American manufacturers and their workers faced repeated layoffs. Economic uncertainty disrupted working-class baby boomers' upward socioeconomic trajectories. For these citizens, achieving the American Dream seemed less guaranteed, despite the reassuring "Morning in America" rhetoric of the Reagan reelection campaign. Blue-collar workers such as Jeanne White could no longer rely on unions' negotiating power—not when their very jobs were at stake.[1]

Jeanne's marriage to Steve Ford, and her family's time in Windfall, did not last. The couple divorced "very amicably," according to Jeanne, in 1983. Instead of mostly disappearing from the children's lives, as their father Wayne had done, Steve remained a constant, calm presence for Ryan and Andrea. He continued to drive Andrea to her skating practices, to take Ryan and Andrea skating, and to help Jeanne with transportation. In her memoirs, Jeanne recalled her relationship with Steve as one of "warmth and respect and fun and a lot of comfort." Ryan likewise recalled Steve's loyalty and friendship, especially after his diagnosis with AIDS. Although they remained close, Jeanne and Steve eventually maintained separate households after the divorce. In 1984, Jeanne moved back to Kokomo with Ryan and Andrea in order to be closer to Jeanne's parents. The small family moved into the Vinton Woods subdivision, settling in a modest house at 3506 South Webster Street.[2]

Kokomo and Howard County had both seen their populations increase significantly during Jeanne's lifetime, especially to the south and the west. The city's population increased 30 percent between 1950 and 1975; the county's rose 64 percent. This part of Indiana was overwhelmingly white—1980 Census figures show that for the Kokomo SMSA (Standard Metropolitan Statistical Area), which included all of Howard and Tipton counties, there were 98,434 whites and only 4,281 blacks. In fact, only two black people lived in all of Tipton County. North-central Indiana was stereotypical middle America, evocative of a John Mellencamp song: white and homogeneous, with drive-ins and bowling leagues.[3]

Overall, Howard County became more urban and suburban, and less agricultural, in the decades after World War II. Kokomo officials responded to the rapid growth by annexing adjacent land. In 1976, the city's area claimed 12.5 square miles, 67 percent larger than its 1950 size of 7.5 square miles. Located on the southwest side, Vinton Woods lay within the "new" part of the city's rapidly expanding boundaries. At a distance of three miles south of downtown, the working-class subdivision rested just minutes away from the Delco and Chrysler plants, and only a mile from the Whites' church, St. Luke's United Methodist. The city of Jeanne's childhood was changing, adding school districts as populations shifted.[4]

Ryan White quickly made friends in his new neighborhood. While Andrea and Jeanne were away at skating practice or competitions, Ryan often stayed behind and played with his friends. Heath Bowen, who lived around the corner on Redwood Drive, had a pool. Another friend, Chris Sadler, lived on the corner of Webster and Redwood, so the three boys often spent time together at Heath's house or riding bikes, skateboarding, and walking in the woods. Wanda (Bowen) Bilodeau, Heath's older sister, remembers Ryan spending days at their home while Jeanne and Andrea looked at new costumes for skating competitions, and recalls Ryan and Heath teaming up to pester her on a regular basis. At twelve-and-a-half, Ryan was smart; he was an honors student when he started at Western Middle School in August of 1984. Western Middle School sits on County Road 250 South in Russiaville, Indiana, about six miles west of Webster Street. Children from Ryan's neighborhood attended Western because, as the city limits of Kokomo expanded outward, the city of Kokomo lacked the capacity for every child to attend city schools. As a result, some suburban children attended county schools.[5]

Despite his good school record, Ryan was not well in 1984. His hemophilia was not the issue—thanks to Factor VIII, he had been able to enjoy an active summer with his new friends—but he had been feeling a bit sluggish. By September, he suffered from diarrhea, stomach cramps, night sweats, and swollen lymph nodes. Jeanne took Ryan to his pediatrician, Dr. Fields, who diagnosed him with both flu and bronchitis, and prescribed antibiotics to no avail. In November, Ryan went for his annual appointment at the local hemophilia treatment center, where staff drew his blood for routine testing. The test brought bad news: Ryan tested positive for hepatitis B, something he had most likely contracted from contaminated Factor VIII. Perhaps that was the reason for Ryan's physical problems, he and his mother thought. But something else made them uncomfortable that day: when they bought a fresh supply of Factor VIII, they noticed a new label on the package. Ryan recounted the moment in his memoir, when he and his mother saw

> a warning about AIDS, like the notice on a pack of cigarettes that says you should know that they're hazardous to your health. I felt funny seeing that— especially since I'd read that Factor was being treated with heat to wipe out the AIDS virus. The sign made Mom uncomfortable too. "I feel like I'm playing Russian roulette with your life, giving you this stuff," she said.

She was right. As of November 26, 1984, 6,993 cases of AIDS had been reported to the CDC since the count began on June 5, 1981. Of those cases, 52 involved people with hemophilia and 93 more were transfusion-associated; there were also 263 adults and 54 children whose risk factors were unknown. The fatality rate for those cases was high: 48 percent.[6]

Blood

On December 29, 1982, Ed Cutter, the in-house counsel for Cutter Laboratories, had written a one-page memorandum to his employer recommending that the firm include an "AIDS warning" in its literature accompanying each vial of Factor VIII. He also advised educating the company's sales staff about AIDS and Factor VIII, as well as mailing a letter to physicians informing them about the new package insert. Cutter Laboratories ignored its lawyer's advice. By the time Ryan and Jeanne read the new warning label on their Factor VIII in late 1984, it was too late to help him—and too late for tens of thousands of other people with severe hemophilia. Ryan took shots of Factor VIII at least twice a week; if he had a bleed in one of his joints, he could receive as much as one shot a day for a month. By late 1984, when Ryan became ill, the blood industry was well aware of the grave threat that their products posed to people like Ryan—indeed, the industry had been cognizant of the danger for years. For its part, the federal government was equally slow in flexing its regulatory muscles vis-à-vis the blood industry. Even though the FDA had licensed all of the plasma fractionators to use heat treatments to kill the AIDS virus in their products by early 1984, the agency did not order a mandatory recall of *un*treated Factor VIII concentrate until 1989. What could explain the actions of the government and the blood products industry? The answer is complicated.[7]

AIDS had entered the national consciousness with a whisper, not a shout. In the summer of 1981, a lone article in the *New York Times* announced, "Rare Cancer Seen in 41 Homosexuals." Obscure as that news may have seemed to the general public, epidemiologists and public health officials at the Centers for Disease Control (CDC) were already taking notice. In their article on AIDS as part of a CDC retrospective commemorating fifty years of the *Morbidity and Mortality Weekly Report* (*MMWR*), Drs. James W. Curran and Harold W. Jaffe, two of the people most deeply involved in the CDC's response to the AIDS epidemic, wrote that surveillance of those early cases was utterly critical. Upon learning about cases that summer of Kaposi's sarcoma (KS—a rare skin cancer) and *pneumocystis carinii* pneumonia (PCP—a rare bacterial infection of the lungs that is not normally fatal) occurring among young men with no other apparent suppression of their immune systems, the CDC formed its "Task Force on Kaposi's Sarcoma and Opportunistic Infections" in order to establish a case definition for surveillance and investigation purposes. The Task Force quickly developed a case definition with two specific criteria, and by the end of 1981—barely six months later—the CDC had already identified 159 cases of Kaposi's sarcoma and opportunistic infections (OIs)—the earliest of which dated back to 1978. Once they began their surveillance and investigation, researchers were able to conclude "that a new, highly concentrated epidemic of life threatening illness was occurring in the United States." And, because it was an epidemic, the number of cases was increasing with each passing month—as were the numbers of deaths.[8]

We know now that the die had already been cast with respect to HIV in the United States for quite some time by 1981. According to microbiologist and epidemiologist Jacques Pepin, the virus arrived courtesy of global commerce—either via contaminated plasma in the commercial market supply for cryoprecipitate production, or via an infected tourist who had most likely contracted it sexually. The virus was already present in 1979 in one-third of IV-drug users in New York City. By 1978, six percent of gay men in San Francisco carried the virus, and it had entered the local blood supply. Evolutionary microbiologists and epidemiologists theorize that the high rate of sexual activity in the city's bathhouses contributed to the virus's quick progress—by 1979, 19 percent of gay men in San Francisco had HIV, a figure which grew to an astonishing 44 percent in 1981. Pepin tells us this phenomenal "amplification" of the virus actually peaked as early as July 1981, with an infection rate of 1.4 percent per month among gay men. He notes that among men with hemophilia, infections have been retrospectively identified in Great Britain in 1979, and in America as early as 1978, with the most intense period of infection occurring in 1981 and 1982. In fact, the virus charted a course in men with hemophilia that paralleled its trajectory in men who had sex with men. Pepin has written that by 1981, "[m]ore than half of haemophiliacs in Georgia were HIV-infected ... as were 85 [percent] of their Californian counterparts by 1984." Globalization enhanced the reach of HIV in another way, by giving it an unprecedented degree of mobility—with the international travel of infected men having sex with men, in combination with the international commercial reach of U.S. blood products—"[f]rom the United States, the virus was re-exported to many parts of the industrialised world." Historian Phil Tiemeyer has a similar analysis of the vital role that air travel played in HIV's geographical expansion—but he specifically correlates the virus's fast and widespread distribution to U.S. metropolitan areas with the 1979 deregulation of the airline industry, and the resulting industry-wide consolidation and adoption by carriers of the "hub-and-spoke" route system. Tiemeyer demonstrates that some of the very same cities that hosted airline hubs at their airports, such as San Francisco, Los Angeles, and New York, appeared as sites of disease clusters for KS, PCP, and other OIs in early CDC studies.[9]

Of course, public health experts in 1981 could not have connected these dots. Instead, they had to rely on their sleuthing abilities to identify and track patterns. The concentration of an immunosuppressive condition within localized communities of gay men, particularly in Los Angeles and New York, spurred researchers to study what links, if any, might exist between the men who were affected by KS and OIs. Drs. Harold Jaffe and Martha Rogers of the CDC conducted a "national case-control study" in early 1982 with fifty of the living patients (gay men with KS/OIs), and a control group of fifty healthy gay men matched for city of residence, race, and age. Jaffe and Rogers found that the men who were sick were "much more sexually active" than the members of the healthy control group. At the same time, epidemiological investigators in southern California, led by Drs. David Auerbach and William Darrow, were able to link many of the patients in that region, and later nationwide, by sexual contact with other patients. All of these findings were evidence that the new disease was sexually transmitted and infectious—not direct evidence, but certainly credible circumstantial evidence. Unfortunately, according to Curran and Jaffe, the "infectious agent causation theory" met with skepticism among scientists and the general public alike. In fact, denial is a common reaction to epidemics. Robert M. Swenson, an infectious disease specialist and immunologist, has identified a predictable "behavioral response of both individuals and society to a given epidemic." According to Swenson, certain attitudes and behavior recur during *all* epidemics: first, denial that the disease is even occurring; second, blaming someone or something else for the epidemic; third, a loss of faith in the competence of physicians and medicine to handle the problem competently (and a concomitant increase of interest in alternative therapies); and finally, the adoption of new laws to prevent or control the epidemic.[10]

Skepticism or no, the epidemic continued on its path, infecting not just gay men but also intravenous drug users and some Haitians new to the United States. The number of new cases reported to the CDC had steadily doubled every six months; the mortality rate was climbing, and an average of one to two new cases were diagnosed every day in 1982. And the new cases now included people with hemophilia: in its *MMWR* for July 16, 1982, the CDC reported three cases of PCP occurring in previously healthy men with hemophilia. These men did not report having sex with other men, nor were they intravenous drug users. The first patient had been diagnosed in late December 1981: two of the three had died by the July 16 date of the report. Lot number checks of each patient's Factor VIII concentrate disclosed no overlapping dosages—in other words, each man had become infected through an injection of concentrate from a different lot number, manufactured from different donors. In the *MMWR* the CDC noted, "although the cause of the severe immune dysfunction is unknown, the occurrence among the three hemophiliac cases suggests the possible transmission of an agent through blood products." The authors of the MMWR also noted that the CDC had notified hemophilia treatment centers about the three cases and had begun "collaborative surveillance" with the National Hemophilia Foundation.[11]

Over the summer of 1982, federal government officials kept in frequent touch with the National Hemophilia Foundation. On July 8, Dr. Bruce Evatt of the CDC called the executive director of the NHF to inform him about those three reported cases of immunosuppression in men with hemophilia. In her history of hemophilia and AIDS, Susan Resnik notes that less than a week later, on July 14,

> the NHF sent out a notice to its chapters in ... *Hemophilia Newsnotes*, entitled "Hemophilia Patient Alert #1." It referred to the three cases reported by the CDC ... as "rare and unusual infections associated with a condition in which there is a decrease in the body's ability to combat disease." It noted that this condition may have developed "as a result of an unknown potentially immunosuppressive agent. One hypothesis that is being investigated by the CDC is that the agent may be a virus transmitted similarly to the hepatitis virus by blood or blood products." The notice emphasized by the use of italics that "it is important to note at this time the risk of contracting this immunosuppressive agent is *minimal*, and CDC is not recommending any change in blood product use."[12]

On July 27, 1982, the Assistant Secretary for Health in the U.S. Department of Health and Human Services convened a meeting of experts from the NHF, the CDC, the blood banks, the Red Cross, the American Society of Hematology, and the blood products industry to discuss the situation—specifically, in the words of some of the attendees, to "review the risks associated with blood-product usage." No consensus emerged from the meeting, perhaps due to continuing skepticism about the blood-borne transmission theory. Resnik characterizes this attitude as a normal part of medical and scientific culture—hypotheses should be proven by independent tests that replicate the results, and then published only after peer review. The CDC did not have that evidence, and it would not have it for at least another year. Then too, the CDC's credibility had itself come under scrutiny during the mid–1970s with its handling of the swine flu vaccine. Experts at the Institute of Medicine (part of the National Academy of Sciences), commissioned by the U.S. Secretary of Health and Human Services in the 1990s to study what had gone wrong with the nation's blood supply during the early years of the AIDS pandemic, noted scientists' reluctance to make definite pronouncements about causation. Even though evidence of blood-borne transmission had clearly been present in 1982 and 1983, the Institute noted, "the U.S. Public Health Service had to deal with a very difficult problem. On the one hand, the ... blood supply was barely adequate to meet the urgent needs of day-to-day patient care. On the other hand, there was growing evidence that a blood transfusion posed a risk of causing a disease that was proving to be fatal for many." While the magnitude of the risk remained unclear, for its part, the NHF saw enough of a risk to reach out to the blood industry.[13]

In November 1982, the NHF sent a written communiqué to the blood products industry recommending that plasma centers screen and/or restrict donors. The warning went unheeded. In early December, the CDC published two more notices in the MMWR that had ominous implications for people dependent on Factor VIII. The first summarized four new cases and one suspected case (since July 16) of hemophilia patients with opportunistic infections—two of those five patients were dead. The report noted, "[i]n most instances, these patients have been the first AIDS cases in their cities, states, or regions," and, like the earlier cases, these patients did not share a common lot number for their infusions of Factor VIII concentrate. Further, two of the new patients were under 10 years old. Taken as a whole, the new information indicated that AIDS "may pose a significant risk for patients with hemophilia."[14]

The second CDC report discussed a case of an infant with "possible transfusion-associated" AIDS in California. The baby had had multiple transfusions, and investigators were able to conclude that one of the 19 donors was later reported to have AIDS. The man was by all appearances healthy on March 10, 1981, when he donated the blood that was given to the baby the next day, March 11. The baby died in August 1982. The CDC again warned that "the etiology of AIDS remains unknown, but … its occurrence following receipt of blood products from a known AIDS case adds support to the infectious-agent hypothesis." This CDC report prompted a San Francisco firm, the Irwin Blood Bank, to stop sending its Bloodmobiles to neighborhoods known as gay enclaves. The CDC report also prompted the NHF to issue Chapter Advisory #5, which echoed the government's increasing concern about blood-borne transmission but, in the absence of a direct link between AIDS and concentrates, only tepidly advised patients to "be aware of the potential risks" and consult their physicians.[15]

It was apparent to scientists by late 1982 that AIDS was transmissible via blood and blood products, in addition to intimate sexual contact. The CDC convened a meeting about the safety of the nation's blood supply at its Atlanta headquarters on January 4, 1983, in an effort to reach a consensus about how best to respond to the threat of AIDS. No consensus emerged from the highly contentious meeting, which was attended by representatives of the American Red Cross, the American Association of Blood Banks, the NHF, the National Gay Task Force, the Pharmaceutical Manufacturers Association (representing the plasma fractionators), the National Institutes of Health, and the FDA. According to Resnik, who describes the meeting most succinctly, "the blood bankers remained skeptical that AIDS could be transmitted through blood; some FDA officials were still unconvinced that AIDS actually existed; and the gay groups called screening out homosexuals 'scapegoating.' … In the end, each group stood by its own agenda, no agreements were reached, and nothing changed." However, over the course of the next few weeks and months, some of the stakeholders and governmental agencies would clarify their positions.[16]

A week after the January 4 meeting, the American Association of Blood Banks, the Red Cross, and the Council of Community Blood Centers issued a statement on donor screening which asserted that "direct or indirect questions about a donor's sexual preference are inappropriate." In late January, the plasma industry (represented by an entity called the American Blood Resources Association) issued its own recommendations for educating donors with brochures, and for screening prospective donors by asking questions to determine whether they were members of high-risk groups. In early March, the federal government made its first official pronouncement on the prevention of AIDS when the Public Health Service issued five inter-agency recommendations in the *MMWR*: people should avoid sexual contact with others known or suspected to have AIDS or with multiple partners; members of the high-risk groups should avoid donating blood or plasma; studies should evaluate the efficacy of screening blood and plasma through lab tests and physical exams; physicians should order transfusions only when medically indicated; and "work should continue toward development of safer blood products for use by hemophilia patients." Finally, on March 24, 1983, the FDA issued a directive to the blood industry, including both fractionators and collection points, demanding that they implement "standard operating procedures to quarantine and dispose of any products collected by donors known or suspected of having AIDS[;] establish educational programs to inform persons at increased risk for AIDS that they should stop donating[;] and ... train personnel who screen donors to recognize the early signs of AIDS." Additionally, the FDA approved heat treatments for Factor VIII concentrate in order to neutralize the threat of hepatitis B in the clotting factor.[17]

Despite the dire implications of its pronouncement, the FDA would not order a blanket recall of all non-heat-treated concentrate until 1989. Infecting people with hemophilia with hepatitis B had long been deemed an acceptable risk, one that patients and their physicians had assumed for years, and infection with the AIDS virus through blood products was still only a theory—albeit one supported by evidence in the form of increasing numbers of patients with AIDS. Nevertheless, Hyland Therapeutics decided on May 11, 1983, that it did not want to gamble when it possessed hard data. The company recalled a single lot of Factor VIII concentrate after connecting the pool to a donor who had later been diagnosed with AIDS. The NHF, which could have used the occasion to sound an alarm and push for more aggressive screening of blood donors, instead reacted weakly by sending a bulletin to its chapters encouraging patients to keep using concentrates and not to change their treatment regimens in response to the recall. Although the NHF lobbied the FDA for a policy requiring the automatic recall of blood products associated with donors who were later diagnosed with AIDS, the FDA did not issue such a directive. Instead, the agency, concerned about both potential shortages of clotting factor and false-positive diagnoses, reviewed each incident on a case-by-case basis. Meanwhile, physicians and patients found themselves in an untenable situation, in which all bets were bad bets. For people with severe hemophilia like Ryan White, there were no viable clinical alternatives to injecting Factor VIII concentrate—the only other options involved time-consuming and painful infusions with cryoprecipitate or fresh-frozen plasma, treatments that could not occur at home. The risks of not treating with clotting factor injections were too great, and they were already well known to both patients and their doctors. The risks of contracting AIDS from clotting factor, on the other hand, were still somewhat uncertain. Most patients with severe hemophilia were, it appeared at that time (despite what we now know), not infected with AIDS. Questions lingered: AIDS was infectious, but could a person develop antibodies to it? Would a patient with the AIDS virus in his blood automatically get sick? Researchers did not yet know. Ryan White was part of a generation of people with hemophilia who enjoyed a quality of life unimaginable to those born in his parents' generation. Stopping the miraculous treatments seemed unthinkable—after all, the fractionators themselves seemed not to be panicking. Their products were still on the shelves. The NHF—the premier advocacy organization for people with hemophilia—recommended that patients continue their treatment. Is it any wonder that across the country, most people with severe hemophilia and their physicians decided to keep using Factor VIII? The consequences of their decisions would become apparent only later. In its post-mortem, the Institute of Medicine cited a 1993 CDC report determining that "approximately half of the 16,000 hemophiliacs and over 12,000 recipients of blood transfusions became infected with HIV during this period [from 1982 to 1984]."[18]

Steel

Americans felt insecure during the early 1980s, and the anxiety was not limited to public health. Voters had elected a new president in 1980 amid economic uncertainty and concern over the industrial and manufacturing sectors. Nationwide, corporations like Penn-Dixie Steel—which was already in Chapter 11, due to its parent company's mismanagement and corruption—faced shaky futures, thanks to an ongoing cycle of recession and recovery, deindustrialization, disinvestment, competition from foreign firms, tensions with labor, and other challenges. In Kokomo, Penn-Dixie president George Downing had warned of impending production cutbacks and layoffs shortly after the firm appeared in bankruptcy court. Downing faced some high-stakes, fateful decisions: Was the Kokomo steel company, and the many jobs it secured, worth saving? Should the firm amass more debt in order to expand operations and better compete in a global market? Or should Penn-Dixie let the bankruptcy run its course, hoping for a buyer to save it from liquidation? Each option carried risks.[19]

Just ten days after Penn-Dixie Industries and Penn-Dixie Steel filed for Chapter 11 reorganization in a New York bankruptcy court, the people of Kokomo endured another shock. On April 17, 1980, the city's three largest employers—Delco Electronics, Chrysler, and Penn-Dixie Steel—announced a new round of layoffs. During the last week of April, the *Kokomo Tribune* reported, those three companies would place more than 7,500 of Kokomo's workers on indefinite or temporary furlough. For its part, the state of Indiana announced that it was in negotiations with Chrysler for a $32 million investment and bailout package in an effort to save Hoosiers' jobs. Of course, the American auto industry's problems were not geographically confined to Kokomo or even to Indiana; nationwide during late April, an additional 27,000 workers found themselves on indefinite layoff. Carmakers blamed their woes on declining sales; by April 1980, sales of U.S. cars were 15 percent lower than the figures for the previous year, while sales of imports soared. That a company like General Motors was laying off its workers by the thousands in 1980 was even more stunning when one considers that just a year earlier, in 1979, the company had recorded its largest workforce ever—618,000 employees.[20]

In the spring of 1980, economists' appraisal of the national economy was grim—the country appeared poised to enter its seventh recession since World War II. The remainder of the year was marked by particular uncertainty in Kokomo, where discussion of the fate of Penn-Dixie Steel seemed to raise more questions than answers. By the end of the year, answers would begin to appear. In early December, a committee of Penn-Dixie creditors approved George Downing's request to spend $500,000 on an engineering study, the first step in a $17 million expansion of the steel plant to include a billet caster and a breakdown mill. The modernization would enable Penn-Dixie to compete in the hot-metal steel production business, as well as reduce its energy costs. While confirming the news of the engineering study to a local reporter, Downing predicted that the steel company would be the only surviving entity left after Penn-Dixie's Chapter 11 process was complete. Purchasers had made "firm offers for all the corporation's remaining cement plants," and Penn-Dixie's creditors had reached a compromise regarding payment of the company's debts.[21]

The beginning of 1981 found William Scharffenberger, the CEO of the Penn-Dixie Industries conglomerate, still working to obtain financing in order to save the steel company. Scharffenberger planned to relocate Penn-Dixie's corporate headquarters from New York to Kokomo, and—assuming the steel firm would survive—to rename it Continental Steel. "We want to wash out the Penn-Dixie name," he told a reporter. "We still have the right to (the name) Continental Steel," a name "still valuable in the steel business." The conglomerate had been able to sell three of its six cement plants for a total of $13 million by early 1981, but it faced a significant unfunded liability for the cement workers' pensions, in addition to the demands of its other creditors and the steel firm's request for a $17 million modernization. The steel company posted a first-quarter loss of $2.5 million. Whether the loss was due to an aging plant, poorly motivated workers, or both was a matter of debate.[22]

A meeting between corporate officials and Penn-Dixie Steel employees in May exposed some of the tensions between workers and management. Although managers told the workers in the May 9 meeting that they were not planning wage cuts, further layoffs, or turning to pension funds to try to make a profit, they stressed that the workforce had to become more productive. W.A. Shively, Penn-Dixie Steel's vice president of employee relations, reported that the week immediately after that meeting, productivity was up $29,000; the second week afterward, the company posted a gain of $31,000. But the third and fourth weeks saw declines of $29,000 and $70,000 respectively. By the end of June, the company had lost $1.2 million on sales of 24,000 tons of steel. Shively forecast sales of only 17,000 tons in July and 19,000 in August, and he put the responsibility for those dismal figures squarely on his workers' shoulders and accused them of sandbagging. Employees "were stretching five-day jobs out to six days, to increase their incomes," he told the *Tribune*. In some cases, "people were working five days when they should only be working four." Penn-Dixie's work force of 1,300, which once produced some 30,000 tons of products each month, now produced only 20,000 tons, according to the paper. At a Saturday meeting in June, Shively introduced the steel company's new president, Thomas Sigler, to about 2,500 employees and their families. "The hardest thing we have to do," Shively told them, "is get you people to believe that we are in trouble." Sigler struck a more diplomatic tone, saying, "I'm very impressed with the people and the community and their interest in Penn-Dixie." Sigler did note that the firm faced stiff competition and warned that the next few years would not be easy.[23]

In September, Penn-Dixie filed its reorganization plan with the bankruptcy court in New York; the company was still awaiting the judge's approval when Howard County Treasurer Elva LaDow announced in October that Penn-Dixie Steel Corp. had paid no property taxes since the fall of 1979, when it had only made a partial payment; and that it currently owed the county over $1.6 million in taxes and late fees. William Scharffenberger, the president of the parent company, could not guarantee when Penn-Dixie would be able to finally pay its taxes in full. Howard County held sixth place in the company's line of creditors. The reorganization plan called for the company to pay all of its back taxes within six years; Scharffenberger indicated that Penn-Dixie might need all six of those years. LaDow told the *Tribune* that even though the economy was doing poorly, Penn-Dixie was the only major local company that owed taxes (Universal Steel had gone out of business earlier in 1981 with a tax delinquency in the $200–300,000 range, while World Color Press, which had moved from Kokomo in 1979, had recently settled its $379,000 debt to Howard County). Of course, since Penn-Dixie Steel still employed thousands, it was in the county's best interest to exercise patience. And the steel company leaders acted as if they did not plan to give up their fight for the company.[24]

In January 1982, Penn-Dixie announced that it had gained concessions from its creditors and the United Steelworkers union, and that it hoped to emerge from Chapter 11 by late February. The *Kokomo Tribune* reported on January 9 that the local steel union leadership had agreed to defer workers' salary increases by a month, subject to the approval of the rank and file. The union bosses' willingness to discuss concessions indicates the fragile state of the nation's steel industry, which in 1982 smarted from an unemployment rate of 21 percent. According to John P. Hoerr's history of the U.S. steel industry in the 1980s, "there was little demand for steel, and foreign producers were taking more than 20 percent of the puny market that existed." To be sure, the dominant narrative during these years cast the U.S. mills as victims of unfair competition from foreign plants which were able to charge significantly less. This narrative served U.S. corporate interests very well, because—as historian William Scheuerman puts it—it "deflect[ed] blame from corporate disinvestment policies" on the part of the conglomerates. Although the "cheap imports" mention may have been good politics, it did nothing to help the steelworkers. In fact, in states like Indiana, the protectionist rhetoric of tariffs that often accompanied complaints of cheap imports backfired when foreign competitors threatened to react in kind by imposing sanctions against U.S. agricultural products. Laborers' interests were thus pitted against those of their neighbors who were farmers, while the corporations they worked for invested elsewhere. In a sense, the workers found themselves holding a losing hand: mill executives across the country had, for decades, failed to upgrade their equipment to keep pace with their foreign competitors' innovations (such as the basic oxygen furnaces). Even were they to spend to make the necessary upgrades, it would take years to catch up. Penn-Dixie was by no means the only company standing on shaky ground in January of 1982; Lloyd McBride, the president of the international United Steelworkers between 1977 and 1983, advised his union's district directors to forward requests for concessions to headquarters, so that the research department staff could evaluate them. At least five such requests had arrived by the end of the month, including Penn-Dixie's.[25]

McBride and other union leaders developed a three-step process for deciding whether to advise locals to negotiate with management: first, assess whether the company truly faced financial difficulty, and if so, the extent to which it needed help; second, establish a procedure for local members to vote on concession agreements; and third, demand a "system of trade-offs," allowing workers to gain compensation (typically, in the form of stock ownership) in exchange for giving up wages and benefits. According to Hoerr, the members of Penn-Dixie's local voted on January 29 to approve concessions that saved the company $2 per hour in labor costs; in exchange, once the company was able to repay the workers, it would do so before it paid any dividends to its shareowners. Agreements such as these alarmed locals elsewhere in the country, because they weakened all steel union members' negotiating positions with respect to wages and benefits. The turbulent market did not abate, though, and the staff at the international headquarters would eventually deal with some 400 requests for concessions throughout 1982.[26]

In March, the bankruptcy judge approved Penn-Dixie's reorganization plan, and within a few months, the company was operating independently under its old name, Continental Steel, with Thomas Sigler at the helm. Sigler faced many obstacles in his quest for profitability, including the scrutiny of the federal government. The steel plant, along with Kokomo's Chrysler operations, faced EPA sanctions for air-quality "nonattainment" during one day in the previous years. Among other ramifications, both Continental and Chrysler confronted the prospect of having to spend millions of dollars on pollution control equipment. Fortunately for both companies, the Kokomo/Howard County Chamber of Commerce formed a task force to study the situation, and determined that farming activity on a dry, dusty day was to blame for the air pollution, not the industries. The EPA had backed down in that episode, but issues with pollution would loom large over not only Continental, but all U.S. steel mills, during the early 1980s. In 1983, the EPA reached an industry-wide agreement to settle disputes with both steel producers and the Natural Resources Defense Council (an environmental advocacy organization) over federal regulations regarding the acceptable limits of waste the plants discharged into waterways. The compromise eased the limits somewhat but would still cost steel mills dearly to implement. For a company such as Continental, already on shaky financial footing, this news only added to the pressure.[27]

By mid–1983, Kokomo's economy suffered under an unemployment rate of nearly 16 percent. Chrysler had regularly shut down its plants for extended periods since the late 1970s, especially during the holidays. Once-bustling shopping malls were now "eerily quiet," according to one observer, who described vacant stores and the families of the unemployed selling "trinkets" at stalls in empty corridors. The city needed every job it could get. Continental invested in improvements to its galvanized wire line, increasing its capacity by 25 percent (wire made up 85 percent of Continental's overall product line), and an April 17, 1983, full-page advertisement in the *Kokomo Tribune* highlighted a new partnership between labor and management. The new relationship featured wages set some 20 percent below those of the "big steel" firms like Inland, U.S. Steel, Bethlehem, etc., as well as stock options and profit sharing. To demonstrate his good faith, Sigler (himself a former mill hand at McClouth Steel, Inc., in Detroit) cut his own salary by 10 percent and passed up an automatic pay raise. Sigler and his board of directors undertook an ambitious modernization program, including a new $18.5 million rod mill set to open in 1984, and a $21 million continuous billet caster scheduled for 1985.[28]

In addition to a pressing need for capital improvements, Thomas Sigler inherited a number of environmental problems when he took over at the steel company. Even as the EPA proposed sanctions for air quality violations, the Indiana Environmental Management Board expressed interest in Continental's dust pile, which had been accumulating in an isolated gravel quarry on the company's property since at least 1980. When the state agency's Land Pollution Control Division performed a routine inspection in August of 1983, inspectors found a 5,000-ton pile of emission control dust. Generated by the firm's electric arc furnaces, the dust was a byproduct of the steel manufacturing process. Since it contained low levels of lead and chrome, it was classified as hazardous waste. The agency feared that those toxic elements would leach into the ground water and end up in nearby Wildcat Creek, but studies showed that the runoff drained into the quarry instead. Nevertheless, Continental, which lacked a permit to maintain hazardous waste, was ordered to remove the pile. The company hired trucks to take the dust to a landfill in Fulton County, and the pile was gone by February of 1984. The state dismissed its notice of violation against Continental in August of that year.[29]

"We came out into a world where we were not competitive," Thomas Sigler told a *Kokomo Tribune* reporter in March 1984. "Everything up to this time has been crisis," he continued. The company's work force numbers reflected that turmoil, fluctuating between 2,700 and 1,000 in the late 1970s and early 1980s, with a 1984 tally of 1,437 salaried and hourly employees and 93 laid off. Perhaps to reassure local residents of its stability and commitment, Continental touted its strengths in a full-page ad in the local newspaper on Sunday, March 25, 1984: "We're part of the mini-mill revolution in steel. The giant, overly-extended steel companies of the past find they have fewer answers for the marketplace, while our specialized and more cost-effective mini-mill is providing new answers. We're totally committed to quality rod and wire production," the ad proclaimed. The twin-strand rod mill, which opened on time in late May of 1984, promised to boost Continental's output to 53 tons of steel rod per hour, with a potential of 400,000 tons of steel per year; that annual figure represented an increase of 100,000 tons over the old mill's maximum production.[30]

As hopeful as those projections seemed, environmental concerns continued to dog Continental. A public notice in the October 31, 1984, *Tribune* announced that Continental was withdrawing a plan it had previously submitted to the state Environmental Management Board. The earlier plan had called for Continental to store its hazardous waste on a long-term basis; instead, the firm now proposed a short-term storage plan that would allow it to accumulate hazardous waste on-site for periods of less than 90 days, or in quantities of less than 2,200 pounds. (State officials routinely sought the public's comments before approving plans to store hazardous waste.) News items like this one illustrated that Continental president Thomas Sigler was responsible not only for managing approximately 1,400 employees, but also for maintaining a facility that spanned nearly 200 acres—and for managing whatever substances had festered in its soil and groundwater since at least 1914.[31]

Sigler was able to close 1984 on an upbeat note, however. His company was finally going to get its long-awaited continuous billet caster in 1985. The continuous caster would replace Continental's slow, six-step method of casting billets and make the plant more productive. In early November of 1984, Continental announced that it had reached an agreement with the North Central Building Trades Council concerning the installation of the multi-million-dollar caster. In a major concession, the Council, which represented building trades unions in a five-county area that included Howard County, agreed to let Continental hire an Italian firm, Danieli, to install the caster. Council president Richard Klein explained that Continental's dire financial circumstances had prompted the unions' conciliatory stance. "These jobs could have been done by Kokomo workers, but we made a commitment with management to let this go through. If anything is done to hold up the installation of this machine, it could mean the end of Continental Steel," Klein told the *Tribune*. The area's laborers had endured many ups and downs of late, and the decision to trade surefire jobs in the present for a chance at long-term economic security could not have been an easy one. Once again, local workers pinned their hopes on the future and sacrificed their immediate income. Unfortunately, the end would come anyway for Continental Steel. Even though both workers and management had shown their willingness time after time to bet on Continental's future, the company would file for bankruptcy in twelve short months. And when management would seek further concessions, steelworkers would mention instances like that involving the billet caster as a reason for not accommodating those requests.[32]

By 1984, the men and women of Kokomo's workforce—especially those in the automobile and steel industries—could no longer count on the same prospects of lifetime employment, generous benefits, and a place in the middle class that their forebears in the 1950s and 1960s enjoyed. But even as the city's main businesses absorbed the twin blows of globalization and deindustrialization and searched for ways to adapt amidst high unemployment, Kokomo's neighborhoods seemed intact. The Brandon Street area around Continental Steel still thrived, and toward the south, in suburban neighborhoods like Vinton Woods—where Ryan White and his family lived—children rode their bicycles, splashed in pools, and ran from house to house. An area like Vinton Woods placed few obstacles in a boy's path, except for the traffic on busy streets. Otherwise, neighbors' doors were usually open to each others' children, who crossed the boundaries of their thresholds as easily as a bikes' wheels glided down the smooth sidewalks.

Ryan White

As Ryan turned thirteen on December 6, 1984, he coughed constantly. Attending school exhausted him. "Mom, you've got to do something," he told Jeanne. "I can't even get off the school bus without being tired." When he spiked a fever of 104 the following weekend, Jeanne took him back to Dr. Fields, who admitted Ryan to the hospital and ordered chest x-rays. The pictures showed that Ryan had pneumonia, but he did not respond to antibiotics (or to oxygen). Dr. Fields suspected that Ryan had AIDS but did not mention his suspicions to Jeanne or to Ryan. Fields arranged for Ryan to travel by ambulance to Riley Hospital in Indianapolis, where Dr. Martin Kleiman, an infectious disease specialist, performed a biopsy on Ryan's lung and sent the samples to a laboratory in Denver for testing. When the results came back about a week before Christmas, Dr. Kleiman told Jeanne that Ryan had *pneumocystis carinii* pneumonia—PCP. In other words, Ryan had AIDS.[33]

Ryan's lungs were so ravaged by the *carinii* microbes that Dr. Kleiman put him on a respirator to help him breathe until he started responding to treatment. Jeanne knew she had to tell Ryan about his diagnosis, but she wanted to wait until all of his tubes were removed and he was able to speak. Due to the AIDS diagnosis, the hospital required his visitors to wear a gown and gloves. In the days before Christmas, three of Ryan's teachers drove to Indianapolis to visit him in the hospital, bringing cards and letters from his classmates. When they asked Jeanne what was wrong with Ryan, she told them, "Well, you know they say he has AIDS, [but] I think they're gonna find out it's something else. You know, we've asked for all the tests to be run all over again." Jeanne went on, "He will be so excited to see you. All you have to do is put on these gowns and gloves and you can go in and see him." When the teachers demurred, Jeanne explained, "No, really, it's for his protection." The teachers left without visiting Ryan.[34]

By Christmas Eve, the staff had removed the respirator and tubes and Ryan was finally able to speak, but Jeanne was reluctant to tell him that he had AIDS until after the Christmas holiday. On Christmas Day, Gloria Hale called her daughter with some terrible news: the Whites' home on Webster Street had been burglarized. All of their presents were gone, along with the family's videocassette recorder and several videotapes of Andrea's skating performances. Jeanne had worked overtime throughout the month of October in order to buy Christmas presents, and they had all been taken. Jeanne's parents stayed and made a report to the Howard County sheriff. The Whites' neighbors, Wanda and Heath, walked over and saw where investigators had taken casts of suspicious footprints that led to the Whites' back door. The house at 3506 Webster appeared to be just the latest target in a spate of burglaries that season: the Howard County sheriff logged seven calls involving breaking and entering and thefts in the Vinton Woods addition between November 14, 1984, and January 1, 1985. Authorities never recovered any of the Whites' missing items. "It was just a very sad time," Wanda recalled. "It was sad for everyone at Christmas time that Christmas presents were taken, but especially with what [the Whites] were going through. Their medical expenses that they had … it was especially difficult on them during that trying time." Word of the Whites' misfortune spread quickly around the hospital, and the staff and some of the other visitors chipped in to get last-minute gifts for Ryan and Andrea; Wayne White also brought some presents with him when he visited that day.[35]

Jeanne told her son about his AIDS diagnosis the next day, when their minister from St. Luke's United Methodist Church, Pastor Harold Williams, was visiting. Jeanne said, "Ryan, you know you've been really sick." When Ryan acknowledged that, Jeanne went on to say, "Well, they say you have AIDS." Ryan asked if he was going to die, and Jeanne told him, "We're all going to die sometime; we just don't know when." Ryan asked whether Laura, his favorite nurse, knew that he had AIDS; he was concerned that she might not want to treat him. Once Jeanne assured him that Laura knew,

Ryan told his mother, "Let's just pretend I don't have it." When Jeanne tried to tell Ryan that that was impossible, Andrea told her, "Mom, that's not what he means." "See Mom, she knows me better than you," Ryan countered. "I just don't want every time somebody enters a room, to talk like, 'Poor Ryan, he's dying.' I just want to go ahead and go on with my life." In Ryan's mind, that included going back to school.[36]

3

"Somewhere, there's going to be that first student with AIDS wanting to go to school"

1985 and the Question of Public Knowledge

Ryan would remain at Riley Hospital until January 24, 1985. On January 10, *Kokomo Tribune* readers encountered a Page Three story by Christopher M. MacNeil headlined "AIDS Case Confirmed." MacNeil's article quoted Dr. Charles Barrett, of the Indiana State Board of Health Chronic and Communicable Disease Control Division, who verified that Howard County's second confirmed case of AIDS was a 13-year-old boy at Riley Hospital in Indianapolis, and that authorities believed he had contracted the disease through a transfusion. The county's only other known case, detected the previous summer, had involved an anonymous adult male "believed to be in one of the at-risk groups." The announcement of his illness made Ryan the 31st reported case in the state of Indiana, a number that led Barrett to observe that Indiana resembled the rest of the country in terms of prevalence. More than 70 percent of the state's diagnosed cases involved gay or bisexual men, followed by IV drug users. The state also reported one Haitian and one other person who had contracted the disease from a blood transfusion. Of the 31 patients, 16 had already died. The article never mentioned Ryan's name, and once Ryan was released from the hospital, the Whites encountered no problems associated with his diagnosis—yet.[1]

In fact, Jeanne White and her son never thought of invoking the privacy to which they were entitled. When asked later whether she had ever considered keeping Ryan's diagnosis a secret, Jeanne replied, "People ask me all the time, 'why did you go public?' I never really thought to hide it." Their natural candor and trust would cost them dearly. By not hiding Ryan's AIDS, the Whites deviated from the practice of nearly every other family in similar circumstances. Their community's reception of the Whites only reinforced the resolve on the part of the majority of those infected with HIV to stay hidden. The question of how much the public was entitled to know about a person with AIDS was also implicated by the media's role in shaping public knowledge about AIDS writ large—as this chapter will demonstrate, the media fed the public a steady diet of speculation and hysteria combined with a smattering of actual facts. Jeanne and Ryan's decision not to hide his diagnosis, however right or natural it may have felt to them at the time, exacted a price. Because the Whites went public, they provided a fearful, ill-informed, and angry public with a target: a teen and his family. By comparison, families in similar circumstances in Massachusetts and New York remained cloaked in privacy, so parents instead directed their wrath at authority figures: school officials and those officials' medical advisors. This chapter explores the tension between public and private information; both the Whites and officials at Continental Steel struggle with whether to share, how much to share, and when to share it—if at all.[2]

As for Continental Steel, 1985 began on a positive enough note, but quickly devolved. Financial and environmental questions went unanswered, as much of the company's fate seemed to be decided behind closed doors. The company tried to keep its mounting troubles hidden from the public, but seismic events—an exodus of top executives, a mass resignation of board members—culminating in a year-end bankruptcy filing undermined its tight-lipped strategy. With each announcement, the firm imparted only the bare minimum of details necessary for a news release, and left its workers, its shareholders, and the public guessing. This closing of ranks at the steel mill contrasted greatly with the openness of the White family as they dealt with their own seismic events that same year.

A second *Tribune* article—this time specifically naming Ryan—followed on March 3. The piece, authored by Steve Marschand and titled "Local Youth Faces AIDS," featured a photograph of Ryan and Jeanne, mentioned the Whites' home address, and told the story of how Ryan had come to be infected with the disease while undergoing treatments for his hemophilia. The story discussed the various opportunistic infections—thrush, esophageal sores, and an intestinal parasite—with which Ryan had recently coped, and then went on to describe Jeanne's response to the concerns expressed by parents of Ryan's fellow patients in Riley's Teen Unit. Regarding the possibility of Ryan transmitting the virus to others, Jeanne White explained that "[a]s long as his blood doesn't mix with anyone else's, and there is no sexual contact there is no problem." Ryan told the reporter that the only precaution the doctors and nurses took while treating him involved wearing rubber gloves when they thought they might come into contact with his blood. As for school, Marschand's article noted that officials at Western Middle School might allow him to study from home and would revisit whether he could return to class in person when the next academic year began. Finally, the piece mentioned a fund established by Jeanne's co-workers at Delco in order to help the family pay for the cost of Ryan's treatment, the Ryan White Foundation. All in all, the article's tone was factual and calm, and contained no hint of the divisions that would rock the community in the months and years to come. But directly underneath it, on the same page, sat another article with a less reassuring headline: "AIDS Test Has Health Officials Worried."[3]

Blood

French researchers at the Institut Pasteur, led by Drs. Jean-Claude Chermann and Françoise Barré-Sinoussi, had isolated the retrovirus that caused AIDS in 1983. Once the CDC was able to confirm those results in 1984, scientists quickly developed two blood tests for antibodies to the virus, the ELISA test and the Western Blot test. The FDA licensed the tests in early March 1985, but as the *Tribune*'s story revealed, local hospital and Red Cross officials were not enthused about the new screening tool for donated blood. Among other concerns, they feared that false-positive results would pose a significant problem, and that "the test might encourage high risk groups, mainly homosexual and bisexual men, to donate blood just to get their blood screened. Consequently, the test's error rate could allow some contaminated blood to slip into the blood system." U.S. Department of Health and Human Services Secretary Margaret Heckler encouraged people who wanted blood screenings to avoid blood banks, and instead to seek the test from private or public health laboratories.[4]

The previous year had ended with the CDC counting 9,920 reported cases of AIDS; the dead numbered 3,665. Most of the afflicted and deceased were gay men, and the linkage between the disease and sexual practices considered outside of mainstream norms proved key to its early social construction. David Black, who wrote two in-depth articles for *Rolling Stone* on AIDS in 1985, recounted some jokes making the rounds that year:

> During his morning radio show on WNBC, Don Imus broadcast a sketch
> which featured a debate between God and an obviously gay Deputy Mayor
> of New York City, in which God, hesitating to shake hands, asked the Deputy
> Mayor, "You got a surgical glove?"

Black also described an editorial cartoon by the *Buffalo News'* Tom Toles, which featured a CDC official conducting a "man on the street" interview and asking the question "What do you think about AIDS?" The responses:

> "I know it can be fatal," says a gentleman in a porkpie hat. "I just haven't decided if I think it's serious yet." "It affects homosexual men, drug users, Haitians, and hemophiliacs," says a woman. "Thank goodness it hasn't spread to human beings yet." [...] "I only hope that scientists are able to discover a cure soon," says a man with a moustache. "But not too soon."[5]

The mentality that both blamed gay men for the AIDS epidemic and labeled them a direct threat to the health of heterosexuals (lesbians were almost always invisible in these rhetorical forays) had been developing for at least two years before Black wrote about Toles' cartoon in 1985. In 1983, the conservative weekly magazine *Human Events* had published an anonymous piece titled "AIDS Epidemic: The Price of Promiscuity." The article, citing the danger posed by the disease to the public blood supply, declared "homosexual activity" to be a threat to everyone's health and imagined that "AIDS victims could deliberately contaminate the blood supply, thus spreading the condition into the general population" in order to force the federal government to increase funding for research and treatment. The piece ended by quoting columnist Patrick Buchanan's admonition that homosexuals "have declared war upon nature, and now nature is exacting an awful retribution."[6]

The Moral Majority, a group founded by the fundamentalist evangelical the Rev. Jerry Falwell, shared Buchanan's view of the AIDS epidemic as a Manichean struggle between a deviant homosexual minority and the forces of goodness. The July 1983 issue of the group's *Moral Majority Report* featured a cover photograph of a man, a woman, a boy, and a girl—all white, and all wearing surgical masks. "AIDS" appeared in block letters above the photo; below it appeared the words "Homosexual Diseases Threaten American Families" (thus implying that gays were neither truly American nor capable of having families). Inside, an article by Dr. Ronald S. Godwin warned that AIDS was a "time bomb." An inset photograph of the fair-haired head and shoulders of the toddler-aged girl from the cover, wearing her surgical mask, illustrated the piece, which alerted the reader to the danger of AIDS spreading to "defenseless heterosexuals whose only mistake was to need a blood transfusion ... or to secretly choose a bisexual mate."

Indeed, Godwin continued, "an entire nation stands essentially defenseless before a malignant minority—unable to take the simplest steps to protect itself" lest it arouse the "powerful" and "influential" "homosexual lobby" and media empire. While the spectral threat of AIDS-stricken gay men intentionally contaminating the nation's blood supply never materialized, the fear of *inadvertent* infection still lingered in 1985, as evidenced by the Kokomo officials' concern about the AIDS screening test.[7]

By the time Ryan went public with his diagnosis in March 1985, scientists knew much more than they had two years earlier about how AIDS was, and was not, transmitted. But the increasing certainty that accompanied the passage of time failed to tone down the media's approach to the subject. After years of relegating AIDS coverage to their back pages, news outlets began to feed the public AIDS panic. Like such right-wing organs as *Human Events* or the *Moral Majority Report*, mainstream publications *Newsweek* and *Life* decided that hyperbole sold magazines and designed their covers accordingly. *Life*'s July 1985 cover screamed to its viewers, "Now No One Is Safe from AIDS." The accompanying story, "The New Victims," informed readers that "the AIDS minorities are beginning to infect the heterosexual, drug-free majority." While not "numerous," the "new cases ... show the same relentless growth as the earlier risk groups: a doubling every year." The magazine warned that "[s]ome private health insurers may collapse under the weight of the epidemic." The article did reassure readers that, unlike the flu virus, AIDS was not contagious through casual contact, and that it required a needle or sexual intercourse for transmission into the bloodstream—but its author also gave serious consideration to the hypothesis that mosquitoes were vectors of the disease. Covers and stories such as these only sowed fear and confusion. By reporting theories for which there was little scientific consensus (such as the mosquito-borne AIDS idea) with the same weight and consideration as concepts on which a majority of scientists agreed (such as AIDS not being transmitted through casual contact), the media deemed both equally worthy of publication and serious consideration. By doing so, writers and editors did a grave disservice to the public.[8]

Newsweek's August 12, 1985, issue featured a blood-red cover, an inset photo of a gaunt, nearly unrecognizable Rock Hudson (whose emaciated appearance on his friend Doris Day's talk show a month earlier had shocked viewers), and the word "AIDS" in three-inch-high letters. Accompanying these images was text designed for maximum impact while the magazine sat on newsstands: "It is the nation's worst public-health problem. No one has ever recovered from the disease, and the number of cases is doubling every year. Now fears are growing that the AIDS epidemic may spread beyond gays and other high-risk groups to threaten the population at large." As with *Life*'s cover feature, the magazine did include some useful factual information. A sidebar listing common myths about AIDS assured readers that "there is no evidence that it is spread through sneezing, coughing, talking or shaking hands." With respect to the belief that gay men contracted AIDS as a result of their own promiscuity, via hundreds, if not thousands, of sexual encounters, the magazine declared that although multiple exposures would increase a person's chance of getting AIDS, "it is still possible to acquire it from a single partner, sometimes referred to as 'meeting Mr. Wrong.'" Even the most measured prose, though, could not obscure the grimness of the news surrounding AIDS in 1985.[9]

In April, the Department of Health and Human Services (HHS) and the United Nations World Health Organization (WHO) hosted the First International AIDS Conference in Atlanta, Georgia. By that point, the AIDS epidemic was becoming a true pandemic: more than 10,000 cases had been reported in the U.S., and countries in Europe and Africa also reported epidemics. In late August, parental objections forced the New York Archdiocese to shelve its plan to place a shelter for AIDS patients in a disused convent located next to a parochial school in the Upper West Side. In September, officials at the Central Indiana Regional Blood Center reported that their blood bank faced "the most critical blood shortage in recent history," owing to the prevalence of the erroneous belief that a person could catch AIDS by donating blood. In November, Boston neurosurgeon Vernon H. Mark suggested that state-owned Penikese Island, which had served as a leper colony from 1902 to 1922, be used to quarantine carriers of the AIDS virus who spread it by "irresponsible" behavior.[10]

As of 1985, then, it seemed that every piece of reliable factual information about AIDS that appeared in the public discourse came with a corresponding expression of hysteria or fear. The federal government offered no unified, reassuring response, no widespread campaign to educate the public. Consumers of the news could pick and choose which information seemed most credible to them, and then filter it through their preexisting prejudices and fears. Uncertainty permeated the public discussion of AIDS in 1985. In this climate, a person with AIDS had every incentive to hide his diagnosis and remain out of the public eye.

Steel

Uncertainty also characterized the fate of Continental Steel. Throughout the year, a disparity would emerge and grow—a widening gap between the company's words and its deeds. Its management and board constantly balanced how much information concerning the true state of Continental's financial and environmental liabilities should be shared with the public and with stockholders. Although its modernization campaign, including the installation of the new continuous billet caster, was well underway in 1985, the firm had exacted concessions from local unions before that work could proceed. For those workers as well as for other citizens of Kokomo, the question remained whether that new equipment would prove to be the answer to the company's problems, as so many hoped.

At the beginning of the year, the Indiana Labor and Management Council and the Kokomo Labor and Management Council—a division of the Kokomo-Howard County Chamber of Commerce—issued a brochure titled "Progress Through Cooperation." The brochure publicized the recent accord between Continental Steel's management, the United Steelworkers, and the North Central (Indiana) Building Trades Council, allowing the Italian firm, Danieli, to construct and install the steel company's modern new billet caster. The job called for highly specialized workers, and Danieli refused to give Continental a warranty on the caster unless Danieli's own employees could perform the installation. As further incentive for Continental, Danieli agreed to finance the $21 million project—a crucial offer, given Continental's heavy financial commitment to its new rod mill. Continental had a powerful bargaining chip to play in its talks with local unions: without the modern equipment, the company would have to shut its doors, costing the union—and the community—1,300 jobs. Of all the factors—the guarantee, the financing—the threatened closure was easily the most persuasive. What choice did the local unions really have?[11]

In April 1985, Continental reported its earnings for 1984. While revenues were up an impressive $14 million, higher production associated with the new rod mill had contributed to an overall loss of $20 million. With the new continuous billet caster scheduled to come online during the second quarter of 1985, however, the company forecast increased earnings. In March, Continental had secured an amended credit line of $26 million from its funder of the past few years, Trefoil Capital of New York, including a $4 million term loan that was not due to be repaid fully until 1990. As far as public perception was concerned, even if the company was deeply in debt, Continental's future appeared stable enough. It seemed to be making all the right moves—modernizing its equipment, securing capital—to enable it to compete.[12]

So the company's news release in the first week of July, announcing that it had dramatically reorganized at the top, came as a surprise. What the firm chose to share with the public was that, effective Wednesday, July 3, Thomas Sigler—Continental's president for the past two years—would step down from his post and remain on "special assignment." In place of a successor, the board named two men to the office of chairman, David Pollak and Pierre J. Stanis. Like Sigler, Stanis, a Florida-based financial consultant, had been affiliated with Continental since its emergence from

Chapter 11 reorganization in the early 1980s. Stanis had been responsible for successfully securing financing from lenders like Trefoil. Neither Stanis nor Pollak lived in Kokomo, but a spokesperson for Continental told the *Kokomo Tribune* that both men planned to spend several days each week locally.[13]

Any hope that reshuffling its executives would produce stability at Continental proved short-lived. In late September, the *Kokomo Tribune* reported that eight members of Continental's board of directors—including its chairman, Howard R. Hawkins—had tendered their resignations. In a news release issued by the company, Hawkins related the mass departures to concerns over liability insurance, and not to the company's "operations, policies, or practices." The company was unable to purchase "directors and officers' liability insurance … on such terms that both made economic sense for the company and its stockholders, and [that] provided coverage that was sufficient to protect the directors." The news release offered no details to explain the directors' concern with respect to their liability— clearly, they felt exposed, but for what reason?[14]

The answer may have lain in the new environmental issues arising at Continental's 183-acre site. Since 1946, the company had been collecting its waste pickle liquor in a 10-acre, 20-million-gallon surface impoundment system. The Indiana Department of Environmental Management (IDEM) had identified chromium, cadmium, lead, and iron from that impoundment in the on-site groundwater during inspections in both 1984 and 1985. According to the Environmental Protection Agency (EPA), residents of nearby areas obtained their drinking water from private wells within three miles of the site. The remediation for such problems would easily run into the millions of dollars—money that Continental did not have. Still, the exact reasons for the departure of Continental's chief and board members remained a mystery. The public only knew what *Kokomo Tribune* reporters were able to unearth and share.[15]

Two months later, Continental made three additional, worrisome announcements. On November 21, it disclosed that it had missed a payment, due November 15, on its continuous billet caster—and that interim chairman Pierre Stanis was to be replaced by a new chairman of the board, Jack R. Wheeler, a former president of Kentucky Electric Steel Company. Stanis, the company announced, had agreed to stay on as a financial consultant. Matthew Chinski resigned from the board but stayed on as vice president for administration and chief financial officer. The next day, vice president of employee relations Doug Brooks announced that Continental would lay off 200 workers effective the week of November 25, and that the layoff would last at least through the remainder of 1985. Brooks told the *Tribune* that the layoffs were unrelated to Continental's missed payment on its billet caster. The layoff brought the total number of idle Continental workers to 325.[16]

Finally, at about noon on November 25, 1985, Kokomo's third-largest employer, the Continental Steel Corporation, filed for relief under Chapter 11 of the U.S. Bankruptcy Code in federal court in Indianapolis. The company's news release cited three reasons for its filing: an "inability … to realize benefits of its modernization program, its higher than expected operating costs, and the heavy burden of its pension and other obligations." Curiously, no mention was made in this statement of any potential costs of compliance with environmental regulations, despite the fact that the issue of pollution had lingered in the background at the Continental site throughout much of the 1980s. Treasurer Richard F. Egge told a reporter that the company had reached a post-petition financing agreement with Trefoil Capital, but the court had not yet approved the deal. Continental was represented both by the Indianapolis law firm of Barnes & Thornburg and by Choate, Hall and Stewart of Boston. The news release maintained an optimistic tone, stating that the recent appointment of Jack Wheeler as president, along with continued production, would ultimately result in "substantial cost savings" that would allow the company to emerge from Chapter 11. The regularly scheduled shareowners' meeting, however, was postponed indefinitely.[17]

At a hearing two days later, Bob Gargill, an attorney from Choate, Hall and Stewart, stated that after investing $40 million in the modernization project, the company was unable to meet its obligations to creditors, and that it had roughly 20 unsecured creditors. Chinski, the CFO and vice president of administration, told the *Tribune* that the company was on track to post losses of $24 million in 1985. In December, the company announced that it had reached agreements with three of its creditors, all utility companies: Public Service Indiana, which provided electricity (and which was one of Continental's top five creditors), the Kokomo Gas & Fuel Company, and the Indiana-American Water Company. Chinski promised that the company would pay its bills in advance on a weekly basis from then on. These agreements would enable Continental to continue its manufacturing operations, and allow the utility providers to keep Continental, a large customer.[18]

Continental Steel was clearly floundering, but by all outward appearances, the company valiantly refused to give up the fight. The venerable firm had been a bastion of local industry for 90 years, and many in Kokomo either had worked there or knew someone who had. Its leaders had displayed tenacity in filing for reorganization, as opposed to liquidation, under the bankruptcy code. As 1985 drew to a close, whether they had chosen the best option was still an open question. With its habit of divulging information via news releases, Continental controlled the narrative and, its officials hoped, public perception. Anyone following the stories in the newspaper would have to wonder whether Continental was being completely open about its situation. Whether Ryan White would be able to attend classes at Western Middle School was also very much an open question.

Ryan White

Once Ryan announced his desire to return to school, Jeanne turned to the National Hemophilia Foundation for support. Years later, she would tell an interviewer from the *Saturday Evening Post* of the disappointing response she encountered, revealing the tension between the Whites and the larger hemophilia establishment about the decision to be open about Ryan's diagnosis. Perhaps when Jeanne and Ryan went public with his AIDS, they threatened the viability of the image that the NHF and the blood industry had worked so hard to promote after years of marginalization: at last, the public narrative had changed, and people with hemophilia could thrive in regular society, not merely survive. The NHF, which represented consumers of blood products, wielded political and economic clout in its sphere of influence and depended on a successful image. And then AIDS surfaced. As Jeanne recalled:

> [w]hen Ryan first became ill, I really got into it with the president of the National Hemophilia Foundation. I was very upset because they didn't come forward to help me out at all. I don't mean with money—I mean support-wise. I couldn't get any help from them when I was trying to get Ryan back into school, because I knew hemophiliacs all had it. They tried to hide [AIDS among hemophiliacs]. I couldn't go to the media and tell them that 95 percent of the severe hemophiliacs now were positive for AIDS, because then I would be hurting all my counterparts. I couldn't do that to the mothers I've talked to over all the years. The president of the National Hemophilia Foundation told me, "Well, we're letting the medical profession fight our battles for us, because we're trying to keep a very low profile." And I said, "We're talking about every child, every hemophiliac here. We're not just talking about Ryan White." I spent two hours one night on the phone with him, and I was just very irate after I finished.

Unlike the Whites, the leadership of the NHF shied away from a public battle. The stakes were too high.[19]

Jeanne was similarly frustrated in her attempts to get an answer from Western School Corporation officials regarding her son's return to classes in 1985. Ryan was healthier, gaining weight, and feeling bored at home. Shortly before spring break, Jeanne called Western Middle School principal Ronald Colby to ask if Ryan could come at lunchtime on the last day before vacation started in order to say hello to his friends. Colby told her to call him back after the break. When she did, according to Jeanne, "he told me that I needed to talk to the local Board of Health, because he said the local Board of Health were—some people had wanted quarantine signs on our door. And he said, 'But you need to talk to them—but Ryan cannot even come to visit school.'" Jeanne recalled, "I was kind of upset, so I called the local Board of Health and they said, 'No, we're not going to put quarantine signs, but we are waiting on some guidelines from the state.' They said the state of Indiana [was] the first state to have to deal with this, and they told me just to be patient and give them a few days to get these guidelines." While the Whites waited, they gradually became aware of their community's sentiments about the situation. Though matters had seemed so promising in the March *Tribune* article about Ryan's diagnosis—the fund at Delco, the probability that he would return to school—the community had already begun to show signs of animosity toward the Whites.[20]

Ryan's memoir includes an account of his family's first visit to church in the spring of 1985, after he had grown healthy enough to go outdoors. Spotting their arrival, a friend of his mother's, whom he called Alice, walked all the way from her seat in the first pew down the aisle, smiled, and gave Jeanne a long hug. But every time Ryan coughed, heads turned in his direction; no one would use the bathroom after he did; and "people shooed their kids away from us" on the way out. A short time later, in the waning weeks of the school year, Ryan's friend Chris Sadler was expelled for three days after hitting a fellow student who joked: "What kind of bread do fags eat? Ryan White bread." Despite that incident, Ryan badly wanted to return to school. "I *like* being at school," he told his mother. "I don't want to stay home alone—I want to be with my friends, just like everybody else."[21]

Dr. Alan Adler, who served as the Health Officer for the Howard County Health Department, recalled that he had declined to certify Ryan's return to school that spring because he lacked sufficient information about Ryan's overall condition. Adler, who was born in nearby Tipton County and had gone to medical school because he felt a calling from God, decided to err on the side of caution: "I think at that time because it was considered an infectious disease, and there was so little known about it … we declined to admit him to school at that point until I could gather some more information." Adler admitted that as a family doctor, AIDS "was not on the radar screen" for him: "I didn't even know what we were talking about when they're talking about an HIV infection."[22]

For his part, Principal Colby recalled no formal decision to keep Ryan out of school in the spring of 1985. He felt that Ryan was better off repeating the seventh grade anyway, due to the length of time he had been away from school because of his illness. Over the summer, though, Western School officials knew that they would need to make a formal decision regarding

Ryan's attendance during the 1985–1986 school year. According to Daniel W. Carter, a German teacher who served as the president of the Western School Board for twenty years, the school corporation put off giving Jeanne and Ryan a definite answer while it awaited word from Dr. Adler at the county health department; Adler, in turn, awaited guidelines from the Indiana State Board of Health (ISBH). In fact, the state had recently hired a new Health Commissioner; Dr. Woodrow A. Myers had begun working at his new post on February 18, 1985.[23]

Myers was only 32 years old when he took command of Indiana's public health service. A native Hoosier, he had graduated from both Harvard Medical School and the Stanford University Graduate School of Business. Before Indiana Governor Robert D. Orr appointed him to the health post, Myers worked as an assistant professor of medicine at the University of California at San Francisco, as quality assurance chairman at San Francisco General Hospital, and as a physician health adviser to the Senate Committee on Labor and Human Resources. Myers was also a former football player, having played well enough to make varsity as a Stanford undergraduate. During his first month as Indiana's Health Commissioner, Myers asked the ISBH's Executive Board to form an AIDS Advisory Committee composed of members from the Indiana State Medical Association, the Indiana University Medical Center, the Indiana Hospital Association, the Indiana Public Health Association, as well as representatives from mental health advocacy groups, the gay community, the state blood banks, the nursing profession, local health departments, the state legislature, and a private citizen. The advisory committee would make recommendations to the ISBH as well as advise the Executive Board of new developments with respect to AIDS. The Executive Board approved Myers' request; thereafter, the AIDS Advisory Committee's report remained a regular agenda item at the ISBH's Executive Board meetings.[24]

At the board's July 10, 1985, meeting, Dr. Robert Hamm gave the AIDS Advisory Committee's report. Since May 8, the Committee had met twice; Hamm reported that "guidelines for school attendance for children with AIDS or AIDS related conditions have been developed and will be compared with guidelines being released by the Communicable Disease Control section of the U.S. Department of Health and Human Services. It is hoped these guidelines can be released by mid–August." In other words, neither Dr. Adler of the Howard County Health Department, nor Carter and the other officials at Western School Corporation in Russiaville, had any state or federal guidelines in hand in early July.[25]

Events in July developed quickly. As Ryan's health continued to improve, he kept up his paper route for the *Kokomo Tribune*, and he felt ready to return to school. On Thursday, July 25, 1985, Ryan delivered a paper in which Rock Hudson publicly acknowledged (through spokespeople, since he was incapacitated in a Parisian hospital) the reason for his shockingly frail appearance—he had AIDS. David L. Kirp, who has studied the attempts of children with AIDS to attend school during these years, writes that Hudson's disclosure proved a watershed event for "middle America," because the media did not explicitly relate the hyper-masculine Hudson's illness to gay sex. "Instead," Kirp observes, the news was "taken as evidence that 'AIDS can reach anyone.'" Jeanne White recalled that the announcement "immediately engaged" the entire country in the AIDS outbreak—and that it gave the press a new angle on the disease. "The media seemed to understand something that nobody in Kokomo had figured out, including me—that this was an important story because it represented the tip of a deadly iceberg. We were having a plague. Not just *them*, but *us*." Hudson's case served as a springboard for the media to present AIDS stories in a new way; importantly, the timing of Western's decision to exclude Ryan White, on the heels of Hudson's disclosure, ensured that Ryan's story would become "Exhibit A" in that new presentation.[26]

It was Western's Superintendent, James O. ("J.O.") Smith, who, on July 30, 1985, made the final decision to bar Ryan from attending school. Kirp, who interviewed Smith for his study, attributed the superintendent's reasoning to the general public's confusion both about AIDS (first it had been a "gay plague"; now was the "general population" vulnerable?) and about how it was transmitted (did finding minute amounts of the virus in saliva and tears mean it was spread by casual contact, despite most scientists' assurances?), as well as to "smart politics." Indeed, Smith's decision turned out to be quite popular locally, and it helped to cement his previously insecure position as Superintendent. In his public statements, however, Smith avoided talk of politics. Instead, he stuck with the theme of erring on the side of caution. "With all the things we do and don't know about AIDS," he told a reporter for the *Indianapolis Star* on July 30, "I just decided not to do it." Smith added that "there are a lot of unknowns and uncertainties, and then you have the inherent fear that would generate among the classmates ... we are also in the habit of keeping kids out who have communicable diseases." He also noted that he was unable to find teachers willing to volunteer to tutor Ryan at home.[27]

Smith's characterization of AIDS as "communicable" implied that, by keeping Ryan out, he was protecting the health of his classmates. For most people—especially in the midst of an epidemic—no great leap separates "communicable" from "contagious." In his essay, "What Is an Epidemic? AIDS in Historical Perspective," medical historian Charles E. Rosenberg explains that "even when ... physicians have questioned the contagiousness of a particular disease, most laypersons have simply assumed that epidemic disease was almost by definition transmissible from person to person and have shunned those who might be potential sources of infection." This natural tendency to assume easy transmissibility was aided, during the early years of the AIDS crisis, by the *Journal of the American Medical Association*'s (JAMA) 1983 article, authored by Dr. James Oleske et al., linking "living in high-risk households"—not sexual contact, intravenous drug abuse, or contaminated blood products—to an increased susceptibility to AIDS in children. Dr. Anthony S. Fauci's editorial in that same issue, which gave serious consideration to the possibility of casual contact, lent the gravitas and prestige of the National Institutes of Health to Oleske's contention. But by the time that Smith made his decision in 1985, however, doctors and scientists had repeatedly and publicly stated that AIDS was *not* spread by casual contact. Nevertheless, the public still tended to conflate "epidemic," "contagious," "communicable," and "infectious." The continued existence of contradictory information—all of it from credentialed experts—proved as likely to undermine public faith in medical expertise as it was to encourage further investigation of the facts. For those already disposed to an opinion on AIDS-related questions—such as whether to deny Ryan White admission to school—just one study, *one* expert opinion, no matter how dated or discredited, justified saying, in effect, "See? We don't have all of the answers about AIDS yet. There are so many unknowns."[28]

School board president Dan Carter recalled that J.O. Smith told Jeanne White on July 30 that he had decided to deny Ryan's attendance because he still lacked government guidelines. Smith told Carter that Jeanne "took it well and seemed to be expecting it. It wasn't what she wanted to hear, but she seemed to be understanding." But Jeanne maintained that she learned about Smith's decision from a CBS television news reporter who called her at work to ask for her reaction to Smith's decision. Jeanne wrote that she "broke down and wept" on receiving the call. "My naïveté, and my total absorption in getting Ryan well, kept me from realizing the truth—which was that from day one, from the time those teachers visited Riley.... Western School District was determined not to let Ryan return." Still, she told an interviewer that "I had not known. You know, they caught me so off guard. That was when I found out." It was also the moment when the national and international media first focused the public's gaze on Ryan White. Over the next several years, that scrutiny would increase, and not cease until well after his death.[29]

National media coverage of the Ryan White story began on the night of Tuesday, July 30, when the Whites appeared in a story on the *CBS Evening News*. The next day, the *Los Angeles Times* ran an Associated Press story under the headline "School in Indiana Bars Boy with AIDS: Officials Fear Hemophiliac Will Spread Disease." Subsequent media coverage across the country continued to associate the city of Kokomo with Ryan's exclusion. The Los Angeles paper quoted J.O. Smith ("With all the things we do and don't know about AIDS, I just decided not to do it"); Ryan ("I'm pretty upset about it. I'll miss my friends mostly"); and a CDC official who stated that there was no scientific evidence that AIDS "can be transmitted by casual contact." The article also informed readers that the Indiana State Board of Health "had issued a report Tuesday [July 30] saying children with AIDS who are well enough should be allowed to attend school." On the morning of July 31, Jeanne and Ryan sat for a live interview on the CBS Morning News. The Whites' telephone did not stop ringing during those early days. Jeanne recalled thinking of the phrase "overnight sensation"—"everybody was calling," she said. From Daniel Carter's perspective, after "word got out that the school had denied him admission to school … the whole country starts swooping down on us, 'How dare you?'" On August 1, a front-page story in USA Today described Ryan's predicament, as well as that of other pediatric AIDS patients. The story quoted some of his would-be schoolmates: "Other kids 'wonder why he can't go to school if everybody else can,' says Blair Britton, 10, who helps [Ryan] with the paper route. The ruling 'stinks' adds James Herron, 11, a sixth-grader at Western." The Whites and Western School Corporation were not the only targets of the sudden wave of media attention. As the Los Angeles Times article indicated, reporters also had questions for the State Board of Health.[30]

The Board's AIDS Advisory Committee had hoped to wait until mid–August to release its guidelines for children with AIDS in school, after consulting with the Centers for Disease Control in Atlanta. Once word of Smith's decision became public, however, that changed. A July 31 article in the Indianapolis Star referred to "a State Health Department report hastily distributed Tuesday [July 30] to those involved in Ryan's case" and noted that the Department "recommends that children with AIDS who are well enough be allowed to attend school." The article mentioned that the Department had withheld the report because the Committee was waiting for the CDC's guidelines, and quoted Dr. Myers: "The thrust is, if a kid is well enough he should be in school. Unfortunately, AIDS victims are sick a lot of times and it's not practical. The child's parents, school officials and doctors are the best persons to make that decision." The Howard County Health Department had received a copy of the report, "Guidelines for Children with AIDS/ARC Attending School, Indiana State Board of Health— July 1985," at 8:45 a.m. on July 30, 1985 (the same day Smith announced his decision). The report, with its nine guidelines, totaled three pages, followed by five more pages of appendices containing medical information. The study acknowledged that "[t]hese guidelines were excerpted and adapted from guidelines and recommendations developed" in two states, Florida and Connecticut. The guidelines painstakingly reiterated the facts of AIDS's communicability, discussed infectious body fluids in great detail, and concluded, "no evidence exists to support transmission of the disease by casual contact or by the airborne route. [...] All evidence regarding the transmission of AIDS indicates that the type of contact between persons which normally occurs in a school setting should not result in the transmission of the AIDS virus." Despite being as close to a guarantee as any official pronouncement would offer, the guidelines would prove ineffective in helping Ryan win his bid to attend school. Having first blamed the *lack* of guidelines for their delay in deciding whether Ryan could go to school, Western officials then used the existence of those guidelines to justify their decision.[31]

In a *Kokomo Tribune* article published August 1, both Daniel Carter and J.O. Smith argued that the guidelines, while incomplete, justified Western's decision to exclude Ryan. Carter pointed out that the report did "not address questions about school swimming pools, drinking fountains, and cafeteria silverware." Smith told a reporter, more vaguely, that "his decision to bar AIDS victim Ryan White from school was based on the health board recommended safeguards in the guidelines." He noted that the guidelines called for schools to have items available in the event of accident or injury at school, including rubber gloves, bleach or other disinfectant, and leak-proof bags; he also told the paper that "[s]eparate restroom facilities also would be required." (In fact, the guidelines did not mention restrooms.) Although the ISBH document thoroughly discussed AIDS transmission and noted no documented cases of healthcare workers contracting AIDS through contact with patients, Carter and Smith said they wanted more. "Until we know a good bit more about AIDS, about how it is and is not transmitted, it's better to be safe than sorry," Carter told a *Tribune* reporter.[32]

Not everyone in Kokomo found the guidelines lacking. On August 2, three days after his department received them, Howard County Health Officer Adler addressed a letter to "All Kokomo-Howard County School Corporations." Adler acknowledged receiving the state guidelines on July 30 and informed his readers that his department "fully supports" them. He went on to pledge the county's support for school systems that requested "assistance in implementing protective measures for both the AIDS victim and their contacts." Adler ended his letter on an equivocal note:

> The Howard County Health Department realizes implementation of the state guidelines may not be practical under some circumstances, and therefore respects the autonomy of individual school corporations to make final

decisions regarding the admission of school-age children diagnosed as having
AIDS and/or ARC.

The *Kokomo Tribune* echoed Adler's confidence in the state's guidelines in an editorial that expressed understanding of Western's decision
while calling for school officials to reconsider. The opinion piece, titled
"Every Right," refuted Carter's concerns about the swimming pool, drinking fountain, and cafeteria silverware point by point, leaving no doubt as
to where the *Tribune* stood on the issue. The editors likened the school's
treatment of Ryan's condition to an earlier era in which children with disabilities, epilepsy, and cancer were also shunned; they urged Western
officials to allow Ryan to attend school; and they argued that "any other
decision just further punishes the child for a situation over which he has
no control."[33]

On the same day that the *Tribune* ran its editorial, Von Roebuck of
the Indiana State Board of Health arrived at the Whites' home to escort
Jeanne and Ryan to a news conference in Indianapolis. At the event, Woodrow Myers explained that there was "no public health reason" to exclude
Ryan from attending school, and that there was "no scientific evidence"
that casual contact with Ryan could transmit AIDS to other students. "The
more important question," Myers argued, "is whether we will allow the
uninformed or the underinformed to dictate our actions." Myers did not
specify whether he counted Western school officials among those groups,
but Superintendent Smith responded quickly to his comments, telling the
newspaper that he "wanted a document signed by health officials saying
Ryan White is healthy to go to school. But they can't do that," Smith added.
Myers conceded that state and county health officials lacked legal authority to order Western schools to admit Ryan. The Whites and the school
were at an impasse; reports circulated that both the Indiana Civil Liberties Union and the National Gay Task Force had offered their lawyers' services to Jeanne and Ryan. Jeanne, asked whether she was considering legal
action, stated that she had discussed the matter with her attorney and was
awaiting his advice, but "I love the people at Western, and I am sensitive to
their concerns and don't really want to do that."[34]

In contrast to Jeanne's diplomatic tack, Western school officials were
incensed that Myers had publicly disputed their decision. Both Colby, the
principal, and Carter, the school board president, were lifelong Howard
County residents who had graduated from Western High School in 1959.
They viewed the Harvard-educated, African American doctor as an inter-
loper in their community. From Colby's perspective, "this Woodrow Myers
flew in from California and the guru of all knowledge concerning this …
[a] very arrogant type individual, well I ended up not even hardly talking to

the man. So, of all of this type of material, he provided us very little assistance, very, very little." Carter, too, made his animus toward Myers apparent: "He went very public, very high profile, pressuring us, urging us to change the decision to enroll him." When asked why he thought Myers would publicly second-guess Smith's decision, Carter alluded to a bigger, conspiratorial picture:

> After all this and during a lot of this, we had the very distinct impression that health people, activists, and the whole country, were just waiting with baited [sic] breath. Somewhere, there's going to be that first student with AIDS wanting to go to school. And we had the very distinct impression that they were hoping it would be someplace in "fly-over" country, rather than on the coasts and big population areas where it happened so they could control how it was portrayed. So that they could set up "good guys" and "bad guys." We had the distinct impression that there was a template already in place for how to portray this in the media, and I have the impression that Dr. Myers was operating ... in consistency with this template, wanting to be a national leader in this matter of AIDS and education.

Carter was convinced that Myers had "gone public" *before* Western School Corporation received the ISBH's guidelines, although the county health department's records and contemporary newspaper coverage clearly indicated otherwise. In Carter's eyes, Myers "got the cart before the horse, and I believe deliberately put us in a negative light in so doing. He didn't even issue those guidelines as he was starting to go public." Carter was further displeased to find that, while Myers sent three staff members from the state health department to Kokomo to meet with Western officials (and their attorney) on Monday, August 5, Myers himself did not attend:

> And he sent these three doctors up without those guidelines, and, in fact, I think here is the ultimate insult and dereliction of duty.... This was the predominant issue before the Indiana State Board of Health at that time, and Dr. Myers did not come himself. Dr. Myers had a duty because of the high profile nature of this, because this was ground-breaking, this was pioneering. In those circumstances, Dr. Woodrow Myers had an obligation as a part of his office, to come personally to meet with us, to discuss it, to give us his reasons, discuss possible alternatives, hear our questions and concerns. No, he did not, he stayed down there in the safety of Indianapolis and sent three subordinates.

Like Smith, Carter felt that the guidelines were insufficient. After Western personnel sent a list of questions to Myers' office requesting clarification of some of the points, he recalls, "it was several weeks before we got answers to those questions and they were inconclusive." The correspondence did not settle the matter for either side. On August 6, three days after telling reporters that she would leave the decision whether to sue the school system in her lawyer's hands, Jeanne White stated she would back whatever action her lawyer, Charles Vaughan of Lafayette, decided to take. Meanwhile, the community was beginning to show signs of division.[35]

On August 3, Mitzie M. Johnson, a neighbor of the Whites and self-described "concerned parent" of a child enrolled at Western's elementary school, circulated a petition supporting J.O. Smith's decision among her fellow residents of the 162-unit Vinton Woods Townhouses. She and her husband obtained 99 signatures from the 102 residences they visited. Johnson reported, "we've gotten calls from others (in the complex) who weren't home wanting to sign the petition and from parents in other parts of the Western district." Johnson hoped the petition would be "interpreted as a vote of Western parents' confidence in Smith and an indication of how we (parents of Western students) feel." The petition expressed "prayers" for Ryan and his family but insisted that "we must back Mr. Smith's decision until more evidence is gathered to guarantee the safety of our children as well as Ryan's." Johnson told the newspaper that she asked local health officials for a guarantee and did not get one, "anymore than state officials could give one to Mr. Smith." Smith, for his part, expressed satisfaction in the support, explaining that he had felt "almost like the villain" during the previous week. But not everyone agreed with Johnson and her cohorts. On August 12, the *Tribune*'s "Streettalk" column reported that four out of six people surveyed during the previous week expressed disapproval of Smith's decision to bar Ryan White from school. Pam Lucas of Kokomo told the newspaper, "I disagree with their attempts to keep him out of school because the only way shown to contact [sic] AIDS is through intimate contact and blood transfusions. It's denying him an education." Betty Cooper, also of Kokomo, agreed: "I think if they educate themselves about how the disease is transmitted they would let him in school."[36]

The pressure on Western officials was increasing, and not simply because of the Ryan White matter. On August 7, school corporation teachers picketed the administration building and burned copies of their contract in protest of what they saw as slow-moving negotiations over binding arbitration. Paula Adair, the teachers' union president, would not rule out a strike. The next day, the Whites' attorney, Charles R. Vaughan, announced that he was filing suit: the Whites would seek an order from the U.S. District Court in Indianapolis compelling Western officials to let Ryan back into school. School board president Carter told the *Tribune* that Western would not reconsider. Choosing to ignore published scientific opinion, Carter stated, "We would like evidence that AIDS is not transmitted casually, and no one can give us that."[37]

Even had Carter and his fellow Western officials accepted the validity of Drs. Adler and Myers' opinions, however, the school system would have remained subject to the emotions of its more vocal parents and employees.

John Wood, an attorney and father of two Western district students, drafted a state tort claim notice which he planned to file on August 13; the notice informed the school corporation, the Indiana State Board of Health, the Howard County Board of Health, and the Howard County Board of Commissioners that he intended to seek not less than $300,000 in damages if a Western student "caught" AIDS. In the event that Ryan was allowed back in school, Wood planned to withdraw his children from the district, send them to private school, and sue the district for reimbursement of their tuition costs. By August 30, some 200 parents, teachers, and employees had signed claim forms like Wood's, even though Ryan was barred from the school. Wood redoubled his earlier stance, offering to pay for Ryan's tuition at another Howard County school, if one would enroll him. "I am sick and tired of the Western School Corp., the superintendent, the principal and board of education being made to look the villains in this situation when other corporations haven't had to face this situation," Wood told the *Kokomo Tribune*. Wood also had words for the participants in the "Streettalk" poll: "It's easy for people to take a position when it doesn't affect them." On the other side of the controversy, listeners of one local radio station, WWKI, heard a one-minute message from a New York organization, the AIDS Medical Foundation, targeting Smith and asking him to admit Ryan. In response to the negative feedback the radio station received after it aired the message, WWKI announced plans to allow Mitzie Johnson to record and run a spot for the opposition. WWKI would run Johnson's piece an equal number of times, station manager Dick Lange said. The rival local stations, WIOU and WZWZ, refused to run the AIDS foundation's spot at all.[38]

On August 12, more than 300 people filled Western High School's cafeteria to share their feelings about Ryan's situation at a meeting organized by Mitzie Johnson. Ronald Colby, Paula Adair, and Dr. Jeffrey Squires, a local pathologist, answered emotional parents' questions. Like Carter, many of the parents wanted absolutely guaranteed answers to their questions. Was Western being used as a "guinea pig?" Could people "catch AIDS through drinking fountains and what about sneezes?" Mitzie Johnson told a reporter, "It [AIDS] is in the saliva. They don't know how contagious it is and unless they can give us a 100 percent guarantee, he shouldn't be in school…. Not that I don't feel for Ryan. I do. But his disease is fatal." Paula Adair, the teachers' union president, told the parents that she had conducted her own research on AIDS, contacting the CDC in Atlanta only to find that "their information is inconclusive, just like everyone else's. It's ambiguous." Dr. Squires explained to the parents that classrooms were not risky environments for contracting AIDS: "[Number one] would be a sexual partner and then would come family members. A classroom is not a high-risk category." But when a father asked him, "Is there a guarantee that my daughter can't get AIDS by helping him?" Squires replied that there was not a guarantee. "Then he shouldn't be in school," the father responded to applause. As Ronald Colby asked the parents not to panic and to express themselves calmly and rationally, Squires tried to tell them that guarantees were "just not available." When parents asked why "contaminated persons" with AIDS were not placed in "isolation," Squires revealed his own mindset in his response: "The common cold is not a gay rights issue. This is. Those are the people you're up against." No one at the meeting argued for Ryan's right to an education; no one responded to calls for the "isolation" of "contaminated" persons; no one explained how scientists had arrived at their conclusions that AIDS could not be spread by casual contact; no one pointed out that there were no absolute guarantees in life, period.[39]

Time magazine's hyperbolic August 12 cover did little to assuage mounting fears. Below the word "AIDS" in 2¼-inch-tall letters appeared the subtitle "The Growing Threat/What's Being Done" against a backdrop of the virus magnified 135,000 times as it destroyed a T cell. A color photograph of a serious-looking Ryan White sitting in front of his computer at home illustrated an article which gave a platform to J.O. Smith's reasons for barring Ryan from attending school, despite scientists' conclusions that the AIDS virus was not transmissible through casual contact. "Smith … points to warnings from the Indiana board of health about the risks of exposure to AIDS-infected saliva and body fluids. 'What are you going to do about someone chewing pencils or sneezing or swimming in the pool?' he asks." *Newsweek*'s August 12 issue (featuring the bright red cover and the photo of an ill Rock Hudson) also mentioned Ryan's case in an article titled "The Social Fallout from an Epidemic." Unlike the *Time* article, *Newsweek* cast Smith's decision in a negative light, stating that Ryan was banned from classes "by a school superintendent who said two dentist friends had helped him decide whether it would be safe to let classmates associate with the boy." Ryan's case served the *Newsweek* report for its value in illustrating the point that "ignorance about the way the disease is transmitted can make pariahs of even the most blameless of its victims." Consumers of news magazines across the country were presented with different pictures of events in Kokomo and Russiaville: Smith's concerns were, according to whom one believed, either prudent or ignorant.[40]

Western's teachers shared the former judgment. At a half-hour-long meeting on August 15, they voted unanimously to support his decision to exclude Ryan from school. Teachers' union leader Paula Adair attributed the resolution, according to the *Tribune*, to a "lack of information about AIDS in general and specifically how it is transmitted. Until we can have some factual information showing that there is no danger to other children,

I don't believe there was any other opinion we could form," Adair remarked. Asked whether teachers would comply with a possible court order to admit Ryan, Adair responded that "we'll do what we can to make every attempt to follow the guidelines.... Of course, it'll be reluctantly, but we would do whatever possible to assure that Ryan is treated as fairly as possible. But," she continued, "we would hope there would be some education (about the disease and its transmission) forthcoming." Presumably Adair was referring to the ISBH. But she need not have worried about Ryan's presence for the first day of school on August 26.[41]

On August 16, the parties in *Ryan White b/n/f Jeanne White v. Western School Corporation et al.* argued Ryan's case before U.S. District Judge James E. Noland, who issued a stay of the federal case because Ryan had not yet exhausted his administrative remedies. Ryan's lawyer, Charles R. Vaughan, had based his case against Western on the argument that the school had violated Ryan's right to an education pursuant to the Education for All Handicapped Children Act (EAHCA), the Rehabilitation Act of 1973, the Civil Rights Act of 1871, and the Due Process and Equal Protection clauses of the United States Constitution. Judge Noland ruled that the EAHCA controlled the case, and that it required a student to exhaust his state administrative remedies before a judge had jurisdiction to review the matter. Without dismissing Ryan's case outright, Noland did issue a stay until Ryan pursued his claim through the local and state administrative apparatus. His ruling meant that Ryan would first have to participate in a case conference/administrative hearing with the school; that decision would then be subject to review by the school superintendent; then, by a hearing officer with the state Department of Education; and finally, *that* decision was reviewable by the state Board of Special Education Appeals. Only after all of those proceedings were concluded would the federal district court assume jurisdiction and be able to review the administrative actions. All of this would take months—and no one knew how much time Ryan had left.[42]

The case against Western schools was not Ryan's only suit in federal court. The Whites had worked with Vaughan earlier in 1985 to file a $2 million civil suit against Hyland Pharmaceutical, a wholly owned subsidiary of Baxter Travenol, the company that made and sold the contaminated Factor VIII product (Hemofil) that had infected him with the AIDS virus. However, U.S. District Judge Allen Sharp dismissed the lawsuit on the grounds that, under Indiana law, Hyland qualified as a blood bank, and was thus immune from liability under the state's product liability statute. This ruling was not unique to Indiana. Across the country, people with hemophilia whose Factor VIII had infected them with the AIDS virus found the courthouse doors slammed shut, courtesy of the "blood shield" statutes that had been passed by 41 states in the late 1960s and early 1970s. Indiana's own blood shield law, passed in 1971, classified the "procurement, processing, distribution or use of whole blood, plasma, blood products, [or] blood derivatives"—regardless of whether any money was involved—as "services," not products, in order to insulate them from responsibility under products liability laws. The statute specified that "no such services shall give rise to an implied warranty of merchantability or fitness for a particular purpose, nor give rise to strict liability in tort." Laws such as these had been passed to limit risk in response to a wave of lawsuits by patients who had contracted hepatitis from blood transfusions during the 1960s; as discussed in Chapter 1, the blood services companies feared that tort exposure might force them out of business. Although Vaughan argued that Factor VIII was a product sold by Hyland, not a service provided by the company akin to that offered by a blood bank, his case was futile.[43]

In a sign of the growing animosity and suspicion that surrounded Ryan's situation in Kokomo, Jeanne White told a *Tribune* reporter that she wished news of the tort action had remained quiet, because she wanted no more "trouble" with anyone in Kokomo: "I had all these people saying I was gonna make $2 million off of Ryan in the first place.... I didn't want to go public and say the lawsuit had been dismissed because I didn't want anyone to think I was hinting that I wanted the city to donate money to support us." Her reticence may have been warranted. Ryan's case had caused a controversy, and the Whites would endure the fallout for years to come. In his memoir, Ryan recalled an incident at an Indianapolis diner as they made their way to a hospital appointment in Fall 1985. When he and his mother asked for glasses of water, the owner gave them cans of Coke instead; when they had finished eating, the owner instructed the waitress to throw away their dishes. The Whites also recounted the rumors swirling around Kokomo, that Ryan had deliberately spat and sneezed on vegetables at the grocery store, or that he spat on people when he was angry at them. What historian Richard A. McKay has characterized as the "old and widely held culture trope" of the deliberate disease-spreader would resurface worldwide in 1987 for AIDS with the story of flight attendant Gaetan Dugas, known as "Patient Zero." Yet, in 1985, central Indiana had its own "Patient Zero" figure in Ryan White—and his neighbors all too eagerly believed those wild rumors. Interviewed by the BBC for its *Witness* program in honor of World AIDS Day 2011, former White neighbor Wanda Bowen Bilodeau described some of the harassment she saw the family endure in their Vinton Woods neighborhood: their house and storage barn were spray-painted with the word "faggot"; their garbage was repeatedly dumped out of its bins; their window was shot with a BB gun; and their house, car, and mailbox were repeatedly egged.[44]

Bev Ashcraft, the nurse employed by the Western School Corporation, attributed some of the community's animosity toward the Whites to the fact that they were perceived as outsiders: "Ryan was new to our school corporation, and there was really not a support group for him in the area," she noted. "He was unknown," she continued, "and part of the problem after he was diagnosed with AIDS was people did not know him and I think the fear of the unknown is huge." Speaking to the mindset of the families whose children attended Western Middle School, Ashcraft remarked, "we didn't know him, didn't know his family, didn't know anything about AIDS and I really feel that played a huge role in how the situation unfolded at Western." Even though Jeanne White was literally born and raised in Kokomo, because the Whites had moved to Vinton Woods from Tipton County, she and her family were viewed as outsiders, an unknown quantity. The Kokomo of her childhood was no longer the welcoming hometown she thought it was.[45]

The issue of AIDS patients' school attendance, of course, did not confine itself to Indiana. On August 30, the Centers for Disease Control had issued guidelines recommending that children with AIDS be allowed in classrooms. As of August 20, 1985, the CDC reported that children under 18 comprised 183 of the 12,599 known cases of AIDS in the United States, a number the agency expected to double in the next year. Significantly, however, none of those children had contracted the AIDS virus in their schools or day-care settings. And, the CDC stated, "based on current evidence, casual person-to-person contact as would appear among schoolchildren appears to pose no risk." This was as definitive a pronouncement as parents would get; but still fell short of the ironclad guarantee that many in Russiaville, and elsewhere, desired. The CDC recommended "for most infected school-aged children, the benefits of an unrestricted setting would outweigh the risks of their acquiring potentially harmful infections.... These children should be allowed to attend school." The report concluded with a call for confidentiality for children diagnosed with AIDS—something Ryan did not have.[46]

Recommendations for confidentiality proved wise, given the state of the public's fears as children across the nation returned to school that season. A Harris poll conducted in September showed that 53 percent of respondents believed AIDS was so infectious that it could be spread through sitting in a classroom with an AIDS patient. A CBS News poll found that 47 percent thought they could get AIDS from a drinking glass, and 27 percent thought they could get it from a toilet seat. Perhaps most worrisome were the results of a *Daily News* poll in New York City that October, which found that 40 percent of residents thought people with AIDS should be quarantined.[47]

An editorial in the October 14, 1985, issue of *The New Republic* dubbed these attitudes "AFRAIDS," for "Acute Fear Regarding AIDS." The piece specifically mentioned Ryan White's situation, along with a similar case in Queens, New York, while reminding readers that in 1983 (the latest year for which statistics were available), the number of people—including students—who had died in school bus accidents (130) was far higher than the number of students who had been diagnosed with HIV contracted at school (zero). Along with citing examples of hysteria-inducing magazine covers such *Life*'s "Now No One Is Safe" issue, the editorial discussed an interview in the September 13, 1985, *New York Times*, in which a reporter asked Dr. Martha Rogers of the CDC why officials avoided making definite statements when discussing the transmissibility of the AIDS virus, and instead spoke in terms of what they believed, or what had been documented. Rogers replied that it was hard to prove a negative; even so, "the evidence thus far indicates that transmission by casual contact will never occur." The *New Republic* editorial observed that experts' "efforts to alleviate panic ... backfired: decisive judgments such as 'never' and 'no risk' have been overshadowed ... by caveats such as 'appears,' 'believe,' 'thus far,' and 'indicates.'" The public, unfortunately, read those contingencies as admissions of a lack of knowledge or confidence, when they were actually part of the standard scientific vocabulary.[48]

To be sure, the lack of a coordinated educational public awareness campaign contributed to the ignorance and fear surrounding the AIDS epidemic in 1985. But who was to undertake such a campaign? The federal government's response to AIDS varied. While agencies like the CDC operated as though an epidemic were truly underway, more visible leaders at the highest levels of government responded with either silence or ambiguity. Surgeon General C. Everett Koop, popularly known as "America's family doctor," was not permitted to work on AIDS—or to speak publicly about it—until well into President Reagan's second term. When Assistant Secretary of Health Ed Brandt created an Executive Task Force on AIDS in 1983, Koop was not invited to join. And when the media questioned President Ronald Reagan directly about AIDS at a news conference on September 17, 1985, his answers were less than forceful.[49]

Asked about his response to a federal scientist's call for "a minor moonshot program to attack this AIDS epidemic," Reagan replied, "I have been supporting it for more than 4 years now. It's been one of the top priorities with us, and over the last 4 years, and including what we have in the budget for '86, it will amount to over half a billion dollars that we have provided for research on AIDS in addition to what I'm sure other medical groups are doing. And we have $100 million in the budget this year; it'll be 126 million next year. So, this is a top priority with us. Yes, there's no question about the seriousness of this and the need to find an answer." Pressed by the reporter to respond to the scientist's characterization of such sums as being not nearly enough to attack the problem, the president answered that "I think with our budgetary constraints and all, it seems to me that $126 million in a single year for research has got to be something of a vital contribution."[50]

In fact, during the first decade of the AIDS epidemic, the United States "financed the lion's share of basic research into a biomedical solution," according to historian Peter Baldwin, with France coming in a distant second. While other European nations spent governmental funds caring for the sick, U.S. federal spending went into "basic biomedical research, vaccine development, clinical trials, and epidemiological surveillance, rather than to public health education and prevention programs." Baldwin calculates that American spending on AIDS during the 1980s was "a hundredfold that of the British and ten times per inhabitant of the Swedes." Even as late as 1993, the U.S. was responsible for "some 90 percent of global governmental AIDS research funding," Baldwin notes. Undoubtedly, the United States government spent millions on AIDS research in the epidemic's first ten years. What is also true is that most American scientists agreed that such an amount was insufficient to fight an epidemic—not enough for research, and not enough for prevention. The Reagan administration, committed to cutting government spending whenever and wherever possible, was not inclined to ask Congress to allocate more funds.[51]

Later during the same news conference, a reporter asked President Reagan whether, if he had young children, he would send them to school with a child who had AIDS. The president responded,

> I'm glad I'm not faced with that problem today. And I can well understand the plight of the parents and how they feel about it. I also have compassion, as I think we all do, for the child that has this and doesn't know and can't have it explained to him why somehow he is now an outcast and can no longer associate with his playmates and schoolmates. On the other hand, I can understand the problem with the parents. It is true that some medical sources had said that this cannot be communicated in any way other than the ones we already know and which would not involve a child being in the school. And yet medicine has not come forth unequivocally and said, "This we know for a fact, that it is safe." And until they do, I think we just have to do the best we can with this problem. I can understand both sides of it.

The president made no reference to the CDC's guidelines and recommendations for children with AIDS attending school, which had been issued less than a month earlier. Had he done so, he might have put the weight and prestige of his office behind the CDC's recommendation that children with AIDS should attend school if they were physically able to do so. Rather than vaguely referring to "some medical sources," he could have paraphrased the CDC's August 30 statement that "casual person-to-person contact as would appear among schoolchildren appears to pose no risk," and reassured parents that he would feel comfortable sending children to school if the guidelines were followed. The president's politic reply acknowledged both sides of the issue without supporting either.[52]

The reporter's question had signaled the prominence that the question of children with AIDS in schools had attained by mid–September 1985. Indeed, Ryan's case was not the only one—but it was the most public in 1985. In August 1972, Mark Gardiner Hoyle was born in Swansea, Massachusetts, a small town located roughly 50 miles south of Boston and 15 miles east of Providence, Rhode Island. Like Ryan White, Mark had severe hemophilia and required frequent treatments with Factor VIII in order to remain active and healthy. In June 1985, Mark was diagnosed with AIDS—but unlike Ryan, his diagnosis did not make the local newspapers. On August 26, Mark's father, Jay, and Mark's hematologist, Dr. Peter Smith, met with Swansea school superintendent John E. McCarthy and with Harold Devine, who was the principal of Mark's school, Case Junior High. Also at the meeting were all of the teachers scheduled to teach Mark in their class that academic year, the school system's lawyer, and the school doctor and nurse. Hoyle and the medical professionals answered all of the questions that school personnel had for them, and the next day, August 27, Mark received permission to attend the 8th grade. Importantly, both the Hoyle family and the school personnel kept his diagnosis confidential, and the matter remained relatively quiet for about a week. Then, on September 8, the *New York Times* ran an article discussing the "epidemic of fear" that surrounded children with AIDS in schools in Florida, New York, New Jersey, Connecticut, California, Indiana, Massachusetts, and the District of Columbia. Of all the cases that the *Times* examined, only schools in New York and Swansea had decided to admit the students. A Swansea physician characterized the Kokomo situation as "appalling … based on misinformation and fear." Although rumors had circulated around Swansea that a student with AIDS was in school, word was now officially out. Parents were not pleased that they had learned about the situation some two weeks after school had already started.[53]

Three days later, Swansea officials held a public meeting at the Case High School auditorium. Speakers included Peter Smith (Mark's hematologist); Dr. George F. Grady, an epidemiologist and associate state commissioner in the Massachusetts Department of Health; Curtis Hall, the regional director of the state Department of Education; Principal Devine; and John McCarthy, the superintendent of Swansea schools. More than 50 journalists attended, as did some 700 parents of children who attended the junior high school. At the meeting, officials explained their decision with respect to Mark's attendance and answered questions from the audience. Smith and Grady advocated for Mark during the long and often contentious meeting. One parent likened letting a child with AIDS go to school to allowing "a kid [to] go around with a match with a gallon of gas." Parents decried the school's decision to announce their policy only after fall classes began; like the parents in Russiaville, many of the Swansea parents demanded absolute guarantees about their children's safety and wellbeing. In contrast to their counterparts in Russiaville, Indiana, the doctors and school officials in Swansea maintained their positions throughout hours of answering questions about AIDS, hemophilia, and school policies—no matter how angry, vocal, and confrontational the audience became, Smith, Grady, Devine, and McCarthy explained their decisions firmly, respectfully, unapologetically, and clearly. Some parents expressed no reservations about sending their children to school with the student (whose full name was never disclosed)—they knew him, or knew his family, and knew them as responsible and mature people. Other parents acknowledged their initial discomfort but considered the meeting beneficial: "A lot of us had so much misinformation. The doctors alleviated most of our fears," said Norma Cote. Still others, like Emily Kiley, remained dissatisfied. She told a reporter, "As a parent, I'll never feel completely assured." In the end, most of the parents supported the school's decision.[54]

The controversy over school attendance extended beyond the United States. On September 16, 1985, parents kept 50 out of 194 students home from the Scantabout Primary School in Chandler's Ford, Hampshire, in England, because of the presence there of a nine-year-old student with hemophilia who had received Factor VIII from a donor known to have died of AIDS. The boy, while not diagnosed with AIDS, had tested positive for the antibody. "Although parents have been assured by doctors and education staff that the disease can be transmitted only by direct blood contact, many still fear their children could pick up the [AIDS] virus," reported *The Times*. At a public meeting on September 18, Dr. Anthony Pinching, identified by *The Times* as "a leading AIDS specialist," addressed the parents and answered their questions. The meeting apparently helped; by the next day, only 21 children were absent. Nevertheless, David Watters of the British Haemophilia Society was worried. He had received anxious calls, as he told *The Times*, from both parents and staff members of several other schools. "We have asked the Department of Education to try to dispel the current wave of unnecessary and unreasonable panic which is building up," Watters said. Watters' concerns were valid; many people with hemophilia feared having to "go underground" about their condition because of AIDS panic. In her memoirs, Jeanne White wrote of her total lack of interaction with other local families of people with hemophilia, many of whom "were fiercely determined not to have anybody know who they were" for fear of experiencing the same backlash that faced the Whites. Against this backdrop, the Whites' decision to be publicly visible seems all the more remarkable.[55]

One other school system made headlines in Fall 1985: New York City. On September 1, New York Mayor Ed Koch publicly stated his opinion that no child with AIDS should attend public school. "I don't believe you're going to have any kids with AIDS ending up in the classroom," Koch told the *New York Times*. "If you can establish that a child would be better off, and the child's colleagues would be equally safe, then we would want to have them in the classroom. I don't believe you can establish that." The mayor's remarks followed on the heels of a city health department recommendation that a panel of experts (appointed by the health and education department heads) decide each child's fate on a case-by-case basis. With several school-aged children in the city known to have AIDS, the panel had some work to do.[56]

In a direct parallel to events in Indiana, New York City Schools Chancellor Nathan Quinones had complained about the lack of guidelines with respect to students with AIDS in an August 15 letter to the city's Health Department. In turn, health officials had conceived of the panel of experts to screen students; this response had come a mere five days before classes were set to begin. Parents were already up in arms; a week earlier, two community school districts in Queens had voted to exclude all children with AIDS from their schools—even as the identities of the children at issue, and thus the schools in which they were enrolled, remained ostensibly confidential information.[57]

In early September, J.O. Smith and Daniel Carter flew to New York for a joint news conference with Queens school board president Samuel Granirer. The educators called for an immediate national moratorium on school attendance by AIDS-infected students until the time when, as Carter put it, researchers had a chance to "get their jobs done." Their statement characterized "health officials" of displaying an "overconfident, cavalier, even casual attitude inconsistent with the care and precautions urged for other less serious and more controllable disease" [sic]. The joint statement also called for a national symposium on AIDS and the schools to be attended by educators, parents, and health officials. Attendees would then develop guidelines and explain their findings to laypeople. Jennifer Brier has pointed out that both school officials and parents (who were united across typical fault lines of race and politics) directed their anger toward a bureaucratic and scientific establishment, rather than at IV drug users or other high-risk groups. The day after the news conference, some 500 parents met at P.S. 63 in the

Ozone Park section of Queens and vocally supported a call to picket the school if officials allowed a child with AIDS to attend. A September 8 article in the *Times* quoted epidemiologists and other experts who expressed concern about an "epidemic of fear" accompanying the AIDS epidemic. The experts reiterated the CDC's August 30 recommendation that children with AIDS should attend school if they were physically able and praised the actions of the Swansea school district. But the Swansea school's decision proved exceptional; elsewhere, from Russiaville, Indiana, to Miami, Florida, educators segregated or barred students with AIDS from attending.[58]

After deliberating over the cases of four children with AIDS, the New York panel of experts decided to allow one, a seven-year-old who had been born with the disease, to attend school. Mayor Koch made the announcement on Saturday, September 7, 1985—two days before school was scheduled to begin. Both the identity of the child and the location of the school were kept secret, but that precaution did nothing to stop school boards in Queens and one other district from threatening a boycott of their schools. Monday, September 9, the first day of school, was a spectacle: parents of between 10,000 and 12,000 elementary and junior high school students kept their children home to protest the decision to allow one anonymous second grader with AIDS to attend school. Parents carried signs that read, "Save Our Kids, Keep AIDS Out"; "Teacher's Aides, Yes; Student AIDS, no"; "Our children want grades, not AIDS"; "Stop the lies: We want the facts"; and "Better safe than sorry." In a display of street theater, one mother placed her eight-year-old son inside a coffin and wheeled him around a picket line in front of P.S. 63. The boycott had faded by the next week, but eventually two school boards—Districts 27 and 29 in Queens—decided to bring suit against the city of New York, the city Board of Education and its chancellor and president, and the city Department of Health and its commissioner of health. The judge in *District 27 v. Board of Education* would not issue a ruling in the contentious matter until February 1986. In the meantime, New York City officials announced the formation of a new expert panel of seven doctors who would decide whether students with AIDS could attend schools, again on a case-by-case basis. This additional measure meant each infected student would now have to undergo a three-step process in order to have a chance to attend school.[59]

Russiaville saw no pickets, since Ryan had been prohibited from attending Western schools. Instead, in the week before classes began on August 26, Indiana Bell installed a dedicated two-way speaker system linking the middle school and the Whites' home. But, because of the hot lights from the television cameras that were now a constant presence at the Whites' home, the family had to keep the windows open. (During the first day of school, more than 50 reporters were present.) Traffic on Webster

Street, a busy north-south artery, kept Ryan from hearing the speakers very well unless his teachers spoke directly into a microphone. While their lawyer pursued administrative appeals, Ryan and his mother asked school officials for headphones. Ryan's setup made the national news; a story in the August 27 *New York Times* featured a photo of Ryan sitting at a desk in his bedroom, phone in hand, while his mother looked on. In response to the poor audio quality, AT&T in Indianapolis sent experts to the school to study classroom acoustics and install new equipment. The new technology, which AT&T donated, resulted in greatly improved sound quality for both Ryan and the school.[60]

The media kept their spotlights on Ryan. On August 28, he and Jeanne appeared on ABC's *Good Morning, America* in New York. While they were there, the Whites visited Roosevelt Memorial Hospital for preliminary blood work to learn whether Ryan could undergo an experimental treatment from France, HPA 23. But Ryan's health took a turn for the worse, and he returned to the hospital the first week of September. As a public figure, his condition was now national news: both *USA Today* and the *New York Times*, in addition to the *Indianapolis Star* and the *Kokomo Tribune*, announced the hospitalization. Jeanne took a temporary 30-day leave from her job as a stockchaser at Delco Electronics so that she could stay at Riley Hospital with her son. Ryan, discharged from the hospital but still battling a cough and a fever, was featured in the "Newsmakers" section of *USA Today* on September 18 in anticipation of the first hearing in his administrative appeals process, a case conference before Principal Colby scheduled for September 19. On his way into the closed-door conference, Charles Vaughan told reporters that he did not expect a favorable ruling. Colby, the hearing officer, was joined by Jeanne White, David Day and Stephen Jessup, attorneys for the school system, Dr. Charles Barrett, director of the State Board of Health's Communicable Disease section, and Bev Ashcraft, the school nurse for Western School Corporation. Colby had ten days to issue a recommendation to J.O. Smith, who would then decide whether to admit Ryan. Smith's decision, in turn, was appealable to the state Department of Education, where a hearing officer could hold another hearing on the matter. Colby ruled against Ryan's bid to return to school; in his written findings issued October 1, he completely rejected the Indiana State Board of Health guidelines as impractical and unenforceable in a public-school setting. He also cited concerns of a hostile school climate, finding that the "potential of social discrimination from Ryan's peers and adults could be devastating." Colby also invoked a by-now reliable red herring, the risk of transmission via casual contact: "we need to know more about AIDS," he wrote, "before Western requires students to come into even casual contact with a person known to suffer from this illness."[61]

Although Colby publicly ruled against Ryan, privately, he had been doing everything he could to research AIDS in the event that Ryan eventually returned to school. In addition to getting information from the CDC, Colby maintained contact with his counterparts in Swansea. With Bev Ashcraft, he participated in conference calls with Martin Kleiman, Ryan's doctor at Riley and an infectious disease specialist. In fact, Colby and Ashcraft had informally begun planning for Ryan's return to school as soon as they learned of Ryan's diagnosis; they had previously worked with Ryan and Jeanne when Ryan enrolled at Western and decided that because of his joint bleeds, he should not participate in P.E. Ashcraft also worked with two nurses from the Howard County Health Department, Jeri Malone and Nancy Mickelson, to write policies for what are now referred to as universal precautions. She also assembled "spill kits" and instructed Ryan's teachers in how to use them. The public remained unaware of these efforts, because they continued behind the scenes while the legal process played out. Perhaps if Colby and Ashcraft had shared their pragmatic and rational mindset with the public, the Whites would have experienced less antagonism. But such openness would have also brought the principal and the nurse into conflict with their supervisors, Carter and Smith.[62]

On October 4, J.O. Smith formally ruled that Ryan, who had since been readmitted to the hospital, could not attend school in person. Charles Vaughan filed an appeal with the state Department of Education, which appointed attorney Kathleen Madinger Angelone as the hearing officer. That same week, the Indiana School Board Association passed a resolution calling for a moratorium on placing students with AIDS in schools; echoing the call in Queens a month earlier, the resolution also called for a national symposium of educators, parents, and health experts on AIDS. These developments occurred as hearings were underway in the Queens school board case in New York, and even as the American Academy of Pediatrics issued a recommendation that most children with AIDS be allowed to attend school "in a normal manner." Ryan remained in the hospital throughout the month of October, while the Goodfellows of Kokomo, a civic and charitable organization, announced that they had established a special fund for Ryan and gave Jeanne a check for $700 to help with expenses.[63]

On November 1, 1985, Department of Education hearing officer Kathleen Madinger Angelone presided over a hearing on Ryan's appeal of the case conference ruling and superintendent's decision. The hearing, which took place in the City-County Building in Indianapolis, was open to the public at the Whites' request. Madinger Angelone had 15 days to announce her ruling; after that, the loser could appeal to the Indiana Board of Special Education Appeals. Once the Board ruled, its decision would be appealable in federal court—in other words, the case could once again reach Judge

Noland. At the November hearing, J.O. Smith testified that, were the matter left up to him, anyone—students or staff members—showing any possibility of getting AIDS would be barred from school. (He did not indicate how he would determine whether someone could "possibly" get AIDS.) The hearing became especially tense when one of Western's lawyers, Stephen Jessup, called Justin O'Brien of Indiana State University to the stand. O'Brien's expertise was in special education, and Vaughan objected to him being allowed to answer a question from Jessup that Vaughan said called for a medical opinion—whether children with AIDS should be allowed in school. Madinger Angelone allowed the question, which O'Brien answered in the negative. When challenged again by Vaughan, O'Brien slapped the court bench with his open hand and countered, "We're endangering the lives of children based on incomplete information, and you damn well know it." Tempers flared again when David Day, another of Western's lawyers, questioned Dr. Charles Barrett of the ISBH. Barrett found himself on the witness stand for two-and-one-half hours answering questions about his agency's guidelines, the prevalence of AIDS in Indiana, and how AIDS was and was not transmitted, among other topics. Perhaps to avoid further outbursts after seven-and-one-half hours of testimony and eight witnesses, Madinger Angelone did not rule at the end of the hearing; instead, she took the matter under advisement and promised to issue a decision by November 27.[64]

Ryan was released from the hospital on November 9. As of November 11, members of the Goodfellows organization reported that they had distributed about $1,700 to the Whites, thanks in large part to donations made by entertainers who had held fundraisers for Ryan during the fall months. That same month, a five-person news team from Japan visited Kokomo, Indianapolis, and Russiaville to film a segment on Ryan. The journalists interviewed Ryan, Ronald Colby, Western students, and Dr. Kleiman. Finally, on November 25, Kathleen Madinger Angelone ruled that Western School Corporation could not bar Ryan from classes. Charles Vaughan held a press conference with his clients on the next day; United Press International covered the event, making the news available to newspapers around the world. Jeanne told reporters that Ryan had called the ruling "a great birthday present" (he would turn 14 on December 6); the journalists observed that Ryan "looked well" as he told them, "I feel great."[65]

Elsewhere in Indiana and the nation, students with AIDS encountered mixed responses. The Hobart, Indiana, school board voted in November to keep one such student out of the classroom and to offer remote instruction similar to Ryan's, instead. Another Indiana student with AIDS—a teenager whose identity remained confidential, in an undisclosed district—was permitted to attend classes. In Lebanon, Pennsylvania, a mostly

Mennonite-Amish community of 30,000 some 20 miles east of Harrisburg, virtually no controversy attended the decision to allow a high school junior with AIDS to remain in school. In New Jersey, a school board refused to obey a state education commissioner's order that a five-year-old girl with AIDS be allowed to attend school. And although Ryan had won the latest round of his appeal, the parents at Western were not about to go down without a fight. On the evening of December 4, about 75 of them attended a meeting at the high school, where J.O. Smith and Ronald Colby advised the parents not to act out the "ignorance and hysteria" ascribed to them by the national media. Interestingly, both Smith and Colby admitted to parents that they now found the State Board of Health's guidelines to be more acceptable than they originally did. Nevertheless, all of the attendees threatened to withdraw their children from Western if Ryan attended, despite Colby and Smith's urging that they avoid a boycott. Although a reporter described the meeting as "generally orderly," parents did express some hostility. A number claimed that their own knowledge about AIDS was superior to that of some experts, while the media came under fire for portraying the concerned parents as "ignorant and refusing to acknowledge that 'we've not been sitting on our cans and have been researching AIDS.'" Parents were upset at health experts for their refusal to issue guarantees about how the virus was spread and, according to one report, they questioned Jeanne White's motives. Speakers also expressed anger at "[c]ivil rights advocates for homosexuals" and at "other unspecified minorities" for "their alleged role in the White case." While Colby continued to prepare for Ryan's return, school board members knew they had a decision to make.[66]

During a December 17 meeting heavily attended by the media, Western's school board voted 7–0 to appeal the ruling to the Indiana State Board of Special Education Appeals. Implying that Jeanne White was a bad mother, school board member Joyce Miller told the *Tribune* that "as a mother, if my child had AIDS, I would want to keep him close to me, let him watch his favorite TV programs, cook his favorite meals, play his favorite games." Saying "the puzzle of AIDS is incomplete," board president Daniel Carter held up a yellow sign resembling a puzzle with a piece missing, and black letters that spelled, "AIDS." During the public comments portion of the meeting, Mitzie Johnson announced that she and other parents had organized into a group, retained a lawyer, and were monitoring the situation. J.O. Smith stated that the school corporation had already incurred over $40,000 in legal fees.[67]

The school board meeting continued to generate public controversy in the days that followed. On December 22, 1985, the *Kokomo Tribune* published a letter to the editor from New Jersey singer Alex Tiensivu, who had

written and recorded "Ryan's Song" to raise funds for the Whites, expressing his shock that Joyce Miller and others would question Jeanne White's
motives. "What would it be called if Jeanne didn't defend Ryan?" he wrote.
"Wouldn't she be letting him down?" Tiensivu recommended that readers seeking facts about AIDS look at an article in the December issue of
Discover magazine, which directly addressed parents' concerns about children with AIDS in school. It is unclear whether scientific opinions or letters like Tiensivu's changed anyone's opinion about Jeanne White's fitness
as a mother for honoring her son's wish to attend school. Most people in
Howard County were silent about the issue. Those opposed to Ryan's school
attendance were most vocal, and most frequently quoted in the *Kokomo
Tribune*, while supporters of Ryan were less likely to voice their opinions
publicly. For her part, Jeanne White tried to remain quiet.[68]

The question remains open to this day: was the community's animosity toward the Whites so much more focused and long-lived because they
provided their opponents with an individual, visible target, as opposed to
the institutional targets in New York and Massachusetts? Unlike in New
York, where parents could sue a school system or a city, parents at Western Schools could zero in on actual people, Ryan and Jeanne White, and
satisfy their human need to find a villain. As Jeanne's comments concerning the dismissal of the Factor VIII lawsuit indicated, she had become
wary of any publicity, positive or negative, about her family. Shortly before
what promised to be a bleak Christmas for a good part of the city's workforce, the *Kokomo Tribune* reported that an Italian television station, RAI
in Rome, had offered to fly the Whites to Italy in February for an interview, to arrange for sightseeing for the family during their visit, and fly
them home four days later. In a city whose third-largest employer was currently in bankruptcy proceedings, an announcement such as that was sure
to cause resentment.[69]

4

Four Months
in a Blast Furnace

December 1985–March 1986

On December 26, 1985, the state Department of Education announced that the Indiana Board of Special Education Appeals would hear Ryan's case on February 6, 1986, and that the hearing would be open to the public at the Whites' request. A few days later, the editorial board of the *Kokomo Tribune* voted Ryan's battle to attend school as its top local news story for 1985. The paper and reporter Christopher M. MacNeil had won the Thomson Newspapers Editorial Award of Excellence for their "thorough and professional coverage" of AIDS and of Ryan White. MacNeil, then just 31 years old, had been with the story virtually from the beginning, initially reporting on news related to AIDS and on Smith's decision to bar Ryan from attending school. He would eventually write more than 100 articles about Ryan during the story's most intense months—from late July 1985 through Spring 1986, when both the events and the emotions that they triggered would reach a boiling point.[1]

The two crises in Kokomo—Ryan's struggle to go to school and Continental's misfortune—exposed fault lines in the community and amplified divisions among residents. In the midst of the legal and economic uncertainty and growing scrutiny of the national media, people separated into camps: employed vs. unemployed, labor vs. management, sick vs. healthy, all as they struggled to redefine their identity and assert their individual power and agency. Not just in Kokomo, but nationwide, what was viewed as the "gay" disease of AIDS, coupled with tenuous job security for blue-collar workers, represented a threat to American manhood, the image of which had been healthy, straight, and gainfully employed—self-reliant and independent, since the early days of the republic. In Kokomo, a group calling themselves "Concerned Citizens and Parents" embarked on a strategy of resisting authority and fighting Ryan's return to school in an attempt to assert some kind of power in circumstances over which they had no control. But their plan backfired: instead of being seen as courageously protecting their children, they were viewed by the wider public as victimizing Ryan White. They were perceived by most Americans as having picked a fight with a single mother and her sick child, not a bureaucratic entity. And instead of coming to the aid of the displaced Continental steelworkers, Kokomo residents largely ignored their plight. This chapter recounts the events of these crucial four months separately because so much of what happened during this time would be used for decades as the basis of the popular narrative concerning Ryan White and the city of Kokomo. The dynamics of power (and its opposite, insecurity) and identity (both of the city and of the archetypal Jeffersonian citizen) help to explain the community's lack of support for both Ryan and for the unemployed steelworkers. And, in the broader context, Kokomo's response was not atypical; a struggle over power and identity manifested itself in reactions to HIV/AIDS nationwide, in legislative chambers and in the media, in early 1986.

Blood

On January 17, the CDC reported that between June 1, 1981, and January 13, 1986, physicians and health departments in the U.S. had notified the agency of 16,458 patients with AIDS. Two hundred thirty-one of them were children under the age of 13. People with hemophilia and other recipients of blood products accounted for 19 percent of those pediatric cases as well as for three percent of adults, but the agency cautioned that six percent of the cases (984 people) had yet to be classified according to risk factors. Just about half, or 51 percent, of the adults had died, and so had 59 percent of the children. Cases had been reported in all 50 states, the District of Columbia, and three U.S. territories. An *Indianapolis Monthly* article from the same month reported 59 cases of AIDS in Indiana, with 30 deaths to date.[2]

In February 1986, the National Association of School Boards met in Washington, D.C. Attendees listened as medical and legal experts recommended that schools allow students with AIDS to continue to attend classes unless their condition or behavior presented a likelihood of transmission to others. Indiana's own Dr. Woodrow Myers addressed the group about his department's guidelines; in a not-so-veiled reference to Western Schools, he observed that it was "very difficult to convince individuals who don't want to be convinced. What the public wants is a one hundred percent ironclad guarantee that nothing will happen to their child, which I can't give…. We cannot ever with any disease give one hundred percent reassurance, so why start now?"[3]

Just as every state counted people with AIDS among its residents, each state's government, it seemed, had a different response. The sexual transmission of AIDS, as well as its association with intravenous drug use, offered an easy avenue for some to register their opinions of homosexuality as well as illegal drug use, and to legislate either tolerance or opprobrium. While some states outlawed discrimination based on sexual orientation, others sought to isolate people suffering with AIDS. For example, after a contentious hearing on January 13, Texas Health Commissioner Dr. Robert Bernstein asked his state's Board of Health to drop its consideration of a proposal to quarantine AIDS patients who, in the state's determination, continued to have sex or share needles. How authorities would have monitored this behavior was unclear. Advocates for gay rights, as well as civil rights organizations, had strongly opposed the measure and argued that education was the best way to stop people from spreading the disease.[4]

Widespread education, which might have helped lessen public fear of AIDS, was not forthcoming; in its absence, public suspicions led to behavior ranging from intolerance to outright gay bashing. In January, gay rights groups reported an increase in both discrimination and violence directed against gays and blamed that increase on fears associated with AIDS. New York City's Human Rights Commission issued a report in March linking widespread publicity about AIDS to a five-fold increase in reports of anti-gay violence, and a doubling of discrimination claims involving sexual orientation, in the previous twelve months.[5]

Fear and uncertainty about an epidemic disease were new emotions for many Americans who had grown up in an era free of such outbreaks. Although vaccinations and antibiotics had relegated widespread death from contagious diseases such as polio to earlier generations, the new "gay plague" seemed to threaten everyone—gay and straight, drug abusers and drug-free. Popular press accounts warned the heterosexual, monogamous, and non-drug-injecting public that they were just one transfusion, one unguarded sexual encounter, away from disaster. As scientists pronounced themselves unable to promise a quick victory over this new virus, impressive technological achievements in other areas of public life also proved all too fallible. On January 28, the space shuttle *Challenger* exploded just 74 seconds into its flight, in front of thousands of horrified spectators at Cape Canaveral; millions more witnessed the event on television. Broadcasters ran the video footage of the disaster over and over again in the days following the incident. A month later, the death of a New York woman after taking Tylenol capsules laced with cyanide, and the discovery of a bottle of tainted capsules in a nearby drugstore, prompted a nationwide warning against the use of that popular painkiller. Authorities' failure to find a motive in the woman's death reminded the public that the deaths of seven people in the Chicago area in 1982, also from tainted Tylenol, remained unsolved.[6]

Media reports of uncontrollable tragedies such as these helped feed individuals' belief that they were powerless over their own safety. News of this type also contributed to public mistrust of scientific and medical information about AIDS, in a decade when trust in key institutions was already declining. Polls conducted by Harris and the National Opinion Research Center (NORC) from September 1981 through March 1986 revealed that an average of only 43 percent of Americans had a "great deal of confidence" in their medical leaders—down from 66 percent in the mid–1960s. More generally, technologies seen as wonders of power and innovation during the early– and mid–twentieth century had, by the 1980s, acquired some tarnish as their consequences became manifest. As psychiatrist Leon Eisenberg wrote in 1986, "we have had to endure radioactive fallout from nuclear tests, degradation of the environment by insecticides and herbicides, congenital defects from drugs, carcinogens in food and water from industrial wastes—the litany is too long to recite." In addition, Eisenberg pointed out that Americans' general scientific illiteracy caused them to suspect answers related to AIDS that were conditional in nature.[7]

Perhaps what people craved most was certainty. Efforts to screen blood donors, and thus shore up the safety of the nation's blood supply, were underway. The tests for antibodies to the AIDS virus had been available for a year. But people still feared AIDS, and they distrusted authorities' assurances that it was not transmitted by casual contact. Even a landmark study published in the *New England Journal of Medicine* on February 6, 1986, showing no evidence of transmission via casual household contact, was not enough to calm some parents' fears about schoolchildren with AIDS. The unwillingness of scientists and medical researchers to issue ironclad, outright guarantees still disturbed many—one reason, perhaps, that a proposal by noted conservative writer William F. Buckley, Jr., that March garnered serious discussion. In a *New York Times* op-ed piece titled "Crucial Steps in Combating the AIDS Epidemic: Identify All the Carriers," Buckley called for tattooing people with AIDS on both the upper forearm and the buttocks, in order to discreetly and privately identify them for the protection of those who would share IV drugs with them or have sex with them. As a counterpoint, the newspaper published an op-ed by Harvard law professor Alan M. Dershowitz, titled "Emphasize Scientific Information," which urged public health policies based on science, not morals or politics. Dershowitz criticized both "moral majoritarians" and gay rights activists for politicizing scientific findings on AIDS and asked both sides to calm their rhetoric so that researchers could impart "objective information" to the public. But Dershowitz's piece contained references to scientific opinions that, while they may have been devoid of moralistic judgments, were nonetheless bound to confuse the public in light of the CDC's pronouncements the preceding year. The professor quoted the opinion of Dr. William Haseltine, of the Harvard Medical School, that "anyone who tells you categorically that AIDS is not contracted through saliva is not telling you the truth," and that "there are sure to be cases of proved transmission through casual contact." Once again, the public found itself in the position of having to decide whom to believe.[8]

Although Buckley's suggestion of forced tattoos provoked much debate, it was not without precedent. As historian Keith Wailoo has pointed out, Nobel Prize–winning chemist Linus Pauling had in 1968 called for tattooing the foreheads of people possessing the sickle-cell gene, in order that, in Pauling's words, "two young people carrying the same seriously defective gene in single dose would recognize this situation at first sight, and would refrain from falling in love with one another." Indeed, Pauling called for legislation mandating "compulsory testing for defective genes before marriage, and some form of public or semi-public display of this possession." That such legislation never materialized did little to change the underlying fact that humans derive comfort from order and from certainty; according to Buckley's argument, the act of tattooing victims of a new and infectious disease would help people cope with the disorder and uncertainty that AIDS had introduced into their lives.[9]

In early 1986, Ryan White and his family also faced uncertainty, of course, about not only his health, but also his chances of attending school with his friends. His immediate academic future was in the hands of the state's Board of Special Education Appeals; he could only rely on Charles Vaughan, his attorney, to persuade the panel to let him go to school. As we shall see, Ryan's insistence on living a normal teenaged life was perceived by Western parents—and by the larger community—as threatening to their health. But his position was also transgressive, because he failed to conform to their expectations of how someone with an incurable, fatal diagnosis should behave. In other words, Ryan did not follow society's prescriptive "sick role."

Michael D. Quam, an anthropologist and public health expert, wrote about the applicability of the sick role theory to AIDS during the epidemic's first decade. According to Quam, the sociologist Talcott Parsons first discussed the notion of the sick role in 1951 as just one of a number of roles to which people in any given society usually conform in order to maintain community stability and harmony. People who deviate from their society's normative expectations for a particular role's performance, therefore, act in ways that disrupt the entire community: for example, one who malingers in order to escape the responsibility to financially support his family can cause an undue burden on the rest of society. The sick role itself, Quam noted, has four dimensions: it confers on its holders the right to be released from expectations that others, who are healthy, must fulfill; others do not hold the sufferer responsible for his condition; others expect that the sick person will believe his condition to be undesirable; and the sufferer is obliged to attempt to improve his condition. While later scholars have questioned the applicability of the *specifics* of this model to modern American society, Quam tells us, they also tend to accept the sick role as a valid archetype— one that helps us understand how societies generally respond to those who are sick. Ryan's refusal to express shame for his AIDS—his unwillingness to remain homebound, his fight to attend school despite his diagnosis; his willingness to travel and make public appearances—defied traditional societal expectations of how a sick teenager *should* behave, and some in his community reacted with discomfort to this state of affairs.[10]

Ryan's nonconformity, coupled with the social construction of AIDS as a "gay" disease, also threatened heteronormative conceptions of what it meant to be healthy, to be male, and to be a citizen of Kokomo. Jobless (mostly male) Continental workers, by their visibility and with their public appeals for aid, likewise threatened to upset Kokomo citizens' self-image as productive, self-reliant individuals. The steelworkers' fates were in the hands of a bankruptcy court, and thus they lacked even the slightest degree of self-determination. In an era of deindustrialization and insecurity (after all, Chrysler had needed a congressional bailout just a few years prior), employees of other companies could not help but wonder if their jobs would be next to go on the chopping block. The future of Continental Steel's workforce was up to the lawyers in the bankruptcy court in Indianapolis in the new year. But the company's fate would be settled very quickly.[11]

Steel

Readers of the January 8, 1986, *Kokomo Tribune* were greeted with mixed news on the paper's front page. One article reported that the nation's unemployment rate was down to 6.9 percent, its lowest mark since April 1980. But the next column told a less hopeful story: officials from Continental Steel had offered the local chapters of the United Steelworkers a settlement that included a $1-per-hour wage cut and a restructured pension. The specifics of Continental's proposal suggested just how dire its financial circumstances were: its provisions also included termination of the existing pension plan; a reduction in the company's contribution from 70 cents an hour to 16; and suspension of dental insurance in order to fund pension contributions. While Continental had negotiated the new offer with the leaders of two affected unions, the proposal was still subject to the rank and file's vote. The smaller union, Local 3601, with only 70 members, planned an imminent vote on the agreement. But John Andrews, the vice president of Local 1064, which represented 950 members, was less accommodating. Andrews's union, he told the *Tribune*, had given Continental wage concessions totaling $20 million since 1980.[12]

On January 21, Local 3601 members voted to reject the company's offer. Faced with the likelihood of an unfavorable vote from the larger union, Local 1064, Continental filed a motion in bankruptcy court asking the judge to reject its 1983 labor contract altogether. Local 1064 members countered with a threat to strike if the judge rejected the earlier agreement; their president, William Collins, cited "pay cuts to ... poverty levels." According to Continental's motion, the company had cut 36 salaried jobs in January, and what remained of its board of directors had cut both salaries and positions for directors in an effort to save money. The company already owed the pension plan some $40 million, its lawyers argued; if it were forced to honor the 1983 agreement, it would lose millions more. Lawyers representing the creditors' committee told the *Tribune* that the creditors wanted to see Continental reorganize—but if they lost confidence in that option, they would ask the bankruptcy judge to instruct the company to file for liquidation under Chapter 7.[13]

On February 5, 1986, the *Tribune* published a letter from James R. Asher of Tipton, who identified himself as a proud member of Local 1064 and explained why he opposed further concessions. Asher had worked at the steel company since 1973, and he blamed the management of that era for the firm's current state: "[if they had] taken some of the profit and put it back into the factory at that time, it would be a booming industry today." Asher cut Continental's current leaders no slack, either. "What do you get when you hire those who are supposed to be 'top notch' men," he asked, "with fat salaries, even though they came from plants that have shut down, even went bankrupt themselves? You get an industry like ours—bankrupt." Asher expressed the workers' side of the conflict in the newspaper; Continental executives would express management's side in court.[14]

By February, it seemed that Continental was running out of viable options. The company closed its Kokomo rod mill and caster operation during the week of February 10. The wire and nail mills were still operational, but only with a skeleton crew of between 325 and 350 workers. That same week, the bankruptcy court heard Continental's motion to reject the 1983 labor agreement. Pierre J. Stanis, the firm's financial advisor throughout much of the 1980s, told the court that Continental had a "favorable

scrap supplier, a good market, modern facilities and a good electric supply." "If you can't make these work, you can't make any steel company work
in this country," Stanis said. His telling omission of the workforce in that
list of assets hinted that in his opinion, the steelworkers themselves bore
responsibility for the mill's failure.[15]

Faulting the workers for the company's lackluster performance was a
recurring theme struck by management throughout the bankruptcy hearings. Under questioning from the steelworkers' lawyer, Andrew Sonneborn, Stanis testified that closing the Kokomo plant entirely, while keeping
Continental's profitable Joliet mill running, would help ease the company's
projected monthly cash-flow shortage of $2 to $3 million. Stanis told the
court that the company had not missed a payroll, although liquidity was
tight. However, everything had to come together for the reorganization to
work—production levels, the labor contract negotiation, effort from both
management and hourly workers, and financing. Additionally, a frustrated
Stanis said, "all the parties need to step back and see what the hell went
wrong." If Continental maintained its current production levels, he contended, it would collapse. Earlier witnesses Doug Brooks, the vice president
of employee relations, and Matthew Chinski, vice president of administration, had also laid the blame for the Kokomo plant's failure on the workers.
Brooks and Chinski had testified that the plant's continuous billet caster
needed to produce 10 to 11 "heats," or ladles, of molten steel a day, but was
only producing seven. Stanis took the same tack, telling the court that the
workers were most productive when personnel from Danieli, the Italian
firm, were on site in September of 1985. Stanis admitted, in response to
a question from Sonneborn, that management had a duty to ensure that
workers were properly trained, and he conceded that the production problems could be management's fault alone. Nevertheless, when Continental's lawyer, Robert Gargill, asked him if the workers were also to blame,
Stanis cited "problems in staffing, work rules and attitudes from this level of
employment." Shortly after the hearings that week, Continental's creditors'
committee filed a motion of their own—to convert the Chapter 11 proceeding to Chapter 7. The court set that motion for a hearing on Wednesday,
February 19, and postponed a ruling on Continental's motion to reject the
1983 labor pact.[16]

On Monday, February 17, 1986—the same week that Ryan White
would return to school—Continental padlocked the gates to its massive
Kokomo plant. The company's financial situation was dreadful: according
to Chinski, Continental's assets of $96 million were offset by $44 million
owed to secured creditors and an additional $62 million owed to unsecured
creditors. The company's indebtedness to Trefoil Capital alone was $19 mil-
lion. For its part, Steelworkers Local 1064 called a general membership

meeting for the evening of the 19th in order to discuss the outcome of the liquidation motion.[17]

As the plant closed its doors, the *Tribune* described a line of "solemn, expressionless" laid-off steelworkers waiting at the Kokomo office of the Indiana Employment Security Division to apply for unemployment benefits. "We've all planned on it for a while," said eight-year employee Don Tackett to a reporter at the scene. Remarked Don Dyer, "[i]t's bad when you work someplace all your life and then it goes down the tubes." Others said they were considering leaving Kokomo to look for work elsewhere. At the hearing on the 19th, Judge Richard Vandivier did not rule on the merits of the creditors' motion, because Continental objected to liquidation and wanted to remain in Chapter 11 (reorganization) proceedings. Instead, Vandivier appointed a trustee, Wayne Etter, to monitor daily operations, examine the situation, and report back to the court by a March hearing date on the Chapter 7 motion.[18]

Robert Haberfield's February 20 letter to the *Tribune* captured the fault lines that had started to develop in the community over the Continental episode. Characterizing the situation as a "fiasco," Haberfield applauded the steelworkers' refusal to agree to further concessions. But Haberfield's letter focused on the cost of the company's failure to taxpayers, to customers of Blue Cross Blue Shield of Indiana, and to Public Service Indiana. Taxpayers had funded a $4 million Urban Development Action Grant for Continental that they would never recoup, and "will also get left holding the bag on the matter of the company's Pollution Control Program," Haberfield wrote. As if to rub salt in the city's wound, the newspaper published a story on the same day reporting that American steel imports reached near record-high levels of over 25 percent in 1985, despite trade agreements that were supposed to restrict foreign imports to 18.5 percent of the U.S. market.[19]

Who was to blame for Continental's failure? Foreign steelmakers? Perhaps it was it the men who called the shots in the executive suite, or the union workers who, as Stanis had implied, were unproductive? In the mid–1980s, the public trusted neither. In 1973, only 26 percent of Americans reported "a great deal" or "quite a lot" of confidence in big business; by 1985, the number had risen only to an anemic 31 percent. Organized labor fared worse: in 1973, 30 percent of respondents had "a great deal" or "quite a lot" of confidence in unions; by 1985, the number had slipped to 28 percent. Such numbers contrasted even more unfavorably with historic survey results; in 1936, an impressive 72 percent of Americans had approved of labor unions, while in 1985, the number stood at barely more than half.[20]

Friday's front page told Continental's story in graphic terms: fewer than 40 workers remained on hand to maintain the idle plant while the parties clashed in bankruptcy court. The company would be able to pay its employees on time for the current pay period. Continental still wished to reject its labor contract and pension plans in order to free some capital; a hearing was pending on that request. The company's creditors, meanwhile, called for a sale of either the Kokomo plant, the Joliet plant, or both.[21]

On February 24, steelworkers set up a picket line outside the colossal, shuttered Continental mill on West Markland Avenue. Its purpose was to draw attention to the uncertain status of the workers' health insurance plan and other fringe benefits. William Collins, the president of United Steelworkers Local 1064, accused Continental of defaulting on its scheduled payments of $100,000 a week to Blue Cross Blue Shield of Indiana to cover the workers' health claims. The next day, Continental agreed with its creditors' request to convert the bankruptcy filing to a Chapter 7 liquidation proceeding, and to sell off its assets in order to make good on its debts. The *Tribune* reported a "stunned silence" in the courtroom, "followed by some crying." "The Kokomo facility is a good facility. There were just too many problems to overturn in a short period of time," Continental president Jack Wheeler told a reporter. The company's decision to no longer oppose liquidation represented a strategic choice to sacrifice the Kokomo plant in hopes of saving its Joliet operation. Wayne Etter, the court-appointed trustee who officially began running the plant on the 25th, clarified that workers currently providing services would still receive their pay, but he made no assurances about the workers' contract, pension plan, or benefits. At his weekly news conference, Kokomo's young mayor, Steve Daily (himself a former part-time Continental employee), said it was unlikely that the plant would open its doors any time soon, or that any future operations there would employ the high numbers of people that Continental had. He listed the city, state, and federal resources his office was marshaling in an effort to help the laid-off steelworkers, including job retraining and financing packages to attract potential buyers to the plant.[22]

As Ryan White started on the path to international fame, a thousand steelworkers agonized over their futures and wondered how they would feed their families. The *Tribune* regularly juxtaposed these two storylines, and in doing so exposed the divisions among the city's residents. The newly jobless could only watch while the blue-collar White family traveled extensively, feted by celebrities. Groups of citizens banded together to oppose Ryan's return to school, yet the cause of out-of-work steelworkers met with much less community enthusiasm. As Ryan's case progressed through the courts and the spotlight shone ever brighter on Kokomo, Jeanne White would find her every move scrutinized, her legitimacy as a mother questioned. Even as the city struggled to recover from the loss of Continental Steel, events surrounding Ryan White reached a crisis point.

Ryan White

While the Whites awaited their February 6 hearing before the Indiana Board of Special Education Appeals, their opponents began to organize in earnest. On January 12, 1986, the *Tribune* reported that a group of Western parents led by Mitzie Johnson had retained attorney David E. Rosselot to represent their interests. The opposition, calling themselves "Concerned Citizens and Parents of Children Attending Western School Corp.," promised to sue the school corporation if Ryan returned to class. Rosselot, a former police officer with a private law practice, had two children in the Western school system, although they were younger than Ryan and would not have shared classrooms with him. He had attended the large parents' meetings held the previous year, and several parents had hired him to appoint their adult relatives guardians of their children to enable their children to attend school in a different district just so they, according to Rosselot, "wouldn't have to sit next to Ryan White in the classroom." While the maneuver may have proved a sound tactic for individual families to employ, Rosselot knew he had to form a larger strategy in order to keep Ryan away from school. He started to plan a lawsuit.[23]

For his part, Charles Vaughan, the Whites' attorney, viewed the upcoming appeal hearing realistically. Calling the Howard County venue "hostile," he had asked the Board of Special Education Appeals to move the hearing from Western Middle School to Lafayette, in Tippecanoe County. The Board obliged and scheduled the matter in the county's Circuit Court. Hostility was also on the mind of New Jersey resident Cynthia Tiensivu (the wife of singer Alex Tiensivu, whose song raised funds for Ryan) when she wrote a lengthy letter to the editor of the *Tribune* in late January decrying the treatment Ryan was receiving from his fellow Hoosiers. "Ryan White is no longer being treated like a human being," she wrote. If local residents shared her opinions, they did not express them in letters to the editor. As Continental Steel's bankruptcy loomed and weeks remained until a definite decision would come in Ryan's case, those who supported him may have chosen to take a wait-and-see attitude.[24]

Parents fearful of the prospect of their children attending school with Ryan were less reticent. Paula Kincaid wrote to Ronald Colby at Western Middle School with a request: "Mr. Colby, I would like to know if my daughter … is scheduled to have any classes with Ryan White. I also would like to know when the information meetings are scheduled for parents." Kincaid included telephone numbers where Colby could reach her. A notation in the letter's margin, "Taken care of 2/1," suggests that the Western Middle School principal tried to respond to parents' concerns.[25]

All three of the Whites traveled to Rome on February 1 for Ryan's appearance on an Italian newsmagazine television show, *Italia Sera*, on February 3. According to an article in the *Tribune*, the Italians' interest in Ryan's case may have been prompted by the fact that their government imported the clotting factor used for treating hemophilia from the United States. The booking was certainly indicative of the international notoriety Ryan—and his hometown—had already received. The Whites' interviewer, Piero Badaloni, told the Associated Press that the purpose of the segment was to "share in the battle that Jeanne White is conducting against the front of sensational news that has been established around AIDS." The Whites experienced much support while they were in Rome. In his memoirs, Ryan recalled "everyone who called in said, 'Stay the course' in Italian.... At the end of the show, the hostess kissed me on the air." The trip to Rome also offered a vacation of sorts for Ryan and his family; while staff members from CNN and NBC took them sightseeing, people who recognized Ryan stopped him on the sidewalk and greeted him effusively. "No one in Rome seemed to be afraid of us," Ryan observed. "We'd almost forgotten what it was like to stroll around a place like anyone else." Equally noteworthy was the reception that greeted the Whites upon their return to Indianapolis on February 5: a clutch of reporters awaiting Ryan's arrival clamored for interviews and took pictures of him walking off the jetway in his "Made in Italy" sweatshirt with Jeanne smiling behind him. A reader of the *Tribune* on the morning of February 6 would have seen that photograph and read about the telegram that awaited Ryan at his home from President and Mrs. Reagan, wishing him a belated birthday and assuring him that he was in their prayers. Ryan's refusal to adhere to the prescribed "sick role," and his international travel, must have been especially disturbing to residents of a city in crisis, who felt that they had little control over their future prosperity and well-being.[26]

The day after their return from Italy, Ryan and Jeanne attended the three-hour hearing on Western's appeal before the Indiana Board of Special Education Appeals in Lafayette. Western School Board president Dan Carter and other school supporters sat in on the proceedings, wearing yellow and black badges that read "The AIDS puzzle is not complete." The panel's ruling, issued later that day, was followed up with a written order and findings signed by the chair, Dr. John P. Mefford, on February 14. The Board characterized Western's decision to install teleconferencing equipment in Ryan's home as "a sincere effort" to educate Ryan but ruled that the decision was "not made upon sound educational information" and was instead "selected as a workable option following the administrative decision to remove" Ryan because of his diagnosis. The Board was impressed that even though Ryan had not physically been in school during the fall of 1985, he had earned average or above-average grades, and that his performance "strongly support[ed] the educational appropriateness for the regular classroom" once Ryan's health enabled him to go to school. Western was legally obligated to educate Ryan in his regular classroom, the Board found, unless he was so ill that he could not physically attend school. The Board also found Colby's concerns about "social ostracism and cruelty by other children" should Ryan return to the classroom to be "unsubstantiated," noting that he regularly attended basketball games and roller-skated with other children.[27]

As for the risk of contagion that Ryan posed to other students, the Board ruled that "there is no medical reason for the student to be excluded from school" as long as Western followed the Indiana State Board of Health's July 1985 Guidelines for Children with AIDS/ARC Attending School. "Medical testimony affirms that the student is able to satisfactorily meet all of the conditions stipulated in these guidelines," the Board noted. Once Ryan obtained a health certificate from local health officer Dr. Alan Adler, as required by the state law governing communicable diseases and school-aged children, he could be readmitted into a regular classroom, according to the Board's ruling. In case any doubt remained, the Board ordered Western Middle School—not the Whites—to request the Certification of Health in order to facilitate his readmission. The Board also ordered the school to complete an Individualized Education Plan for Ryan's instruction, to develop a plan for implementing the State Board of Health guidelines, and to ensure that both plans were in place by the time Adler issued the health certificate.[28]

Both Adler and Woodrow Myers declined to discuss Ryan's case until they had reviewed a written order. Dan Carter told *Tribune* reporter Chris MacNeil that the Western School Board would meet in executive session to discuss the matter. Others, however, had plenty to say about the Board's decision. David Rosselot, the attorney for Mitzie Johnson's Concerned Parents organization, complained to *Tribune* reporter Christopher MacNeil that the Board had focused only on Ryan White's right to attend school, and in doing so had ignored the "health and welfare" of other Western students when it ruled that Ryan could return to the classroom. According to MacNeil's article, while Rosselot appreciated the moral support the Concerned Parents group had received, both he and Johnson "stressed the need for contributions to a checking account opened at Union Bank & Trust Co. to help pay legal expenses to challenge White's return to school."[29]

The Indiana Board of Special Education Appeals would not have the last word in Ryan's case. Russiaville resident Becky Graves responded directly to Cynthia Tiensivu in a letter to the *Tribune* on February 9. "I didn't appreciate a comment from the lady in New Jersey that our community is being judgmental and teaching our children to be prejudiced,"

Graves wrote. She added that she and her family had prayed for Ryan daily, but pledged not to change her position on Ryan's school attendance until authorities issued a guarantee. Graves continued, "we don't need criticism from outsiders who haven't walked in our shoes." It was clear to anyone who read Graves's letter, let alone the comments of Rosselot and Johnson, that even if Ryan obtained a health certificate from Dr. Adler, his path back to the classroom would not be a smooth one.[30]

On Monday night, February 10, Western School Board members held a three-hour-long, closed-door meeting to discuss Ryan's case. Stephen M. Jessup, an attorney representing the school system, helped the board members draft a four-page letter to Dr. Adler to be delivered the next morning, just days before he was to examine Ryan and decide whether to issue the health certificate. J.O. Smith, Western's superintendent, signed the letter, which advised Adler that the school planned to hold him legally accountable for his decision and would name him in any resulting lawsuits. The board also asked Adler to address a series of points, conditions, and situations in his certificate—including whether Ryan's presence in a classroom would pose any risks to students or staff members, as well as to Ryan's own health. After the media publicized the letter, Carter and Jessup expressed surprise that some had interpreted it as an attempt to influence or threaten the medical officer. Their protestations of innocence did little to convince the Whites' lawyer, Charles R. Vaughan, who expressed his deep disappointment in school officials' actions and pronounced their approach "unethical." While the lawyers sparred in the press, Ryan was at Riley Hospital for Children in Indianapolis, being examined by Dr. Martin Kleiman. Adler had selected Kleiman, the infectious disease specialist, to examine Ryan and to make a recommendation regarding his fitness for the classroom. Adler promised to render a decision within days.[31]

That same week, the five-week trial concluded in the Queens, New York, case, *District 27 Community School Board v. Board of Education*. On February 11, New York State Supreme Court Judge Harold Hyman ruled against the two school boards who had sued the city of New York to prevent an anonymous second grader with AIDS from attending public school. Notably, Hyman found that both the federal Vocational Rehabilitation Act and the Fourteenth Amendment's equal protection clause protected the child against automatic exclusion from school. He also upheld the city's case-by-case system for determining whether AIDS-infected children should attend school and found it consistent with existing state statutes on communicable diseases, which (like Indiana's) had been drafted in the decades before the AIDS virus was known to exist.[32]

Hyman's opinion specifically addressed the argument that, because medical and scientific authorities would not issue ironclad guarantees regarding the transmissibility of AIDS, infected children should be excluded from the classroom setting. "The testimony reflects," he wrote, "that it is not in the nature of medical science to be governed by a 'no-risk' standard." Hyman expressed sympathy for parents concerned "for the health and welfare of their children within the school setting," but wrote that the court was "duty bound to objectively evaluate the issue of automatic exclusion according to the evidence gathered and not be influenced by unsubstantiated fears of catastrophe." Instead of reacting to the court's decision with hostility, the Queens school boards and parents' associations worked to get accurate information about AIDS (in the form of flyers) to parents of local schoolchildren. A social worker from the Brooklyn Jewish Hospital offered training for teachers seeking to learn how to clean up after children with nosebleeds or injuries, and parents in both districts amassed and delivered supplies for spill kits—bleach, gloves, paper towels—to teachers and school officials. With that, all of the parents who had previously kept their children out of school returned them to classes.[33]

Any hope that cooler heads and similar legal interpretations would also prevail in Kokomo and Russiaville following Dr. Adler's decision proved unfounded. On February 13, 1986, Adler examined Ryan for 35 minutes and determined that he was fit to attend classes but recommended that he wait one week due to an influenza outbreak in the area. The brief delay would also give Western School Corporation officials time to train their personnel in universal precautions. Adler's written certification specifically referenced his consultation with Dr. Kleiman. It also cited a section of Indiana's communicable disease statute, Ind. Code 16–1–9–8, as the source of his legal authority to permit Ryan to attend school despite his AIDS diagnosis, something Adler characterized as "a communicable disease under limited circumstances." Significantly, the statute had been enacted in 1949, well before the AIDS virus was discovered. Its preceding section, Ind. Code 16–1–9–7, prohibited persons having custody of a child infected with a communicable disease from attending school or even from appearing in public. Section 8, the law Adler cited, required teachers to exclude children infected with communicable diseases unless a health officer issued a "written permit to attend." Adler's certification also conditioned Ryan's return upon Western's complete obedience to the Indiana State Board of Health guidelines issued the preceding year.[34]

Adler's issuance of the permit made both local and national news. In Kokomo, the story appeared on the front page above the fold, with the headline "Ryan's schooling is medically OK" (while a smaller headline below the masthead optimistically announced that a "[Continental] Adviser says closing would solve cash flow: Thinks firm can work"). The *New York Times*, headlining its story "Indiana School Told to Readmit

14-Year-Old Student with AIDS," quoted J.O. Smith as saying, "I don't see any way we can keep Ryan from attending school. That doesn't mean he ought to be there but I don't think we have any grounds for keeping him out." The *Tribune* followed up the next day in greater depth, with Smith reiterating his 1985 talking point about incomplete information, despite all that had transpired since the previous summer: the issuance of state guidelines, Dr. Adler's ruling, the *JAMA* article on casual contact, and the court's recent decision in the very similar Queens, New York, case. For his part, Adler explained that he had conducted a thorough review of the literature in order to determine that it was safe for Ryan to attend school. He also told reporters that he believed Ryan would be able to handle the "antagonism" that all parties—Ryan, his mother, school officials, and health officials—expected would accompany his return to middle school and characterized the teen as "very mature for his age." Jeanne White described for reporters the conditions under which Ryan had agreed to return to school. The agreement included stipulations that went above and beyond the precautions dictated in the State Board of Health's guidelines and included using a separate restroom and eating with disposable utensils. Jeanne also told the *Tribune* that she was proud of what her son had accomplished, especially if his public struggle helped other hemophilia patients with AIDS. Ryan told reporter Christopher M. MacNeil that he was "very, very happy" to be returning to school.[35]

The local fallout from Adler's decision continued. J.O. Smith told the newspaper that the school would be ready for Ryan's return and that the school corporation planned no further legal action, although he admitted to concerns about whether the parents in the Western school district would accept Adler's determination. Attorney David Rosselot informed reporters that he was conducting research and investigating all possibilities in order to present the parents' group with options when they met the following week.[36]

Instead of resisting the new developments, Western Middle School principal Ron Colby continued to prepare for Ryan's return. On February 13, he talked with Gerald Vasconcellos, the assistant principal at Joseph Case Junior High School in Swansea, Massachusetts, about how that school had handled Mark Hoyle's attendance. Vasconcellos mailed Colby a copy of a booklet titled "AIDS: Public Health Fact Sheet and School Attendance Policy," which Case officials had mailed to every parent in the fall of 1985. A letter from the Commonwealth's Department of Public Health, addressed to the superintendents of each Massachusetts school district, accompanied the booklet. In it were the names and telephone numbers of state officials in the departments of public health and education who could answer educators' (and, presumably, parents') questions about the policy. Such examples of interagency cooperation and coordination stood in stark contrast to the events in Indiana. At the Western School Board meeting on February 18, an angry Dan Carter called on Woodrow Myers to resign, demanded that he apologize to the people of Kokomo, and insisted that the Indiana Board of Health owed the school corporation $50,000 in legal fees. According to a report in the *Tribune*, Carter said all of this even as he urged the community to cooperate with the Board of Special Education Appeals' mandate to readmit Ryan to school: "Cooperation 'will show a side of the community that has always been present, but not always shown ... the upbeat, positive side.'"[37]

Carter himself was anything but upbeat and positive in his views toward Myers. With the rest of the school board members, he voted to send a letter outlining their grievances to Governor Robert D. Orr, who had appointed Myers to the Board of Health post. Instead of calling on Western to allow Ryan to attend school, he told reporters, Myers should have issued a health certificate for Ryan during the previous summer, thus saving the district time and money. Carter also accused Myers of negligence for not issuing the guidelines for children with AIDS in schools sooner than late July, a decision that, in Carter's mind, prevented Western officials from making an educated decision about Ryan's school attendance. Finally, Carter accused Myers of pursuing a strategy that "backed Western into a corner." For his part, Myers told reporters that he thought he knew why Carter was so vitriolic: "I certainly can understand why a person like Mr. Carter can be frustrated. He now has to justify the $50,000 the school spent in legal costs when it could have gone for education." Myers repeated his claim that his office had offered to help Western officials implement the guidelines, but that the school had declined that offer. His staff remained ready to assist Western, Myers insisted, in what appeared to be a conscious effort to remain detached and calm in the face of Carter's invective.[38]

At the same school board meeting, Carter announced to the members of the media that they would not be permitted inside Western Middle School on Friday, February 21, when Ryan returned. Instead, Western officials would hold a press conference in the elementary school's gymnasium at 10:00 that morning, in an effort to avoid disruptions to classes at the middle school. The national news media continued to focus on Ryan's case: the drama generated by the September 1985, meeting in Swansea had long since died down, and even the situation in Queens had quieted since Judge Hyman's carefully reasoned decision. On February 17, while Western teachers underwent training at Adler's direction, Ryan, his mother, and his lawyer were booked to appear on both *The Today Show* and the CBS *Morning News*. Ryan's friend and neighbor, Heath Bowen, made the trip to New York with the Whites and Charles Vaughan. The *New York Times* published a UPI report on Ryan's interviews on the two morning news programs; the piece informed readers that Ryan was nervous, but ready to go back to school. Ryan told his television audience that he hoped "to be treated like everybody else" and that he thought those who still opposed his attendance would "come around" in time. Jeanne was far less sanguine, telling interviewers that "I think there's going to be a long, major problem" in seeking acceptance for Ryan from his schoolmates' parents.[39]

Jeanne was prescient. On February 19, 1986, parents of Scott Bogart, Chad Gabbard, and Nicole Williams filed suit in the Howard Circuit Court against the Howard County Board of Health, Dr. Adler, the Whites, Western School Corporation, and the Indiana Department of Education to prevent Ryan from returning to school. Paragraph Two of the complaint referred to the plaintiffs as "representatives of the Concerned Citizens and Parents of Children Attending Western School Corporation"—the group spearheaded by Mitzie Johnson and represented by David Rosselot. In an affidavit accompanying the complaint, the six parents stated that they had "researched, examined data, and/or been informed by others concerning the A.I.D.S. virus"; that they believed "said virus to be fatal to those infected and to be communicable in nature. And a virus for which there is no known cure or treatment"; that they believed "every possible method of transmission has not been medically proven or eliminated"; and that "Ryan White may transmit the A.I.D.S. virus to their children within the classroom setting and since there is no known cure, the harm or damage done to their children will be immediate and irreparable." The plaintiffs requested that Judge R. Alan Brubaker issue a temporary restraining order that would prohibit Jeanne from allowing Ryan to attend school.[40]

In an *ex parte* proceeding attended by about 50 Western parents, Rosselot, and attorneys for both Western schools and the county Board of Health (but not the Whites), Judge Brubaker heard arguments from Rosselot and from Western Schools attorney Stephen Jessup. Jessup told the judge that it had been the position of Western for some six to seven months "that this boy should not be returned to the classroom but it's in his best interest and that of the school corporation that he attain his education at home." He noted that since Adler had issued his certification of Ryan's health during the preceding week, indicating that Ryan presented no threat to the health of others, Western would allow Ryan to return to school on Friday. During his arguments before the bench, Rosselot introduced the plaintiffs to the judge and outlined the substance of his complaint. Brubaker declined the parents' request for a preliminary injunction and set the matter for a hearing on Friday, February 21, at 2:30 p.m. In denying the preliminary injunction, Brubaker said, "You're not going to convince this court by having a group of parents parade in and tell me what they read in *National Enquirer.*" Pressed for her reaction to the lawsuit and hearing, Jeanne said, "I thought it was going too smooth."[41]

As the people of Russiaville and Kokomo prepared for Friday, the *Tribune* published letters critical of their treatment of Ryan. On February 19, two Indiana-born residents of Killeen, Texas—Jacqueline K. and Jeffery L. Fetz, Jr.—signed their names to a strongly worded letter expressing their disgust with the situation. "It makes us sick the way the people of his own community treat him," they wrote. They observed that Ryan had to travel to Italy "to even be treated as a human being."[42]

The next day, the *Tribune* published a letter signed by Tammy Collier and accompanied by the signatures of 50 of her fellow students at Ball State University in Muncie, Indiana, favoring Ryan's return to school. Collier identified herself as a graduate of Western High School and noted that she had "witnessed ... the everyday gossip of a small school...." Referring to the education she had received about AIDS at college, Collier emphasized that the disease was not transmitted by casual contact and wondered why Western's parents and administration were more concerned with "closing their minds and believing myths" than finding factual information. She urged readers to remember Ryan's "ultimate fate," and hoped that he would not be isolated any further.[43]

Opponents of Ryan's return to school proceeded with their plans. On Wednesday night, February 19, a crowd of 350 concerned and energized parents met with attorneys for two hours at the Western Middle School gym. Two large glass jars sat on tables to collect donations for legal fees, and reporters watched as parents filled them with dollar bills and checks. Approximately 100 parents indicated they would not send their children to school on Friday when Ryan returned, even though such an action was against the law. One mother, Faye Miller, complained to a reporter from the *New York Times*, "All our children have to give up their right to a safe education for him." Another, Barbara Bourff, who worked as a nurse's aide, told the reporter she planned to keep her three children home because "at the hospital, the doctors tell me there's a 75 percent chance of him spreading AIDS."[44]

Several parents expressed hostility toward both the media and outsiders. David Rosselot characterized Judge Brubaker's denial of the preliminary injunction as "strike one," telling the crowd that if the judge denied a restraining order at Friday's hearing, that would be "strike two." As if such rhetoric were not inflammatory enough, Rosselot disclosed that he had researched the possibility of having Ryan declared a ward of the Howard County Welfare Department—in other words, a strategy that formally accused Jeanne White of abuse or neglect—in order to prevent the teen's attendance at school. In the *Tribune*, Christopher MacNeil reported that

Rosselot had talked with Joseph Scionti, a lawyer representing the welfare department, on Monday, February 17, to learn whether such a legal move would even have a chance. "I simply answered that all the medical evidence points to this child not being in danger in the classroom," Scionti told Mac-Neil. After completing his research, Rosselot concluded that the move would be a losing strategy, so he filed the lawsuit instead. Learning of this development from MacNeil, a shocked Jeanne White could only ask, "They tried to take him away from me?"[45]

The next day, February 20, Rosselot filed a motion to remove Dr. Adler, the Howard County Board of Health, and the Indiana Department of Education from the lawsuit. This meant the only remaining defendants for the Friday afternoon hearing were Western School Corporation and Jeanne and Ryan White. As of February 20, three students had already transferred out of the Western School Corporation to Kokomo Christian School, where tuition was $120 a month. Since many of the area's public schools would not accept transfers after the beginning of a semester, Kokomo Christian had started a waiting list in order to handle transfer inquiries. As Rosselot fine-tuned his legal strategy and Western officials prepared for a media onslaught, the Whites did what they could to prepare for Ryan's return to school on Friday. It would be a very long day for all parties.[46]

February 21, of course, was the same day the people of Kokomo learned from their local newspaper that Continental Steel was operating with only a skeleton crew, that it was on the brink of liquidation, and that its creditors wanted to find a buyer for the facility. On that morning, a photo of a smiling Ryan White sitting on his bed amid textbooks appeared on the front page of *USA Today* under the headline "AIDS boy back to school." But inside the newspaper, on page 3A, an article by Cheryl Mattox Berry carried the headline "AIDS victim's return to class resisted." The article quoted Mitzie Johnson: "If they let AIDS in one school, they'll let it in all the schools." "Ryan won't be treated like a leper," Ron Colby told Berry, whose article nevertheless described the special conditions to which the Whites had agreed in order for Ryan to return to school for the first time in 14 months, including using paper cups instead of drinking directly from the school's water fountains.[47]

Colby faced a wave of absences that morning. Out of 360 students, 151 stayed home, an absentee rate of 43 percent. (The school would later revise this figure downward to 141, 82 of whom explicitly stated they stayed home because Ryan was back in class.) In the two weeks prior to Ryan's return—weeks that included the influenza outbreak—absences had ranged from 10 to 15 percent. Seven students withdrew from Western School Corporation the morning of Ryan's return. Some parents wrote to Colby seeking excused absences for their children: Donald A. Ozogar of Kokomo explained that he and his wife kept their daughter home "because of concerns for her physical safety following reports in Thursday's *Kokomo Tribune* about the possibility of picketing and violence related to the return of Ryan White to school." Ozogar added that "rumblings from the community indicated the possibility of violence over this emotional issue." "Since no mention was given in the newspaper report about any extra measures taken to protect the children," he continued, he and his wife felt it was wise to keep their daughter home.[48]

Susie White and her husband likewise cited the media's role in their decision to keep their daughter home: reporters, she wrote, "did not paint a very pretty picture of the expectations of the day, and we felt like the stress of the occasion was not conducive to a good educational setting." They also mentioned concerns about their daughter "sharing a classroom with a student with a possible communicable disease or perhaps being subjected to irate parents." Several other correspondents echoed these concerns—Linda Cauble's letter openly stated that she kept her son home "because I was afraid for his safety. I do not feel Ryan White's return poses as great a threat to [my son's] safety as do the parents and people who oppose his return. I wasn't sure just what their course of action would be Friday," she explained. Other parents, however, blamed Ryan for their children's absences. Shirley and Michael Crites, for example, wrote "that Ryan White should not be back in school at this time. There are, we feel, still too many unknowns about Aids [sic]." "Our hearts ache for Ryan and his family because of this horrible thing," they continued. "But our first concern is our children."[49]

Ryan's neighbor (and his friend Heath Bowen's older sister) Wanda was one of the majority of students who did attend Western that February morning, which sparkled brightly after a fresh snowfall the night before. Wanda saw picketers carrying signs that read "Faggot," "Go Home Gay," and "Go Home to Die." She also encountered demonstrators who wore surgical scrubs and masks, as well as Halloween masks, outside the school. Inside, however, she saw some people welcome Ryan. The *Indianapolis Star* also reported mixed responses: Ryan and Andrea's ex-stepfather, Steve Ford, drove them to school that morning in his Ford pickup truck, and he walked them into a back entrance to the building. As Ryan walked to his locker, some of his classmates patted him on the back. Other students, who arrived on school buses at the front, shared their reactions with reporters. Georgia Wheeler, a seventh-grader, said, "I think most of us understand about AIDS," but sixth-grader Trevor Cooper was less certain: "I don't know. I'm scared ... a little." Linda Rayl, another seventh-grader, told the *Star*, "I have mixed feelings. I don't want him in school with that disease, but I guess he does miss his friends." The newspaper reported that three Western High School students protested Ryan's arrival, including senior

Don Hochstedler, who held a sign reading "STUDENTS AGAINST AIDS" outside of a side entrance. Hochstedler told the *Star*, "I feel sorry for everyone else in the middle school," and worried that AIDS would spread to the high school. The *New York Times* ran a photograph of a grim Hochstedler, sporting a moustache and mirrored sunglasses that obscured his eyes, holding the sign in the midst of other bystanders in its February 22 edition, directly underneath a photo of a smiling Ryan flanked by Ron Colby and Steve Ford.[50]

Colby recalled that the media had begun setting up telephone and power lines in the school's parking lot the night before—he estimated some 40 to 50 different mobile facilities for television and radio stations. Although six to eight inches of snow had fallen overnight, Colby decided to go ahead with school as planned on Friday, partly to avoid having to deal with the assembled crowds of reporters yet again. Colby, his secretary, and Bev Ashcraft, the nurse for Western Schools, held the 10:00 news conference across the street at the elementary school's gymnasium. Colby told the crowd of roughly 60 reporters that there had been no picketing (despite the pictorial evidence to the contrary that would appear in the day's papers) and that he observed nothing untoward inside the school, either. Colby told his questioners that Ryan's day would run from 8:00 a.m. to 12:45 p.m., that it would include classes in math, science, English, social studies, and health, and that he would not participate in any activities involving swimming. Once Colby felt that reporters' questions became redundant, he ended the session. The rest of the day proceeded smoothly until the afternoon's hearing on the Concerned Parents' request for a court order to keep Ryan out of school. Ryan had only been back at school for a total of four hours and 45 minutes.[51]

Rosselot's Amended Complaint was now captioned *Bogart et al. v. White et al.*, and that afternoon—unlike the proceeding the Wednesday before—Charles Vaughan and the Whites were present and ready to contest the matter. The courtroom was filled with spectators. Representing the plaintiffs and charged with the burden of proof, Rosselot went first. He began by calling to the stand twelve-year-old Scott Bogart, a student at Western Middle School, to prove that Ryan attended public school with other children. After Scott testified, the judge heard from his parents, Daniel R. and Pamela Bogart. Rosselot then called Nicole Williams, another student, and her parents, Tom and Jacquelyn Williams. The last student to testify was Chad Gabbard, Ryan's former friend and neighbor, whom Rosselot called as a witness to establish that Jeanne had custody of Ryan. Chad's parents, Larry and Brenda Gabbard, testified next. Then Rosselot called Ryan's pediatrician, Dr. Donald Fields, to the stand, to testify about Ryan's ability to attend school.[52]

Fields would later recall that he worried about the repercussions of his testimony for his medical practice—Judge Brubaker's daughters were patients in his office, as were Stephen Jessup's children. Mitzie Johnson's mother was one of his receptionists. His associate, Dr. James A. Tate, was "completely anti-going to school," Fields knew—so their lunchtimes were especially uncomfortable. Yet Rosselot had subpoenaed Fields to appear in court that day, and he had no choice in the matter. Sometime after he testified—either that Friday evening or the next morning—Fields returned to his office to find something amiss: on the building's exterior, someone had placed a small pile of trash at the corner and turned off the main electrical switch to the building. "Somebody was just making a gesture, I'm sure," Fields decided. "Somebody's expressing their dislike of what we're doing." Rosselot also called Dr. Adler to the stand to testify about his certification that Ryan was fit to return to classes. Next up was Jeanne White, whom Rosselot called to establish that she planned on letting Ryan go to school. Finally, the plaintiffs called Ron Colby as their last witness before resting. Charles R. Vaughan, Ryan's lawyer, then moved for a judgment on the evidence, arguing that the evidence presented thus far was insufficient to make the plaintiffs' case. The crux of his argument was that AIDS was not communicable in a classroom setting—that it was akin to a disease like hepatitis—and that Ind. Code 16-1-9-7 should not apply to Ryan's situation. Judge Brubaker denied Vaughan's motion.[53]

Vaughan called only one witness, Dr. Charles Barrett, whom he presented as an expert witness. As the director of the Chronic and Communicable Disease Control Division at the Indiana State Board of Health, Barrett specialized in public health. He testified about the current state of scientific and medical knowledge about AIDS, including that it was not communicable by casual contact, as far as researchers could determine. The normal scientific qualifiers and cautious wording marked his testimony on both direct and cross-examination—for example, Rosselot was able to get Barrett to admit that "the evidence is not all in yet" with respect to research on AIDS—but Barrett never wavered from his basic position that Ryan's presence in the classroom posed little, if any, threat to others' health. The defense rested, and Judge Brubaker allowed closing arguments.[54]

Rosselot argued that there were still "unknowns" about AIDS, and that the plaintiffs would be irreparably harmed if the judge permitted Ryan to continue attending classes in person. He characterized that harm as "the contraction of a no-known-cure fatal disease." Vaughan argued that the statute, which had been enacted in 1949, should not apply to Ryan's situation. He also pointed out that all three physicians who testified during the hearing had said Ryan belonged in the classroom, and that the judge could not overlook the medical evidence. In his response, Rosselot relied on the statute, arguing that the law was on his side. Jeanne White would be violating Ind. Code 16–1–9–7 by sending Ryan to class; the only way to stop that violation, he argued, was for the court to issue the restraining order.[55]

The wording of the 1949 law itself was deceptively simple: "Persons having custody of any child, infected with such a communicable disease, shall not permit him to attend school or appear in public." Would Judge Brubaker find Vaughan's arguments more persuasive, or Rosselot's? In announcing his ruling from the bench, Brubaker characterized the statute as "antiquated," "a statute that is not, that's simply not meeting the needs of today's society." He expressed the "utmost respect" for Drs. Adler, Fields, and Barrett, and then returned to the problematic statute. While Rosselot had stuck to only one section of the law, Ind. Code 16–1–9–7, Vaughan had urged Judge Brubaker to read Ind. Code 16–1–9–7 together with Ind. Code 16–1–9–8 (the section that conferred authority on Dr. Adler to issue a medical permit for Ryan to return to school after an examination) and Ind. Code 16–1–9–9, which read in pertinent part, "all pupils found to be ill in any degree shall be sent home and kept there until the local health officer gives a certificate of health. After he receives a certificate of health, the pupil may be readmitted." In making that argument, Vaughan had invoked the well-established legal doctrine of statutory construction known as *in pari materia*, which allows a statute to be read together with its surrounding sections (and thus in context). Instead, Brubaker chose to read section 7 in isolation from the sections that followed it—as if sections 8 and 9 did not exist. And he appeared to ignore the constitutional aspects of the case that his counterpart in New York, Judge Hyman, had cited. Like Hyman, Brubaker could have invoked the Fourteenth Amendment to declare section 7 of the Indiana statute unconstitutional. Indeed, while not binding, Brubaker could have used Judge Hyman's ruling in the Queens school board case as a guiding precedent in upholding Ryan's constitutional right to attend school. The two statutes in issue (New York's and Indiana's) were of similar vintage. Instead, Brubaker made no mention of that case, or of the state or federal constitutions—despite the fact that Article 8 of Indiana's constitution had, since 1851, declared a right to education and that the schools "shall be … equally open to all." He granted the temporary restraining order in open court, which prompted a "loud, continuous outburst from spectators" in the courtroom as onlookers cheered and applauded. Judge Brubaker would go on to be reelected for several terms; in fact, he presided over the Howard Circuit bench until 1994, when, in July of that year, he was arrested and charged with Dealing in Cocaine, Patronizing a Prostitute, Theft, Conversion, and Official Misconduct. Brubaker, who had been regarded as one of the state's leading child advocates before his arrest, was charged with attempting to sell cocaine to an undercover police officer posing as a prostitute. He allegedly took the cocaine from his own court's evidence safe. In October, he pled guilty (pursuant to a plea agreement) to Dealing in Cocaine, a Class B felony; to two felony counts of Theft; and to two misdemeanor counts of Official Misconduct. The terms of the plea agreement called for him to resign from the bar and to serve a sentence of ten years, four of which would be served under house arrest.[56]

In Brubaker's courtroom in 1986, Ron Colby, who attended the hearing along with school nurse Bev Ashcraft, felt "disgusted" and extremely disappointed—after months of preparation for Ryan's return (which Colby had viewed as inevitable), he and Ashcraft could only sit, stunned. An officer of the court offered to show them out of the courthouse via the back way in order to avoid the crowds and the media. Most of the spectators exited the courtroom from its main door, of course, including Marcia Rosselot, David Rosselot's wife (and legal secretary), who emerged beaming, with two thumbs up. The jubilant crowd notwithstanding, David Rosselot soon came to feel that he had represented a minority viewpoint. "The group of people who were on my side ... or favorable to my position, I never knew how small a group that was until after that decision.... After that decision, that was it. The rest of the world hated us." Rosselot was right: that day, the city of Kokomo's image had reached a crucial turning point. The next day, readers across the country opened their newspapers to see two photos: the jubilant image of a victorious Marcia Rosselot juxtaposed with that of a downcast Ryan White.[57]

"I'm upset," Jeanne White told the *Tribune* after the hearing. "I think anybody that was there would have to be upset. I was stunned. Ryan is very disappointed. He really enjoyed school today," she added. Jeanne vowed to keep trying to get Ryan back in the classroom and shared that Ryan seemed to handle the adverse ruling well enough, sticking to his usual Friday night routine of skating at a local roller rink after receiving supportive telephone calls from classmates and their parents. But Jeanne remained disturbed by the events in the courtroom. "I prayed I wasn't hearing clapping and yelling," she told MacNeil. "Dear God, what kind of people find something to cheer about in a case of a child with AIDS?" she asked.[58]

One explanation for the Concerned Citizens and Parents' celebration may have been simply that they won. The legal system, their attorney, and the judge had all empowered them at a time when external crises, such as AIDS and deindustrialization, made them feel disempowered. The *New York Times* hinted at a generational difference in local responses to Ryan's return to school. In its summary of the day's dramatic events, the *Times* reported that "Ryan's classmates said their families were split on the issue and that they welcomed his return. 'Just because he has AIDS, he shouldn't be that different from us,' said Wendy Rayl, a seventh-grader." Yet the powerful contrast between spectators' joy and Ryan's sadness as they left the courtroom doubtless overshadowed Rayl's expression of tolerance in the mind of the general public. The *Times* also quoted the reaction of Ryan's lawyer, Charles Vaughan, to the court's order: "I think the world knows that statute's terrible, but our Legislature passes a lot of bad laws every day," he told the newspaper. A few days later, the *New York Times* published an editorial titled "AIDS in Queens and Kokomo," comparing the two cases of children with AIDS going to school. "Ryan White, a normal Indiana kid except that he has AIDS, is being kept out of school because some adults aren't learning about the disease fast enough," the editorial board wrote. After discussing the outcome of the Queens case, they ended with a call for compassion for "kids like Ryan" as well as "for the parents who fear him and whose distrust of medical authority is understandable; and for school officials who must consider the consequences for Ryan and his schoolmates, whatever they decide."[59]

The events in Kokomo during the week of February 17 marked the point of no return for both the city's image and for Continental Steel. Going forward, Continental Steel would never again reopen its doors. Instead, its identity would be transformed from that of a generous community institution into an unsafe producer of toxicity and danger. And because the Concerned Citizens' legal action and vocal opposition toward Ryan White generated drama that drew media from all over the nation to the story, Kokomo would emerge a city divided against itself and reviled by much of the outside world. As it happened, the people of Kokomo had feared the wrong thing.

5

"He's the good guy, and I'm the bad guy"

February 1986–May 1987

Inside Kokomo, conflict continued and division deepened after the events of February 1986. The displaced steelworkers did not receive the sympathy and finality they had hoped for; instead, uncertainty and finger-pointing followed the immediate aftermath of Continental's closing. Meanwhile, the Whites found themselves turning increasingly outside of Kokomo for support and encouragement, because their own community had failed them. As its title implies, this chapter deals with contrasts: it traces the developing narrative that cast Kokomo as a bully and Ryan White as a victim. Indeed, Ryan White had emerged from the metaphorical blast furnace as a hero-in-waiting, forged from Judge Brubaker's ruling excluding him from school. The nationally published photos of students picketing against Ryan's attendance, and media accounts of cheering spectators exiting the courtroom juxtaposed with a forlorn Ryan White, cemented Kokomo's role as the antagonist in the narrative. Just as important, Ryan's experience gave the media a new perspective on the AIDS story, one of sympathy for its suffering victims. Although negative angles about AIDS, stigma, and division still dominated the national news during 1986 and 1987, we can see the story around Ryan start to pivot from one of sickness, infection, and health to one of outcasts and oppressors. Reports of Ryan's legal travails, as well as the latest news of his health, slowly began to replace frightening headlines and baseless speculation about AIDS. These months represent the very beginning of a transition from the vilification to the commodification of the disease of AIDS, and the body of Ryan White helped to serve as the vessel for this change.

Closer to home, while the people of his community contributed to the developing national narrative by continuing to treat Ryan and his family as if they were toxic, a preliminary inspection of the abandoned Continental Steel site by the EPA and IDEM would uncover the truth about what was actually toxic in Howard County: the mill's hulking campus was a polluted mess that threatened to contaminate the surrounding neighborhoods and compromise people's health—if it was not already doing so. The community's perspective on Continental Steel also pivoted during these years as that realization began to sink in: the narrative slowly shifted from one that pitted laborers against managers to one that cast the abandoned mill itself as the threat, and the community as its victim.

Blood

In the national arena, the remainder of 1986 continued as it had started, as different officials tried varying approaches to both AIDS and people with AIDS. Of all the controversies surrounding the states' diverse reactions to the growing epidemic, California's was perhaps the most visible. In March, ultraconservative Lyndon H. LaRouche had gained nationwide political traction when two of his adherents won surprise victories in the Illinois Democratic primaries for Lieutenant Governor and Secretary of State. LaRouche-backed candidates in May primaries (including Indiana's) were not as successful—but, thanks to the stunner in Illinois and LaRouche's own four failed presidential runs, his had become a familiar, if marginal, name by the time he entered California AIDS politics. On June 24, 1986, the California Secretary of State's office announced that his group PANIC (Prevent AIDS Now Initiative Committee) had gained nearly 700,000 signatures on its petition to place an AIDS initiative on the state's November ballot. The measure, known as Proposition 64, proved extremely controversial; public health officials, along with many physicians and gay rights groups, strongly opposed it on the grounds that it might force mandatory blood testing for every Californian—as well as quarantines. Backers of the proposal openly stated that their goals included the assurance that no one suspected of carrying the AIDS virus would be allowed to attend or teach school, or to work in a restaurant.[1]

In a July 12 interview with KGO-AM radio station in San Francisco, LaRouche blamed the Soviet Union for its role in "the AIDS conspiracy." He also alleged that the virus was spread by mosquitoes, which he said explained its prevalence in Africa, the Caribbean, and southern Florida. Despite the skepticism of physicians and scientists, such claims still found fertile ground in the minds of fearful Americans, including the Californians who LaRouche hoped would support Proposition 64. Opponents of the measure held rallies to protest the initiative and wrote opinion pieces on the state's editorial pages in an effort to convince voters to vote against the plan. Even normally reticent corporations, such as Pacific Bell, joined the battle to fight against the initiative.[2]

On October 6, federal authorities raided LaRouche's headquarters in Virginia. Hours later, a federal grand jury in Boston indicted ten of his confederates, alleging that they had used fraudulent credit cards to fund political activities, including California's Proposition 64. A month later, Golden State voters defeated the initiative by a greater than two-to-one margin—71 percent to 29 percent. That LaRouche's group was ever taken seriously— not to mention successful in its effort to get a draconian proposal on a statewide ballot—suggests the fear with which the American public still regarded AIDS in 1986. Would California voters truly find their existing public health apparatus so inadequate that they would endorse mandatory testing for AIDS, publicly naming those who tested positive, quarantines, and overt discrimination in education and employment? In the end, it turned out not to be even a close call, but advocates for both sides took the fight seriously, in part because of public uncertainty over the proper response to AIDS.[3]

William F. Buckley's March 1986 *New York Times* op-ed calling for tattooing individuals with AIDS had sparked much debate over the proper bureaucratic response to people with the new disease. Without going to the extreme of requiring tattoos, the U.S. government nevertheless did authorize discrimination. In June, Charles J. Cooper of the Justice Department's Office of Legal Counsel issued a written opinion (subsequently known as the "Cooper memorandum") announcing that employers and public health officials could lawfully discriminate against people infected with the AIDS virus who were asymptomatic, as long as they could prove their actions were necessary to prevent the spread of the disease. In other words, federal civil rights laws written to protect the disabled—such as the Rehabilitation Act of 1973—would still apply to someone who was actively sick with AIDS, but would not apply to people who were, in today's terms, HIV-positive. According to Cooper, a person with the AIDS antibody in his blood could lawfully be fired from his job based merely on an employer's fear of his "real or perceived" ability to spread the disease—in effect, the worker was considered so powerfully unclean that his very presence might contaminate the entire workplace. The Justice Department's interpretation of federal law caused much dismay among scientists and federal health officials and contradicted the Public Health Service's own guidelines, which advised against segregating or firing people with AIDS. Even as federal health officials promoted testing as one of the best means of controlling the disease's spread, the legal opinion effectively encouraged workers to go underground in order to keep their jobs and homes—to avoid testing, and to pretend they were not sick.[4]

People with AIDS faced discrimination not only from their employers, but also from health insurance companies that refused to pay claims on the grounds that AIDS was a preexisting condition. The stigma associated with the disease was so great in 1986 that many doctors falsified death certificates to list "respiratory failure" or other vague ailments in place of AIDS as the official cause of death. "I have a tendency not to put AIDS on the death certificate," one San Francisco physician told a *New York Times* reporter. "That is public information, and if the wrong person sees it, it could be a problem for the family." Another news report gave the example of a Boston doctor's subterfuge after his patient, a young gay man, died of AIDS. "His mother, who was taking the body back to a small town in Indiana for burial, was concerned that the funeral home would get a copy of the death certificate and the information would become known in town. The Boston doctor did not list AIDS as the cause of death, but rather an opportunistic disease associated with it. An alert researcher would know the victim died of AIDS, but most laymen would not." Doctors also cited instances of life insurers refusing to pay claims for AIDS deaths, and of funeral homes refusing to embalm people who had died from AIDS or refusing to allow wakes with open caskets.[5]

Despite the federal government's mixed messages, some state and local administrations around the country stood out for their support of the rights of people with AIDS. In June, New York City's sanitation department suspended 40 workers who had refused to work with an AIDS-infected colleague after he returned to work from an extended medical leave. The Georgia Task Force on AIDS, established by the state's Department of Human Resources, issued recommendations over the summer in favor of allowing children who had AIDS or who were seropositive to attend school under the guidelines established by the CDC and the American Academy of Pediatrics. The Task Force also recommended against excluding seropositive individuals from the workplace and advised against mandatory testing (except in the case of convicted prostitutes). The National Educational Association issued revised guidelines for dealing with AIDS in schools in the summer of 1986. The new rules severely limited administrators' discretion to decide whether an employee with AIDS could remain at work; they discouraged schools from testing employees for antibodies to the virus; and they kept in place the NEA's recommended case-by-case approach to deciding on students' attendance.[6]

Even with these hopeful signs, AIDS continued to polarize the country in the summer of 1986. The U.S. Supreme Court's decision in *Bowers v. Hardwick*, upholding the constitutionality of a Georgia law that criminalized sodomy, prompted gay rights and public health advocates to worry that gay men would retreat further into the closet and refuse to seek testing for AIDS. Thomas Stoddard, the executive director of the Lambda Legal Defense and Education Fund, called the decision "our Dred Scott case," while the Rev. Jerry Falwell of the Moral Majority applauded the court for "recogniz[ing] the right of a state to determine its own moral guidelines," and for issuing "a clear statement that perverted moral behavior is not accepted practice in this country." The stigma attached to gay men stuck to everyone with AIDS—including people with hemophilia. In 1986, the disease was steadily taking its toll in that community, whose members found themselves as likely to face discrimination as any other AIDS patients. By year's end, the *Journal of the American Medical Association* (JAMA) reported a finding of the National Hemophilia Foundation that more than 95 percent of persons with severe hemophilia had tested HIV-positive.[7]

In all, 1986 brought little good news for people with AIDS. It was clear that AIDS would not be a condition like polio or smallpox, against which one could receive a vaccination and about which one would not have to think further. It was a complex disease, and reactions to it based on fear and misunderstanding caused complex social problems. The year would prove no better, and no less divisive, for Continental Steel.

Steel

While the state of Indiana pledged $10 million to help attract a buyer for the bankrupt Continental Steel, its trustee, Wayne Etter, worked to compile a sales package for prospective buyers of both the Kokomo and the Joliet plants—separately or together. Steven Ancel, the lawyer representing the creditors' committee, explained to the *Kokomo Tribune* that since the proceeding had converted to Chapter 7, the steelworkers' pension plan had been "terminated." The company's union employees and retirees, now creditors themselves, worried whether they still had active health insurance and reliable pension checks. Salaried employees soon found themselves in the same situation; they planned to meet on March 2 to discuss whether to file claims as creditors for severance pay, vacation pay, and health and dental benefits. Meanwhile, female employees and wives of Continental workers set up a women's group to offer moral support, to share information along with used children's clothes, to discuss babysitting arrangements, and to pray.[8]

A bit of good news arrived in early March: a federal agency, the Pension Guaranty Benefit Corporation (PGBC), had agreed to provide security for Continental's pension plans. It would honor the commitments, but not necessarily at 100 percent. Dependent on employer contributions, the PGBC was also one of Continental's creditors. Continental was some five years behind in its payments to the PGBC—it had missed millions of dollars' worth of premiums. Still, the PGBC would attempt to pay something to pensioners according to a formula that factored in their age, length of employment at Continental, and the specific terms of each employee's contract. On March 3, the North Central Indiana Private Industry Council announced it would seek funds from the U.S. Department of Labor to retrain and re-educate former Continental employees. And on March 4, the *Tribune* reported that officials of Interlake, Inc., of Oakbrook, Illinois, had expressed interest in buying part of Continental's Kokomo operation after reading in the *Wall Street Journal* of the bankruptcy's conversion to a liquidation proceeding.[9]

Any optimism surrounding the fate of Continental came to a halt the next week, when Etter, the trustee, filed a petition to abandon the Kokomo plant. The petition foreshadowed the catastrophic extent of the pollution and danger that lurked behind Continental's bankruptcy filing. According to a *Tribune* report, Etter asked the court's permission to take that drastic measure after learning that he faced costs of $17 million to properly close down the steelworks in compliance with the EPA's requirements. If the court allowed Etter to abandon the facility, Trefoil Capital would then own the property and incur the liability for its cleanup—and Kokomo would have an empty, polluted steel mill on its west side. Naturally, the city opposed the petition.[10]

On April 16, the *Tribune* published a letter from a resident of the neighborhood bordering a quarry that Continental had used as a dump. Barb Haberfield of Kokomo described the poor air quality that resulted in stains, pitting, and apparent rust on many of the homes in the area, as well as the "many occasions when I could not see the sun for the pollution coming from the melt shop of Continental Steel." She admitted that until now, she had made a deliberate decision not to complain about the pollution, because she did not want to jeopardize the livelihood of her friends and neighbors who worked at the mill. With Continental's closing, however, Haberfield wondered whom to trust: the firm's seemingly inept management, its creditors, or "the EPA which … should have had more to say about the pollution from its melt shop?" In Haberfield's opinion, there was plenty of blame to go around. Indeed, by that time, EPA and IDEM investigators had found "soil, sediments, surface water and ground water contaminated with volatile organic compounds[,] PCBs[,] and several metals, including lead," on the massive campus. Inspectors also found lead contamination in "nearby residential soils," according to the EPA. But answers to Haberfield's concerns would not come quickly.[11]

Letters published in the *Tribune* during the spring and summer of 1986 reveal a community divided in its responses to the Continental bankruptcy. Some correspondents, such as Mrs. Larry Causey of Kokomo, wrote that they were "fed up" with all of the complaints about the cost of aid to the steelworkers. In those letters, writers had expressed resentment at the "handouts" given to displaced workers. Causey wanted readers to know of the real hardships that the plant's closing had caused her own family—their car had been repossessed, and they had had to move from a trailer they had been planning to buy to an apartment in an undesirable neighborhood. Canned food drives had helped her family, and their monthly wait at the welfare office yielded $79 in food stamps for her family of four. Grateful for a home and food, Causey nonetheless felt compelled to ask, "what is wrong with helping people?"[12]

The state tried to help, but its aid had limits: Lieutenant Governor John Mutz, traveling to Kokomo in August to highlight job training programs, bluntly remarked that steelworking skills were simply not transferable to other jobs. More than 1,000 former Continental steelworkers qualified for state and federal "dislocated worker" funds to help them train for new skills, further their education, take advantage of job placement services, and learn to write résumés. Mutz made a point of stating that such programs were not charity, but "self-help" programs. He reiterated the state's offer of $10 million in assistance to any purchaser of the Continental Steel plant. The property was scheduled for auction in October.[13]

Continental found some success with its sister plant in Joliet, Illinois. On August 30, Sheffield Steel, a Sand Springs, Oklahoma-based mini-mill, announced that it had purchased the company's Joliet Bar Mill Division. The Joliet plant would get a new name—Sheffield Steel Corp.-Joliet—and Matthew E. Chinski, the former board member, vice president for administration, and chief financial officer of Continental's Kokomo plant, would be the firm's vice president and general manager. The news was not as good for the Kokomo steelworkers. On September 23, picketers outside of Continental's padlocked front gates carried hand-lettered signs that read, "We Were Lied Too [sic]," "Our Rights are Being Denied by Bankruptcy," and "Pay Our Benefits Now," as well as others that mentioned "jail" and called for an immediate investigation. The impetus for the laborers' action was a decision from the Pension Benefit Guaranty Corporation to deny pensions to more than 300 steelworkers. A month later, Judge Richard Vandivier refused to allow a delay in the scheduled auction of the Kokomo plant's assets, meaning that efforts to find a buyer for the shuttered facility would end. Cargill Steel & Wire of Houston, Texas, had purchased Continental's fence mill for $730,000 on the last day of the auction, October 15, along with various other pieces of equipment. But buying the facility and reopening it were two very different ventures; Cargill's board of directors would have to approve the latter action, and it was not close to coming up for a vote.[14]

Speaking to the *Tribune* about the future of the site late in 1986, Mayor Daily was realistic. "We think the day will come when the trustee (Wayne Etter) will abandon and the city will be [left] here" to deal with the buildings and property, he told the paper. The closing of the year brought with it little hope for Continental's former steelworkers—or for its neighbors, who had started to wonder just how poisonous the idle colossus was. Letters like Haberfield's and Causey's, the picketers' signs, and Daily's grim remarks demonstrated the trauma that Continental's demise had inflicted not only on Kokomo's industrial sector, but on its self-esteem as a community. Workers who had once defiantly refused to make concessions to Continental Steel now found themselves without pensions and dependent upon government programs for their survival—but castigated by their neighbors for taking part in said programs. Their fellow citizens had shown themselves to be more willing to donate money to keep Ryan White out of school than to help out their newly jobless neighbors.[15]

Writing of the impact of deindustrialization in Youngstown, Ohio, Sherry Lee Linkon and John Russo discuss the importance of a community's "constitutive narrative" to the meaning that its residents give both to the place and to themselves. The people of Youngstown, itself a prosperous steel center until its mills shut down, proudly remembered their city as a valuable contributor to the regional and national economy, as well as an important site in the history of workers' rights. Once the mills closed, however, longstanding divisions over race and class surfaced, and the narrative broke down—unity and pride vanished as conflicts came into the open. Kokomo's constitutive narrative was its identity as "The City of Firsts"—a place that innovators, inventors, and industries called home. Penn-Dixie's extended takeover of Continental Steel, as well as the subsequent fraud and two painful bankruptcies, damaged that narrative and threatened the city's identity. So did the rocky path of the domestic auto industry; its own ups and downs in the 1970s and 1980s meant that a manufacturing job like Jeanne White's no longer guaranteed a stable and secure livelihood. The condemnation brought to bear on the city from the Ryan White case occurred simultaneously with this threat to Kokomo's identity and made the closure of the mill sting even more.[16]

Ryan White

On Monday morning, February 24, Ryan once again sat at home and listened to classes via remote telephone conference. His lawyer, Charles Vaughan, filed a motion for a bond that morning, explaining to reporters that the law required plaintiffs who win temporary injunctions to post bonds in order to indemnify them in case defendants are later able to prove that they were damaged by an order that was issued in error. If Vaughan were to get the restraining order overturned, the bond money could be used to relieve the Whites of the responsibility of paying for his legal fees, expert witness fees, and court costs. Judge Brubaker heard the matter the next day and ordered the Concerned Parents to pay a $12,000 cash bond to the clerk of the court for damages to the defendants. At the hearing, Vaughan testified that he had already put in $7,000 worth of work (at a rate of $150 an hour) on the case since the plaintiffs filed it the previous week. Stephen Jessup, Western's attorney, made it clear to the court that his client was not asking for a bond. A combative David Rosselot accused Vaughan of padding his expenses. Brubaker agreed with Vaughan, however, ruling that since the plaintiffs had brought the case, they bore responsibility for the costs associated with it. They would have until Monday, March 3—less than a week—to post the money with the clerk. Rosselot spoke with reporters after the hearing, telling them he thought the plaintiffs would be able to raise the funds in the allotted time.[17]

Mitzie Johnson and some 50 other members of "Concerned Citizens and Parents of Western School Corp." hit the streets almost immediately after Judge Brubaker ordered the bond, standing at corners with buckets and knocking on doors seeking donations. In the first day alone, they raised $800. "I've found that the people in the community always seem to come through when there's a challenge to be met and when their hearts are in it," Rosselot told the *Tribune*. Ryan's case was also getting plenty of attention from people outside the community, however, and those people had strong opinions. On February 27 alone, the *Tribune* published four letters about Ryan's case—all supporting Ryan, and all from out of town. Thales Kaster of Chicago likened Ryan's treatment to that of a leper, urged people to pray for him, and also to pray for their own fears to moderate. Margery Gilcrest-Hesse of Lansing, Michigan, asked residents to ease their fear of AIDS, citing the example of her son, who lived with a friend who had AIDS and did not contract the disease. Elsie Ward of Columbus City, Indiana, chose to focus on Ryan, calling him one of the most loved and admired people in the world. The final writer, Jeff L. Hayward of San Francisco, was more openly hostile as he referred to the "brutal treatment of Ryan White," he wrote. "For Shame."[18]

Jeanne White was also upset on February 27, when a local radio talk show devoted an entire hour to the question of whether Ryan should be allowed to go to school. In an interview with Chris MacNeil, she complained that the guests and hosts on the show "moaned" about Ryan returning to school with certain precautions in place if his presence did not threaten the health of others. "Apparently they didn't read or see on national TV that the conditions they were talking about were suggested by Ryan and me and not demanded by the school." The Whites had indeed offered to abide by more restrictions than Principal Colby had proposed, and that approach had backfired. MacNeil noted that people remained skeptical of the reason for those conditions (the disposable utensils, the separate restroom facilities, etc.): why have them at all if Ryan did not pose a threat to others' health?[19]

Others asked the Whites that question more directly. Following the show, Jeanne White received an anonymous letter, signed by "A friend of mankind" and postmarked Kokomo, February 27, 1986:

> Dear Mrs. White, I am listening to WWKI and the parents discussing AIDS. I do not even live close to Western or have children in school, but I certainly understand their problem. Mrs. White, it is very difficult for me as a nurse to understand why you insist your son exposing so many innocent children. Plus, the important problem for you would be to protect your son, due to him having no immune system. There is [sic] so many bugs out there, why would you want him exposed? And then possibly come down with something that would shorten his young life [...] even if you do not care of [sic]others, don't you even consider your own? Every time I see Ryan on TV, I feel for him being made a spectacle by his own mother. You may think you are trying to prove a point but at the cost of his life and others? [...] I pray, Mrs. White, you'll try to reconsider this serious situation. These young parents are so afraid that they are having to raise money for needless court fees. Oh, if only that money could be used for education. It makes me very sad. As a nurse, the medical field does not have all the answers. Please won't you help protect others and Ryan?

The Whites would soon learn how other members of their community felt, because the Concerned Citizens needed help raising the bond money. Johnson and her allies had deposited $1,600 in the group's bank account on Thursday, February 27—all of it raised in one day—but they still needed about $10,000 more to satisfy the bond amount. Would the people of Kokomo and Russiaville support the group, even as their neighbors who had worked at Continental Steel wondered how to feed their families?[20]

Two local businesses stepped up to answer that question over the weekend. KS & Co., a beauty salon, and Westside Auto Parts held special events to raise money for the Concerned Citizens group. The salon held an all-night "tanathon" between 6:00 Saturday evening and 6:00 Sunday

evening, offering 20-minute tanning sessions for $4, and donated its reve-
nues to the group, raising about $500. The auto parts store donated all of the
proceeds from a day's sales of used parts—nearly $600—to the concerned
parents' group that Saturday. On Sunday, the Concerned Citizens hosted
an auction and yard sale at the Western Middle School gymnasium. Marcia
Rosselot told a reporter before the event that she hoped for a "large turn-
out." She got her wish. The group exceeded its goal, with the auction raising
$9,822.85 and donations and concessions bringing in another $3,549.79.[21]

But the Concerned Citizens' biggest asset was local celebrity Dick
Bronson. Bronson, along with Charlie Cropper, hosted a two-man radio
show, "Male Call," that Ryan White, in his memoir, called "an institution" in Kokomo. The daily morning call-in show was a staple for drivers
stuck inside their cars and for workers at the local factories, including the
Delco plant where Jeanne worked. At the height of its popularity in the
1980s, WWKI broadcast the show live every Friday morning from Kokomo's Markland Mall, and audience members often drove in from other cities to see the show in person. Bronson, with his stocky build and narrow
eyes, and Cropper, with his lanky frame and glasses, were opposites in tem-
perament as well as appearance. "He's the good guy, and I'm the bad guy,"
Bronson told a reporter for a lengthy profile piece in Kokomo's *Our Town*
magazine. The laid-back Cropper worked as a more sympathetic foil to
Bronson, who often insulted and argued with listeners who called in to the
show. Although their routine worked well to bring in listeners and spon-
sors, Bronson and Cropper dropped the yin-and-yang shtick every year
before Christmas in order to raise funds for their annual "WE CARE" campaign. Bronson had started the project shortly before the holidays in 1973,
when a laid-off autoworker called the show worried that he was unable to
provide for his family. The "WE CARE" campaign took on a life of its own,
outliving both Bronson (who died suddenly from a massive heart attack in
2002) and Cropper (who passed away in 2009, after 40 years at WWKI).
Over the years, the successful campaign had raised money for many worthy causes and families, including the Whites, who had received help with
Ryan's medical expenses in the 1970s. But with Ryan's fight to go back to
school, everything changed.[22]

"I not only oppose him going back to school … I think he should be
quarantined, and I've said it on the air many times," Bronson told a reporter
for *Indianapolis Monthly* magazine in 1986. Bronson said he had offered to
help the Whites financially if the Whites dropped their legal claims to Ryan
attending school, by using his radio show to raise funds and give Jeanne air
time to garner the community's support. The Whites never took Bronson
up on his offer. Although Jeanne had repeatedly stated that Ryan's wishes
dictated her actions, Bronson viewed her as the driving force behind the

lawsuit that had turned the nation's gaze toward Kokomo. He questioned how one 14-year-old's desires could be allowed to affect the lives of hundreds of students. Bronson had equally harsh words for *Kokomo Tribune* reporter Chris MacNeil, whom he criticized for "hanging his community out to dry."[23]

Commenting on his own family's move to the district a few months after the *Indianapolis Monthly* interview, though, Bronson said that he did plan on sending his six children to Western schools, while praying they remained healthy. With "Male Call" and its many listeners arrayed against them, the two funds set up to help the Whites had raised only $2,500 in the past 18 months—a far cry from the thousands that the Concerned Citizens were able to raise in just one weekend.[24]

Marcia Rosselot walked into the Art Deco Howard County courthouse in downtown Kokomo on Monday, March 3, with a cashier's check for the full $12,000 bond. Even as the bankruptcy trustee worked to find a buyer for some or all of Continental Steel, Rosselot reported that the Concerned Parents organization still had $6,000 left over in the bank—but that the balance would not suffice to cover her husband's attorney fees, only his expenses. Meanwhile, the media relentlessly pursued the story. The *Chicago Tribune* reported on the growing resentment felt by the people of Kokomo over the media presence. In his March 4 story headlined "Kokomo Bristles Over Publicity on AIDS Boy's Plight," reporter Rogers Worthington quoted Western Middle school parent Leslie Wells, who complained, "We're all kind of angry that it has turned around to where we're the bad guys." "We're tired of it because it tends to create a great deal of mixed emotions in everybody," Mayor Steve Daily explained, before going on to point out that Western Middle School was not actually in Kokomo, but Russiaville. Ron Colby was less diplomatic than the mayor, telling Worthington that "you're dealing here with a community that was caught up in a situation where they were made to sound like a bunch of country bumpkins." Worthington's account did little to reverse that image. Rather than focus on the majority of reports that firmly concluded AIDS was not transmissible by casual contact, he wrote, concerned Kokomo residents had elected to emphasize the "unknown, the exceptional, the speculative, and the apocryphal." He quoted a local history professor, Victor Bogle: "what is happening here is pretty typical of a community for a disease for which there is not much precedent.... And they are scared." Scared, yes—and also divided.[25]

As ex–Continental Steel employees waited for food stamps and sought help at local emergency pantries, Gentry's, a local nightclub, announced it was holding a wet t-shirt and briefs contest in order to raise funds for Crisis Center of Kokomo's aid program for the newly jobless. The steelworkers' fundraising efforts stood in sharp contrast to the ease with which the

Concerned Citizens had raised the bond money in their case against Jeanne and Ryan White. And letters to the *Kokomo Tribune* made the ruptures in the community more apparent with each passing day. As Kokomo residents Elmer and Emma Jean Gunnell praised a local physician, Dr. Pratap Gohil, for his offer to care for unemployed steelworkers without charge, Mrs. Pendu Miller could not understand why her neighbors were ignoring the plight of other unemployed residents such as her husband, who had been laid off from Carnation for so long that his unemployment benefits had run out. Why wouldn't people in her husband's position move to the front of the line when jobs became available, ahead of the Continental workers?[26]

Correspondents continued to criticize local citizens' behavior toward the Whites. David A. Parrish of Kokomo, who identified himself as a former Western student, expressed his disappointment with the "interfering of the disc jockeys" at WWKI and inveighed against the Concerned Citizens as well for their actions. H.D. Waterman of Beech Grove, Indiana, a suburb of Indianapolis, invoked a higher power in his reference to the courtroom cheers. "Two thousand years ago another crowd cheered at the decision handed down against an innocent party," Waterman wrote.[27]

But Kokomo resident Carla Leffert would have none of the criticism: she had two daughters and planned to send them to private school unless she received an absolute guarantee that they would not get HIV. Leffert assailed Jeanne White's parenting skills and wondered why she would hasten Ryan's death by sending him to a public school. Russiaville resident Ron DeGraaff addressed critics' accusations of un–Christian behavior head-on, by characterizing the Whites' defenders—in particular the ACLU—as "ungodly, un–Christian, and un–American as any group can get," he argued.[28]

Homer and Gail Trammell of nearby Greentown wrote to the *Tribune* to compliment Dan Carter for his handling of the whole situation, calling him a "Christian gentleman [and] competent leader...." Over at the middle school, Ron Colby received an "attaboy" letter of his own in March from J.O. Smith and the entire Western School Board. The brief letter conveyed the Board's "appreciation of the manner in which you have handled the difficult problems this year related to our Ryan White case," and added Smith's personal thanks. "Your steady positive influence has certainly been noticeable."[29]

As Western's principal, Ron Colby was the recipient of a less pleasant letter that month. An anonymous writer sent a clipping of a column by John Krull from a March edition of the *Fort Wayne Journal*. Western's angry correspondent had annotated the opinion piece, which was titled, "Brutal irony behind the tragedy," with comments such as "Shame ON ALL OF YOU! How Can You Live with Yourselves" and "Stupid-Ignorant-People." Krull's column had expressed understanding for parents who continued to fear their children might get AIDS from Ryan, even in the face of experts' reassurances to the contrary. But Krull had no understanding for, or tolerance of, what he labeled the "mean-spirited and nasty excesses of some of these terror-stricken parents—and their children." The anonymous writer had underlined "mean-spirited" and "nasty excesses" for the reader, as well as Krull's statement that "all of that ugliness and inhumanity has been directed at one sick 14-year-old-boy." The "brutal irony," as Krull saw it, was that all of the negativity, "anger and violence" directed at Ryan "probably have convinced other AIDS victims that it's better not to report that they have the disease or its symptoms."[30]

Colby also received a letter from Louise Fritz and her friends in Oregon, who asked him to please give an enclosed Easter card to Ryan. Fritz mentioned watching television news stories that showed an excited and happy Ryan entering school on February 21, as well as the boy's "rejection" at the hands of townspeople. Fritz hoped "the card will let Ryan know that people, even far away, are thinking of him." She added a postscript to Colby: "I grew up in Illinois and know how dismal the winter can be for a shut-in—the kid is an unsung hero."[31]

While each day brought more impassioned letters to the *Tribune* about both the Continental steelworkers and Ryan White (eight letters on March 6, six on March 7, for example, and on all sides of the issues), other news continued to unfold. On March 6, David Rosselot announced that he was running for Howard County prosecutor—he had previously run unsuccessfully for judge in 1980. Reports in the paper's March 9 edition detailed the efforts of Continental steelworkers to obtain insurance from Blue Cross and Blue Shield of Indiana as well as news of another fundraiser for displaced workers—this time, donations to a fishbowl at the local Home Show would go to the Crisis Center's efforts to buy food and pay utility bills for the ex-workers. But perhaps most interesting was a feature by Chris MacNeil about the situation in Swansea, Massachusetts.[32]

In an interview with MacNeil, Joseph Case Junior High School principal Harold G. Devine, Jr., explained that the students had already been in school before the fact of Mark Hoyle's attendance became public knowledge. That gave school officials a chance to educate the students, who in turn helped ease their parents' fears with factual medical information. Devine believed that the administration's compassionate approach toward the parents helped to defuse the situation and disarm the parents. Mark Hoyle was known publicly only by his first name; MacNeil described his fellow students' treatment of Mark as "just another kid." "Parents in Swansea do not circulate petitions or raise money for a bond to keep the pupil out of school," MacNeil wrote. "Instead, they raise money to help the victim's family and defend the right of an AIDS victim to a classroom education." MacNeil reported that, although one woman had circulated a petition to keep Mark out of school, she collected only 43 signatures, half of which proved to be invalid because the signers lived outside the school district. Out of a student body of 3,000, parents removed only two students—and the removal proved to be temporary.[33]

As the *Kokomo Tribune* continued to publish strident and heartfelt letters to the editor from writers both near and far (including one from Tom Hale, Jeanne's father and Ryan's grandfather), and as lawyers wrangled over hearing dates in Ryan's case, Kokomo mayor Steve Daily pondered how best to address the city's growing public relations crisis. Daily suggested a fund drive for AIDS research, to be held in the summer, and asked the local clergy to support him. Daily proposed that the city raise funds for donation to a special fund at Riley Hospital for Children in Indianapolis in an effort to portray Kokomo in a more favorable light to the rest of the country. The hospital had already established the Ryan White Fund for the Care of Childhood Infections with money that Jeanne White received from a national magazine whose readers sent donations after reading about Ryan's plight. While the local clergy studied the mayor's proposal, Ryan continued to attend school remotely. His seventh-grade science teacher, Frances Sempsel, made national news in March when she visited him at home in order to be his lab partner when the class dissected a grasshopper. For that class meeting, the students experienced what it was like to listen and try to learn through a telephone speaker. Sempsel, a lifelong educator who taught in the Western schools from 1974 to 2003, later recalled that she thought it would be fruitful for the students' roles to be reversed, so that his fellow students could appreciate the extra effort it took Ryan to learn from a distance. Sempsel arranged for Ron Colby to cover her classroom while she worked from Ryan's home that period.[34]

On March 12, Ryan's attorney, Charles Vaughan, filed a motion for a change of venue from the Howard County Circuit Court, and Judge Brubaker granted it with dispatch. "There's too much talk and prejudice in the community. I want a neutral court," Vaughan explained. After the parties struck judges' names from a list, they selected the Clinton County Circuit Court in Frankfort, Indiana—only one county to the west and thus a short drive—and Judge Jack R. O'Neill. Vaughan's sense of the hostile mood in Howard County was probably correct. In the pages of the *Tribune*, as the editor continued to publish some of the many letters that arrived from all around the country, local readers fought back. On March 20, for example, Kay Smith of Kokomo wrote to respond to a letter the paper had run from one Daniel Fry of Alamogordo, New Mexico. Whether Mr. Fry ever read Ms. Smith's response remains an open question, but it is clear that a daily diet of opprobrium from letter writers near and far had struck a nerve in Kokomo, and that people like Ms. Smith were on the defensive and felt compelled to respond with a letter of their own.[35]

A week later, the Kokomo ministers' group met to discuss Mayor Daily's proposed fundraiser for AIDS research and announced to reporters that they had approved of a community fund drive. The group also challenged Daily to act to control pornography and asked the media to use better judgment in their reporting of Ryan White's case. Asked for her response to the mayor's idea, Jeanne White was cautious; although the community had to start somewhere to repair its image, she felt the fundraiser idea was not the solution. In her mind, outsiders perceived the problem as Kokomo's response to Ryan White, not Kokomo's response to AIDS. MacNeil wrote that the city had been "moderately successful in weathering [the] generally negative opinion" the nation held toward Kokomo—"until Feb. 21." That was the day of the afternoon court hearing when Judge Brubaker had granted the temporary restraining order to keep Ryan out of school. According to MacNeil, the tipping point came when television cameras and newspaper photographers recorded the victorious parents and their supporters leaving the "courtroom cheering and flashing thumbs up." "Almost immediately," MacNeil reported, "generally hostile letters from around the nation flooded the city." Kokomo's mayor, he pointed out, had not commented publicly about the situation until the week of March 10, when he submitted his idea for a "'lavish, classy'" fundraiser for AIDS research. Such a benefit did not materialize that year, at least not in Kokomo.[36]

But in New York, a splashy affair led by Elizabeth Taylor was already in the works for late April. The gala aimed to raise $1 million for the organization Taylor had co-founded with Drs. Mathilde Krim of New York's Sloan-Kettering Institute for Cancer Research and Michael S. Gottlieb of the UCLA Medical Center, the American Foundation for AIDS Research (amfAR), after her friend Rock Hudson's death a year earlier. A publicist for the event explained to Chris MacNeil that Ryan had been invited because he was a "very courageous man." MacNeil reported that Jeanne and Andrea would also travel to New York with Ryan, who was very excited to attend the event. As amfAR's first major fundraiser, the event had already attracted the support of the cosmetics and fashion industries, along with celebrities from the worlds of entertainment, sports, and medicine. It is not difficult to imagine the resentment that some in Kokomo may have felt at this news. As steelworkers wondered how they would pay their bills and as layoffs threatened the auto industry, the Whites crossed class lines and mingled with the glitterati, which only added to the community's division.[37]

The following weekend, on Easter Sunday, the Whites and the Hales went to St. Luke's United Methodist Church, as was their custom. Jeanne had attended St. Luke's her entire life and had worked as a Sunday school teacher for ten years. As Ryan described the day's events in his memoirs, the whole congregation customarily shook hands with each other on Easter Sunday, beginning with the minister shaking hands with the people in the front rows and saying, "Peace be with you," and ending with the back row. The Whites sat in the back of the church. When the family in the pew in front of them turned around, Ryan recalled, "I held my hand out—to empty air. Other people's hands were moving every which way, in all directions away from me. No one in the whole church wanted to shake my hand and wish me peace on Easter." When their car's transmission failed in the church parking lot (after the Hales had left), not one person would assist them. Finally, a stranger drove over from an auto parts store across the street, helped them push their car to one side, and gave them a ride home.[38]

On the legal front, Judge O'Neill set Vaughan's request to dissolve Brubaker's injunction for a hearing on April 9. O'Neill also allowed the Indiana Civil Liberties Union (ICLU) to file an *amicus curiae* ("friend of the court") brief on April 8, over the objections of both David Rosselot and Stephen Jessup. Rosselot and Jessup objected to the ICLU's inclusion of medical and scientific references in the *amicus* brief in lieu of expert testimony at the hearing, but according to one report O'Neill replied, "the court needs all the friends it can get."[39]

As the lawyers prepared for the pivotal hearing on April 9, tensions in Howard County remained high. On April 4, the *Tribune* published a letter from Sylvia Payne that exemplified the level of anger and suspicion toward disapproving outsiders that some residents felt. Kokomo was a caring city, Payne maintained, and she denied that the community had mistreated Ryan White. As for Kokomo's image, she wrote, "I suggest we let the mayor know we like our image, and we don't want to be another L.A., New York or San Francisco."[40]

As Payne wrote those words, people in other cities expressed relief that they did not live in Kokomo. Writers to the nearby *Fort Wayne Journal Gazette* conveyed outrage at Ryan's treatment. "I'm glad I don't live in Ryan's community and have to face the hypocrisy of the adults who are ostracizing Ryan, yet trying to teach their children to love thy neighbor," wrote Miriam E. Stewart. David Kaufman had even harsher words for the people of Kokomo. "This is a letter directed to some of the citizens of the Kokomo area. I am appalled at your treatment of Ryan White, a person with AIDS. Ryan poses no health threat to you or your children. So why this despicable behavior on your part?" he asked.[41]

The people of Kokomo would have another chance to display their character after the hearing in Clinton County on Wednesday afternoon, April 9. Depending on how Judge O'Neill ruled, Ryan White would either return to classes at Western or continue to study at home. The next day, O'Neill announced his ruling: he dissolved the preliminary injunction and found that "there was no evidence of irreparable harm to plaintiffs presented at the February 21, 1986, hearing to warrant the issuance of a preliminary injunction to enforce the provisions of I.C. 16-1-9-7 in derogation of the entire chapter dealing with the Prevention and Control of Communicable Diseases." He further clarified his reason for vacating Judge Brubaker's order keeping Ryan out of school: "The Court, being cognizant of the principles of statutory construction, would note that it would be impossible for a child with a communicable disease and a written permit by the appropriate health officer to attend school without the persons having custody of such child being in violation of I.C. 16-1-9-7 and believes that such was not the intent of the Legislature." In O'Neill's view, his Howard County counterpart had misconstrued the statute by reading one section (-7) in isolation from all of the other sections in that same chapter. In effect, Charles Vaughan's reasoning had finally carried the day: the judge read all sections of the statute together. Although his ruling meant Ryan could return to school immediately, O'Neill did not grant Vaughan's motion to dismiss the plaintiffs' entire case. Nevertheless, David Rosselot was incensed. Some 25 years after the hearing, he told an interviewer:

> I felt that I had done all that I could the day that the judge in Clinton County dissolved the injunction … even though the law was on my side, even though I had done the right thing, even though Judge Brubaker had done the right thing, by that point in time, again with the help of the media, we were so unpopular in our cause and the result that there was just no overcoming it. I was beat, I was beat by the attitude, I was beat by the outside feelings of people, I was beat at that point. The law wasn't enough, does that make sense? It just wasn't enough. And the judge made the absolute wrong decision legally in Clinton County, OK, that he could have made, but I know why he made it. Because he didn't want to be part of us, he didn't want to be part of the spear-chuckin' ogres that were out to get this kid. I know why he did it.

If Rosselot was disappointed, Jeanne White sobbed with relief and hugged her son. "I love it. Is it really over? We finally won something," she told reporters after the hearing concluded. There were only about 30 people in the courtroom that morning, most of them reporters. Jeanne and Ryan made it to Western Middle School in Russiaville by 10:30, just one hour after Judge O'Neill announced his ruling. Ryan had been scheduled to fly to California that morning to meet with *Tonight Show* host Johnny Carson, but he missed the date in order to spend his second day in school in more than a year.[42]

Word of the decision traveled quickly—27 dismayed parents came to Western that day and took their children home. Ron Colby met with the group of reporters who had assembled outside of the school after he walked Ryan to his mother's car. "I really feel things went very well," Colby told the media, adding that he had not asked the children who left—or their parents—why they were leaving school that day. "Tomorrow may be something different," he said. "I think if the media would leave us alone, the situation would remedy itself," he told reporters. He also made it clear that he supported Ryan's bid to remain in classes: "As the principal of the school, I don't see any reason why Ryan shouldn't be in school. I don't think he poses a threat to anyone."[43]

Debbie Hill, a mother who took her son out of school that day, saw things differently. Judge O'Neill's swift decision had surprised her, she told a reporter. Hill's son Bryan was one of Ryan's classmates, and he told a reporter that he wanted to be in school, but "not Western...." Bryan's friend Marty Johnson said he was not in any of Ryan's classes, "but was afraid to walk the same halls as Ryan." Other students also encountered Ryan in the halls, and in his memoirs, Ryan described their actions as they "backed up against their lockers when they saw me coming, or they threw themselves against the hallway walls, shouting, 'Watch out! Watch out! There he is!' Maybe some were putting me on. I think most of them were acting like that just to get to me, to make me mad mainly," Ryan wrote. "But it hurt that no one wanted to get close to me."[44]

As the "angry and frustrated" plaintiffs vowed to appeal, Mitzie Johnson, the leader of the Concerned Citizens and Parents of Western School Corp., complained, "We didn't get our day in court." Rosselot remarked to the press that he was considering filing for a stay of O'Neill's ruling pending appeal, which if granted would mean the injunction would be back in place and Ryan out of classes. He also told a reporter that he was checking into whether one of his expert medical witnesses, a physician, had "political ties" to the extremist Lyndon LaRouche, who advocated quarantines for people with AIDS. As Rosselot mulled over his legal strategy, Ryan returned to school on April 11 for just the third day since August of 1985. The *Tribune* cited an absentee rate of 14.5 percent, or 53 absences out of 364 students. Ron Colby suspected that 30 of those absences were attributable to Ryan's presence, but the percentage of missing students was well below the 40 percent absentee level Western had experienced on Ryan's first day back in classes in February. The April 11 issue of *USA Today* quoted a student whose mother kept her out of school as asking, "If people with chicken pox and measles can't come, why should Ryan?" It is noteworthy, though, that contemporary reporting on the story never cited the fact that a majority of parents chose to keep their children in class—albeit a slight majority in February, but an overwhelming one in April.[45]

Over at Western, Ron Colby received a letter dated April 11, 1986, from

Sister Julia Delaney of Corpus Christi, Texas, that was inspired by the news accounts of Ryan's latest court battle. "Dear Mr. Colby," she began. "I am torn apart every time I read something new about Ryan White." She went on: "I have come to love the child and his winning smile, brave despite all the rebuffs and the disappointments. The same goes for his mother. They are both so very brave." Then she turned her attention to recent events. "And now today, in the *N.Y. Times* I am reading 'Mr [sic] Colby walked Ryan to his mother's car after school.' I would not expect less, but I am nevertheless moved by your commonsense stance, as well as your compassion." Sister Julia had less kind words for Kokomo. "Ignorance continues to abound in the matter of AIDS. It is almost primitive. One does not expect to find such enclaves of it in the great U.S.A." Like so many correspondents, she asked Colby to relay a message to Ryan for her: "Please tell Ryan that I admire him more than any child of this century; that I love and care for him even at this distance and that I pray daily that he will never lose his cool, his patience, or his great sense of humor. He walks tall," she remarked.[46]

Mayor Steve Daily was keenly aware of the hit his city's image was taking nationally—whether in the press, on television, or in the minds of people like Sister Julia. The Friday after Ryan's return to school, the mayor met with Kokomo's business and community leaders to strategize ways to improve the city's tarnished image. Not everyone was receptive to his idea of an organized fundraising drive for donations to AIDS research and education. Dale Tetrick, the president-elect of the United Way of Howard County, felt a fund drive would not work to repair the city's image. "We can't generate enough publicity … to offset the publicity Ryan White gets every day," he told a reporter. Other citizens also voiced their concerns about Kokomo's image. In a letter to the *Tribune* published on April 15, five people (Noel and Dianna Vandevender, Jerry Lee Henry, Daphne Antrim, and Ray Antrim, Jr., all from Kokomo) wrote to express their disappointment in Ryan's treatment by their fellow citizens. Such letters did nothing to sway the Concerned Citizens and Parents group, however, nor did they make Ryan's life easier.[47]

On Monday, April 14, Jeanne White returned to work at the Delco plant. She and Ryan had planned on Ryan taking the bus to school, but Ryan chose to have his grandmother, Gloria Hale, drive him instead. His bus driver, Dale Etherington, expressed puzzlement to a reporter for United Press International (UPI). "I have assigned him a seat with a wastebasket," the driver said. "I'm going to tell him if he blows his nose and puts the tissue or anything else in that wastebasket to let me know because I'm going to throw it out right away." If the fact that he was the only person on the bus to have an assigned seat and to have his garbage treated as hazardous waste dissuaded Ryan from riding the bus, we do not know—Etherington said the prospect of Ryan as a passenger on his bus did not bother him—and had not appeared to bother the other students on his bus. However, 35 students were absent from Western Middle School that Monday. Like Ryan's bus driver, the families of those absent students seemed convinced that one young teen weighing less than 80 pounds could contaminate an entire school. Indeed, some "Concerned Citizens and Parents" would go to great lengths to avoid sending their children to school with Ryan—even if it meant establishing a separate school.[48]

On April 17, the *Tribune* published a notice informing parents of sixth-and seventh-graders of a meeting that evening at Western High School to discuss enrollment in a home study group. J.O. Smith, the superintendent of Western schools, was not only allowing the parents' group to hold meetings in his facilities—he also planned to attend the meeting to answer parents' questions. The notion of creating a special school evoked the "segregation academies" that disgruntled white parents had established in reaction to court-ordered school integration a generation earlier. The Western parents intended to hire one or more teachers to staff the alternative school and split the cost among themselves, with a goal of having a student-teacher ratio of 20 to one. "It's the only alternative we have," Mitzie Johnson told a reporter. Larry Gabbard, one of the plaintiffs in the lawsuit that sought to ban Ryan from school, told the Associated Press that he expected the group would hire two teachers full-time, with two more acting as substitutes when needed, and that the school would be housed in a former American Legion hall—rent-free. The teachers and students would use Western School Corporation textbooks and lesson plans, according to Gabbard—further evidence that, while Ron Colby did his best to accommodate Ryan, his colleagues elsewhere in the school system did their best to undermine his work.[49]

National and international wire services reported news of the separate school, as they had the arrangements made by Ryan's bus driver. The *New York Times* published an item from UPI with the headline "Special School Planned to Avoid AIDS Victim," and quoted Mitzie Johnson as saying some 15 students would attend a "makeshift school" in Russiaville, rather than Western Middle School, because "AIDS is there." In her steadfast refusal to mention Ryan's name, Johnson seemed to conflate Ryan, the teenager, with the virus itself. Ryan White was AIDS, and AIDS was Ryan White—his identity was completely merged with his illness in Johnson's rhetoric.[50]

Speaking to an interviewer from the Howard County Historical Society in 2011, Johnson expressed no regrets concerning her actions. In Queens and Kokomo alike, she felt, parents and others who protested actually deserved credit for prodding the government to conduct more research on AIDS:

My children are proud of what I've done, that I stood up for what ... we believed in, and spoke out backing the school board and asking for more information. I think my children realize that probably the parents of Western School Corporation are probably very responsible for the amount of information that we do have about AIDS now. Because we stepped out and we said we want answers and said we want ... information, ... answer our questions.... I think that my children realize that, not me, but the parent group that was there at that one time ... if it weren't for us, how far would the research have gone.[51]

If people outside of Kokomo were searching, like Diogenes, for one virtuous person, they might have found her in Arletta Reith. Yet hers was a story that the wire services did not pick up. Reith worked at Delco from 1968 to 1998 and was a coworker of Jeanne's; her brother worked with Jeanne's father at the Kroger store, and the two men were fishing buddies. After reading the story about Ryan's AIDS in the *Tribune* in March 1985, she introduced herself to Jeanne: "I just went to Jeanne and told her who I was, how I knew who she was, and how badly I felt about her son having AIDS." The two women became friends, and Reith visited occasionally at the Whites' home. The lawsuit to prevent Ryan from attending school inspired her to design buttons that read, "FOR Friends of Ryan White, Kokomo, Indiana, 1986." Reith planned for people to buy the buttons for $6 each and wear them to show their support for the Whites. In this way, she felt she could help to repair the city's damaged image as well as benefit the Whites. She also ordered heart tokens printed with the inscription "Ryan Thanks You from the Heart," for the Whites to give to their supporters. Reith imagined using the revenue from button sales to help Jeanne with her aging car, or to get Ryan bunk beds, or to buy the family a new television. In the end, however, she sold only five or six of the buttons.[52]

Despite the apparent lack of support from within his community, Ryan had famous allies elsewhere. On April 20, Olympic diver Greg Louganis gave Ryan the gold medal he had won at the recent U.S. Diving Indoor Championship platform event in Indianapolis and made national news in the process. "I heard about Ryan as I traveled around the country," the gold medalist told a reporter for the Associated Press. Meanwhile, the amfAR benefit in New York quickly approached. Readers of the *Tribune* read Chris MacNeil's story noting that Ryan would miss five days of school in order to attend the function on the same day that an article appeared on David Rosselot's filing of a Notice of Appeal and Motion for Stay of Order Pending Appeal. Judge O'Neill set the matter for a hearing on April 30; if he granted the stay, Ryan would be forced out of school once again. MacNeil's story explained that Ryan, Jeanne, and Andrea would leave on Thursday, April 24 to start a fund drive that would culminate in the gala on Tuesday. Elizabeth Taylor and Calvin Klein co-hosted the benefit. According to MacNeil,

Jeanne "braced for criticism" for taking Ryan out of school after fighting for months to get him into school but hoped people would consider the charitable purpose of his trip. Jeanne praised Ron Colby for having a flexible attitude toward Ryan's attendance. MacNeil's article gave a partial list of the celebrities who were expected to attend the event, in addition to Taylor and Klein: Dustin Hoffman, Brooke Shields, Marlo Thomas, Paul Simon, Bernadette Peters, Bob Mackie, Donna Karan, Vidal Sassoon, Helen Gurley Brown, and Gloria Steinem. Although his opponents fought hard to keep him away from school, these celebrities considered Ryan's presence an asset. While his neighbors shunned him, the rich, famous, and beautiful sought him out as a fundraiser.[53]

As the letters to Ron Colby and the editor of the *Kokomo Tribune* attested, consumers of news nationwide had formed mostly negative opinions about the people of Kokomo, and they also viewed Ryan White with sympathy. Although we now know that most other boys with severe hemophilia also had HIV by this point, because Ryan was publicly "out" about his condition, he became the poster child for AIDS. By lending his name and his image—innocent, "blameless" in his nonsexual means of infection—he helped along the process by which AIDS became a "cause." Ryan's participation in the New York fundraiser marked the beginning of this progression.

The *New York Times* reportage of the benefit mentioned such luminaries as Grace Jones, Bianca Jagger, Oscar de la Renta, Perry Ellis, Carolina Herrera, Norma Kamali, Dina Merrill, Twyla Tharp, and Andy Warhol in the same vein as Ryan White and his family. "I was surprised from the first day that this event could be so big," Jeanne told the reporter. "All Ryan wanted to do was to go to school." The *Kokomo Tribune* featured an Associated Press story about the affair, along with a photo of a smiling Ryan and Andrea backstage on Broadway with cast members from the musical *Cats*. The morning of the benefit, Ryan appeared on the ABC morning news program *Good Morning America*, with David Hartman. Press accounts of the appearance quoted Ryan as saying that his fellow students had treated him favorably. He also shared that he understood why the students who left upon his return were frightened, "but with all the facts, I don't really see why." Ryan admitted that he, too, got "pretty scared" sometimes, and when that happened, he sat with his mother and talked.[54]

On April 30, Judge O'Neill denied the motion to stay his order lifting the injunction; he also denied Charles Vaughan's request to increase the bond. While Vaughan told a reporter that he was happy with O'Neill's decision, Roger Miller, co-counsel for the plaintiffs along with David Rosselot, was less gracious. According to the news report, Miller asked the judge why Ryan had not been in school for the past several days if attending classes was so important to him. Miller said the reason for the trip was "an exploitation of a young man." Later, Miller refused to tell reporters whom he believed was exploiting Ryan. Elsewhere in that day's *Tribune*, Chris MacNeil treated readers to the Whites' account of their trip. Ryan mentioned meeting actor Tom Cruise at the gala, as well as New York mayor Ed Koch. Ryan, who returned to school on May 1, looked tired as he exited his flight the afternoon of April 30, according to MacNeil, but took time to tell MacNeil about their helicopter tour of the city and visit to the offices of Marvel Comics.[55]

Ryan's attendance as Greg Louganis's guest at the diving championship, like his hobnobbing with A-list celebrities at the amfAR benefit, transgressed powerful social norms. The ire that attorney Roger Miller expressed before Judge O'Neill no doubt matched that of many in Kokomo who resented the Whites—not only because the blue-collar family traveled to glamorous destinations and mingled with celebrities, but also because Ryan failed to adhere to the "sick role" discussed previously, and by doing so, he threatened their understanding of the status quo, how society was supposed to work. Others saw in Ryan someone whose refusal to accept quietly and passively his community's ostracism brought condemnation on their beloved "City of Firsts." If only the Whites had accepted J.O. Smith's decision, the rest of the nation—indeed, the rest of the world—would not have focused its attention on Kokomo. (As early as 1986, Ryan was receiving mail from correspondents all over the world.) If only the Whites had accepted Judge Brubaker's ruling as the last word on the matter of Ryan's school attendance, the Concerned Citizens and Parents' group would not have been forced to raise five figures' worth of bail money, and their fellow Americans would not have been outraged at the spectacle of the community's response. Many in Kokomo felt that the nation's attention was focused on them for all the wrong reasons.

In late June 1986, Dick Bronson, WWKI's "Male Call" on-air personality and nemesis of the Whites, received a special citation from President Ronald Reagan at the White House honoring his years of charitable work with the "WE CARE" campaign. As Bronson received his accolades, Ryan learned that he would be prohibited from swimming in several of the local pools over the summer. As if to offset that piece of bad news, the Second District of the Indiana Court of Appeals handed the plaintiffs in Ryan's case a crushing defeat on July 17 when the court denied the concerned parents' appeal and dismissed the case. That same day, the parents' group driving the litigation announced that they had decided to end their legal quest to keep Ryan out of classes. The dismissal did not mean that the parents had had a change of heart. Rather, David Rosselot told reporters, the group had run out of financial support. And on November 24, 1986, the parties to the federal case the Whites had filed in August of 1985 filed a Joint Stipulation of Dismissal, which Judge Noland granted on December 1. Ryan would never again appear in court.[56]

Another noteworthy development occurred during the summer of 1986: the byline of Chris MacNeil, the award-winning reporter who had written more than 100 articles about Ryan White and matters related to AIDS since early 1985, stopped appearing in the *Kokomo Tribune*. Mac-Neil's name would not be seen in the paper's coverage of Ryan from May 1 until December 7, 1986. One hint of the reason for the hiatus may be found in the July 1986 story on Ryan White that Steve Bell wrote for *Indianapolis Monthly*. By that time, MacNeil, a lifelong Kokomo resident, had worked at the *Tribune* for eight years. MacNeil related to Bell that he had received death threats for his coverage of the Ryan White story and AIDS. Asked whether he was biased, MacNeil had a rhetorical question for Bell: "What's going on here? A very sick little boy is going to die ... does there have to be sides?" But Bell, who described Kokomo as a "finger-pointers' paradise," noted that MacNeil's stories had been picked up by the wire services and published nationally, and that MacNeil had also written for *Newsweek*—activities that earned him the praise of his fellow journalists, but the condemnation of Kokomo. In fact, life was becoming so miserable that MacNeil was contemplating changing careers and moving away. "This doesn't feel like home anymore," he told Bell. But in the more immediate future, he was concerned that he was getting too close to the story. He related to Bell that Ryan had started calling him "Uncle" at some point, and "in the last few weeks, he's started calling me 'Dad.'" John Wiles, who had edited the *Tribune* since 1981, told MacNeil that some in the community perceived him as taking sides. Wiles recalled that MacNeil had been seen on television hugging the Whites at the airport in Indianapolis upon their arrival from a trip. "And so I told him that if it happened again, we'd have to pull him from the story," Wiles recalled. Within a year of that episode, Wiles remembered, MacNeil moved away from Kokomo.[57]

Beginning in the summer of 1986, Kay Bacon was the reporter whose byline most frequently appeared in articles about Ryan for the *Tribune*. Aside from writing about the action in the Clinton County Circuit Court, Bacon mainly wrote about Ryan's return to classes—this time as an eighth grader at Western High School. J.O. Smith had required a new health certificate for Ryan's admission to the 1986–1987 academic year, so Dr. Adler obliged. He examined Ryan on August 21 and issued the certificate. More than 900 students attended the high school, in contrast to the 350 at the middle school. Charles Wolf, the high school principal, told Bacon that he had a son in Ryan's grade, that he hoped to keep everything calm and that he expected no problems. Wolf and Bev Ashcraft, the school nurse, had met with the high school staff at least twice in anticipation of Ryan's attendance and covered subjects ranging from medical emergencies to proper use of the spill kits that had been added to first aid kits in every classroom and office. Ashcraft also instructed the returning high school students about AIDS and its transmission in preparation for Ryan's first day. Ryan would attend under the same restrictions at high school that he had followed at middle school: a separate bathroom stall, a separate drinking fountain, and a disposable cafeteria tray and silverware. Wolf also conducted a one-on-one orientation with Ryan, showing him around the building and answering his questions.[58]

While Wolf hoped to keep Ryan's return to school quiet, the media would not oblige. Ryan's attendance at high school was reported from coast to coast. The *New York Times* described Ryan as "bounding off the bus" on his first day, excited to return to school. The paper also noted that the restrictions on Ryan's attendance—the separate facilities and disposable food service items—were not medically necessary. Reporters also interviewed Ryan's fellow high school students to get their reactions. "It doesn't mean anything," freshman Jack Smith told the press. "It kind of bothers me, but all the scientists and everything say it's OK for him to come to school." While there were "no protesters or disturbances," according to the *Los Angeles Times*, Doug Wescott, a junior, told a reporter he was against Ryan attending school in person. "He's at our school and there's nothing we can do about it," Westcott said. "It wouldn't be a bad idea to keep him out of school just to be safe." Speaking to an Associated Press reporter on August 26, senior Sabrina Johnson had a warning for Ryan. "We've fought it and fought it, and it's over now," she told a reporter. "As long as he keeps his distance ... he's OK." The wire services also reported that the Concerned Citizens had pledged to work for legislation to exclude people with AIDS from school once the Indiana General Assembly convened, and that Mitzie Johnson was spearheading a new organization called the Foundation Supporting Homebound Education for Students with AIDS, Inc. News accounts such as these only reinforced Kokomo's image as an intolerant place, one that would begrudge a fatally ill teen his only wish.[59]

In fact, none of the Whites had an easy autumn. In her memoir, *Weeding Out the Tears: A Mother's Story of Love, Loss and Renewal*, Jeanne White summed up Ryan's experience in the eighth grade rather tersely: "Every minute of the short time that he was there was hell." Jeanne told of an incident at the school involving Ryan's locker—someone had opened it and written "Faggot!" and "Get butt-fucked!" on his folders—and related that no one wanted to sit next to Ryan in class. "When he walked down the hall," she wrote, "the kids would flatten themselves against the walls and yell, 'There he goes! The AIDS kid! Stay back!'" "Or they'd run up and touch him, then touch other kids and say, 'Now you've got it,'" Jeanne continued.

"I began to feel completely paranoid about my fellow citizens. I didn't know whom to trust—so I trusted no one." William Narwold, the Dean of Students at Western High School when Ryan attended, differed in his recollection. "Ryan always had a crowd of people that sat at his table. He interacted with them. There was a social stigma attached to him by, certainly that was a very minor group of people and never did I see anybody do anything to him that I would consider taunting or teasing or any of those kinds of things while he was in my sight, nor did I ever, was I ever able to validate any of that."[60]

Ryan's neighbor, Wanda (Bowen) Bilodeau (Heath Bowen's older sister), was one of the people who sat with Ryan at lunchtime; Heath was still at the middle school. "We made sure he wasn't harassed," she told a reporter. But Ryan was ostracized, according to Wanda. In the cafeteria, Wanda witnessed students staring at Ryan, pointing at him, making comments, and taunting him by "bang[ing] up against the wall" and saying things such as "Don't touch the AIDS boy's trash," when Ryan dumped his tray after eating lunch. Although Wanda saw Ryan shrug his shoulders and try to laugh it off, she believed such incidents hurt him. Wanda also believed that other factors played a role in Ryan's unhappiness at Western. His closest friends, including Wanda's brother Heath, were younger, and still in the middle school building. "And then there were others who were just frightened," she observed. Wanda also tried to watch over Ryan in high school because he was frail—something that Narwold also mentioned. Even with the normal jostling of a high school hallway, they both worried for his safety. But Wanda suffered repercussions for her support of Ryan, as did her younger brother. Older boys on the school bus would call Heath "gay," and Wanda, who worked on the school newspaper, found that someone had carved "bitch" and "faggot lover" into her table at the journalism room. Another Western High School student, Chantel Kebrdle, recalled a classroom incident in which the other students refused to sit next to Ryan.[61]

How was it that William Narwold saw and heard nothing abusive directed toward Ryan, while Wanda and Chantel witnessed incidents of harassment firsthand? Was Ryan misleading his mother when he told her about his folders and other incidents of bullying? While the answers to such questions might seem obvious to anyone who has experienced high school culture, the situation also reflects a more general tendency for those in power (in this case, school administrators) to construct a narrative of events differently from those who are powerless (students). James C. Scott's concept of "public" and "hidden transcripts" reminds us that the boundary between what is public and hidden is forever shifting, due to the "constant struggle between dominant and subordinate." It should come as no surprise that Narwold witnessed nothing he believed was untoward.[62]

Across the country, in Swansea, Massachusetts, Mark Hoyle began ninth grade at Case High School (he had not been held back a grade, unlike Ryan) as Ryan started at Western. The two youths' experiences were similar in that neither participated in physical education classes or in study halls, so their days were shorter than most other students.' Further, recurring bouts of poor health prevented both teens from attending school regularly. Both boys' health declined in the fall of 1986: Ryan was hospitalized for five days in September, and Mark entered the hospital on October 3 because he was having trouble breathing. Mark Hoyle died in the hospital on October 26, 1986, at the age of 14. His death served as a catalyst for his community to recognize his brave spirit and help his family, as had his illness.[63]

While Mark was alive and attending school, his fellow students made banners and sent cards whenever he was hospitalized. The most impressive support for Mark and his family came from three concerned mothers, Susan Travers, Linda Nahas, and Robin Sherman, who had no history of any community activism but who wanted to help. Aware of the toll Mark's hospitalization was taking on his parents and younger brother, they started an organization called "Friends of Mark," and arranged for help cutting the Hoyles' grass, raised gas money, and made sure the Hoyles had hot meals every night with enough left over to take to Mark while he was in the hospital. The mothers also worked with students to organize a dance fundraiser called "That's What Friends Are For," named for the 1985 Dionne Warwick hit.[64]

Friends of Mark opened a post office box to receive donations and mail for the Hoyles and staffed a booth at the Swansea Mall where they sold balloons to raise money. They later helped pay for funeral expenses. The Case Junior High School choir sang at Mark's funeral, and the school's administrators, faculty, and staff planted a tree at the school in his memory. Supporters started the Mark Gardiner Hoyle Scholarship Fund; the mothers' group donated their leftover cash to the fund and held a fundraising dance in October of 1987. But perhaps the greatest tribute to Mark's short life materialized some time later, when the community named an elementary school after him: Mark G. Hoyle Elementary School educates children from pre–K through second grade.[65]

In marked contrast to Swansea, Ryan's greatest support came from outside of his own community. Elton John flew the Whites to California in early October; they attended John's concerts and went to Disneyland, where the star pushed a still-weak Ryan around in a wheelchair. Later that same month, Jeanne White and Ron Colby attended the fall meeting of the Indiana Associated Press Broadcasters Association and reflected on the media coverage of Ryan's case. Jeanne told the assembled reporters that she sometimes felt "the news media blew the case out of proportion and violated her family's privacy. But in general, she said, reporters have 'done a good job of handling a sensitive issue.'" Colby believed "the coverage that was given really helped Ryan … go back to school." He felt the media focused unduly on the relatively few students whose parents withdrew them from Western Middle School instead of the majority of students who stayed. "Showing the fight by a small group of parents was 'lending credibility to what these people are doing,'" Colby pointed out. For Colby, though, the media onslaught was over—Ryan was no longer attending the middle school, after all.[66]

Ryan's failing health did not allow him to attend Western High School much at all. On November 3, he returned to Riley Hospital with a high fever, coughing up blood and keenly aware that his counterpart Mark Hoyle had died less than a month earlier. Dr. Kleiman tried to get him approved for treatment with Burroughs-Wellcome's new drug azidothymidine (AZT), but was unsuccessful. Ryan remained in the hospital for two weeks. Fortunately, he was able to return home before his fifteenth birthday in early December. And as the year closed, he found that the subject of his life had once again been voted the top news story in Indiana of 1986.[67]

Ryan made the news again in early February 1987, when he and Jeanne spoke at an "AIDS in the Heartland" conference organized by the Indiana State Board of Health. More than 800 health and education professionals attended the Friday and Saturday conference in downtown Indianapolis on February 6 and 7, where they heard from officials such as Indiana's Woodrow Myers, Dr. David K. Henderson of the National Institutes of Health, and Western Middle School's Ronald Colby. Colby spoke at a Friday workshop on coping with AIDS in schools, telling some 50 educators in attendance that "fears among students and their parents were 'soothed' after the school adopted an AIDS policy," which included equipping each classroom with a spill kit containing bleach and rubber gloves. Ryan and Jeanne spoke on Saturday at a session called "Hoosiers Speak Out," along with the mother of a man who had recently died from AIDS and a Fort Wayne man living with an AIDS diagnosis. "Whatever you do, please don't isolate us," Ryan told the crowd of 900 who had come to hear his panel; the audience responded with applause. Ryan and Jeanne also read a letter they had received while they were in the midst of the legal fight to attend Western Middle School the year before. Before Jeanne began reading aloud, she told the audience, "I am sure the person who wrote this doesn't feel the same (now)." Then she read the letter to everyone there:

> Mrs. White, I can't believe you are such a puke. We all in Kokomo are so sick of your fat, ugly face in the (Kokomo) Tribune and on TV. You are not thinking of the welfare of your son. …can you imagine what is going on through your son's mind?

Jeanne told the crowd that Ryan laughed at the letter and jokingly called her a "puke" for days afterward, although she found it more difficult not to be discouraged. Even though Ryan was more upbeat in the face of abuse and ridicule than his mother, all of the Whites found life in Kokomo increasingly hard to tolerate.[68]

In the early morning hours of Saturday, March 14, 1987, someone fired a shot through the Whites' front storm window. While the shooter appeared to have used only a BB gun, the incident still disturbed the family—especially Andrea, who told Jeanne that she did not want to live there anymore. Ironically, the next day's issue of the *Tribune* featured two stories whose juxtaposition seemed especially ironic: above an item about the Ku Klux Klan marching in nearby Delphi, a small city some 35 miles northwest of Kokomo, was a story about a song. Two men concerned with Kokomo's image, Jack Welker and Roy Bowen, had composed a song extolling the city's positive features—a "happy little town" where the "people are friendly"—in order to counteract the negative publicity the city had received over Ryan White's efforts to attend school. The lyrics to "Kokomo, My Home Town," included the verse, "When you're really feelin' down and your spirits get low, You'll dance your troubles away when you come to Kokomo."[69]

All of the Whites were under pressure that spring. Ryan's health seemed to be fading fast; he was able to attend school for only three and one-half days that second semester at Western High School. Andrea was terrified by the gunshot in their living room window. Even Jeanne's parents were hurt by the unrelenting criticism of their daughter's parenting skills and constant rumors about how Ryan "really" contracted AIDS (some people said he did not really have hemophilia, but that he had contracted the disease as a result of Jeanne's supposedly perverted lifestyle). And Jeanne White herself knew that her family had to leave Kokomo in order to survive. But how would they afford it? Where would they go—where *could* they go? Everyone knew who they were and that Ryan had AIDS.[70]

6

"I am ashamed to admit that I even live here!"

Stigma and Transformation, 1987–1990

Jeanne White was able to move her family away from Kokomo only because of the interest she received from producers wanting to turn Ryan's story into a made-for-TV movie. At least three production companies approached the Whites and Charles Vaughan, the family's lawyer, seeking the rights to the story of Ryan's battle to attend school. Jeanne chose Linda Otto of Landsburg, an independent producer not affiliated with a major studio, in part because Otto had come to see the Whites at their home in Kokomo. The company sent Jeanne a check for $25,000, and a move away from the City of Firsts suddenly seemed plausible. In her memoirs, Jeanne recalled staring at the check for a full two weeks in wonder. She resolved to use the money to make her family's life better, and soon started looking for a house.[1]

Jeanne's main criterion for selecting a new place to live was simply that the new house be "somewhere else." Even if Ryan never went back to school, Jeanne thought, she wanted a place where they could lead quieter lives. After locating a home two counties to the southeast in the tiny town of Cicero, Indiana, Jeanne sought financing. While she had received, in addition to the check from the rights to Ryan's story, a $10,000 loan from Elton John, she was in a difficult financial position—committed to buying a new house, while not yet having sold their current home. Who, she feared, would want to buy "the AIDS house," as the home on Webster was known? Even though a community leader in Kokomo asked for volunteers to "help scrub the house until it was spotless," it would end up on the market for quite some time before someone bought it for use as a rental property. Determined to relocate despite the unsold home, Jeanne notified the local health department and the administration of the Hamilton Heights High School that her family would soon arrive; she did not "want to be seen as sneaking into Hamilton County." The Whites moved to Cicero on May 15, 1987.[2]

Cicero, Indiana, is a town of a few thousand people near Morse Reservoir, nearly halfway between Indianapolis and Kokomo. The reservoir attracts those who want to live on the water and offers recreation as well as lakeside vistas. Driving from Kokomo to Cicero, one passes through Tipton and miles and miles of flat, open farmland. The local high school, Hamilton Heights, is located in Arcadia, a five-minute drive to the north from Cicero. Jeanne's strategy of forewarning local officials of her family's arrival reflected her awareness of small-town life—people know each other's business, and word travels fast. Indeed, she found a community already anticipating her family's arrival. The *Heights Herald*, the area's weekly newspaper, put the story of the Whites' move above the front-page fold of its May 7, 1987, issue, beneath the headline "Whites moving to area." The piece featured a photo of Jeanne (identified as "Jean White") informing the Hamilton County Community Task Force on AIDS that she, Andrea, and Ryan planned to move to Cicero. "I am here today to ask the support and encouragement of your group," Jeanne told the Task Force. She continued: "We need to stop these fears right off the bat. Kokomo was the first city to have to deal with this situation and unfortunately they were misled and misinformed. We want the community to accept us and we need your help in educating and informing the community." Jeanne explained that Ryan had "been through so much. He needs to get away. We all need to get away," she continued, "to someplace that is quiet." Noting bluntly that she was unsure whether Ryan would be able to attend school in the fall, she tried to assure the audience that she did not want trouble: "Let me say that I am not intending to throw the Hamilton Heights school system into a panic. Ryan will not attend if he is not healthy enough," Jeanne continued; "We chose Cicero because it is a nice quiet community.... We needed a bigger house, too, and when Ryan saw the house, he loved it." The article mentioned the television production deal that had enabled the Whites to relocate, although Jeanne declined to disclose the amount that producers had paid her family for the rights. During the same meeting, the *Herald* reported, the Hamilton County Health Department issued a news release welcoming the Whites to the county and offering assistance; the announcement also included an offer to educate the community about AIDS with workshops and printed material. Jeanne reacted with tears of gratitude, according to the article, and thanked the task force members for their "optimism and encouragement."[3]

The following week's edition of the *Heights Herald* signaled that Ryan's attempt to attend school in his new community might face resistance: under a headline reading, "School board OKs plan to evoke [sic] law," the front-page article reported that "if AIDS victim Ryan White enrolls at Hamilton Heights this fall, school officials said during their May 4 meeting they will not voluntarily welcome the 15 year-old as a student." Hamilton Heights School superintendent Bob Carnal told the board that he planned to rely on a newly passed state law that empowered him to exclude any student with a communicable disease until the Indiana State Board of Health determined whether other students were at risk under normal conditions of contact. If the State Board concluded that Ryan was not a threat, the article explained, "the system will be forced to accept the student." Carnal advised the school board that he did not think such a scenario would come to pass, however, because Jeanne had told the school nurse that Ryan was currently too sick for even homebound instruction. Carnal also reported that he had spoken with his counterpart at the Western School Corporation in Russiaville and learned that Ryan attended just three-and-one-half days the second semester of the 1986–1987 school year, and only 53½ days the entire school year. "I honestly don't think he'll enroll," the paper quoted Carnal as telling the board. "He has already outlived his life expectancy." But should Ryan prove fit to come to classes in the Fall of 1987, Carnal was going to be ready. He had planned an early dismissal for a May afternoon in order to conduct an in-service training on AIDS for school employees. If not Ryan, Carnal reasoned, then someone with AIDS—a student, or perhaps a staff member—would, at some point, enter one of his schools, and he wanted to be ready.[4]

By 1987, many educators' attitudes toward students with AIDS had undergone a transformation: pragmatism, such as that displayed by Carnal, had replaced reactionary exclusionary policies. This chapter focuses on both transformation and stigma: in the years 1987 through 1990, unfortunately, as the experiences of the Ray brothers, Dwayne Mowery, and Shawn Decker attest, stigma still governed the lives of many people with AIDS, including those with hemophilia. Prospective immigrants and would-be airline travelers found themselves subject to new laws and prejudicial corporate policies, even as radicals injected a newfound militancy into the public discourse around AIDS and sought to transform the narrative from one of victimhood to one of conflict. But stigma also arrived full force in the city of Kokomo, Indiana, thanks to the changing themes in media coverage of AIDS and continuing publicity of Ryan's plight. The public's view of Continental Steel likewise underwent a transformation during this time, as their realization of the extent of the environmental damage left behind began to eclipse the finger-pointing about who was to blame for the mill's demise. The campus itself, littered with festering, contaminated barrels, pits, and chemicals, was like a literal stigma, a physical wound to the land-scape, one that would take decades to heal.

Back in Cicero, as school personnel planned to receive Ryan, so did his new neighbors in Shorewood Estates, the subdivision where the Whites would soon live. What kind of reception would their new neighbors give Ryan, Jeanne, and Andrea? Within this small community, a disease its members had only read about was suddenly hitting home in a very tangible way in the spring of 1987. Outside of Cicero, however, some AIDS patients and their advocates displayed a newfound radicalism, a willingness to be contentious and combative in the face of what they saw as official inaction and discrimination.

Blood

In March 1987, the Food and Drug Administration (FDA) formally approved the use of the first anti–HIV drug, Burroughs-Wellcome's Ret-rovir (zidovudine), commonly known as AZT (azidothymidine). While FDA approval represented a positive development for people afflicted with AIDS, it could not alleviate one enormous problem: the drug's cost. At an estimated $10,000 for a year's worth of treatment, AZT was simply too expensive for many AIDS sufferers. Most patients would quickly reach the limits of both their health insurance coverage (if they had any) and their personal funds, and the decision of whether to use taxpayer funds such as Medicare or Medicaid to assist patients had been left to each state. Burroughs-Wellcome, for its part, reported having invested some $80 mil-lion in the development and exclusive patenting of AZT and informed the media that it had only enough of the drug to supply 15,000 patients. The company needed to charge such a high price, it reasoned, in order to sustain the drug's production. The situation offered fertile ground for a growing power struggle, and AIDS patients had a new voice in early 1987: ACTUP.[5]

ACTUP, the AIDS Coalition to Unleash Power, had been founded in New York by playwright Larry Kramer and others in March 1987. The group combined guerrilla theater, street protests, and civil disobedience in a way that had not been seen before in the AIDS crisis. Just a week after the FDA approved AZT, a group of some 250 demonstrators blocked traffic on Wall Street in reaction to Burroughs-Wellcome's price points. The group hung an effigy of the FDA's commissioner, Frank Young. Seventeen of the pro-testers, arrested by police, went limp and forced officers to drag them to the jail wagon. The protest was effective: it called attention to the intractable situation in which those in need of AZT found themselves and prompted the *New York Times* to publish an editorial the next day decrying the cost of the drug. Just days later, more than 3,000 protesters assembled at New York's City Hall to call attention to what they considered the city's inadequate handling of the AIDS epidemic. Police arrested approximately 200 of the crowd whom they accused of blocking traffic. This demonstration, the city's largest thus far in response to the AIDS crisis, lasted for three hours.[6]

ACTUP staged even more dramatic events the following year. On October 11, 1988, more than 1,000 demonstrators vowing to "Seize Control of the FDA" disrupted business at the agency's Rockville, Maryland, headquarters. The protesters demanded swifter approval of experimental drugs and a streamlining of the rigorous drug development process for people with AIDS. Their protest lasted for nine hours; although it was mostly peaceful, authorities did arrest 176 people—and, media reports made a point of noting, police wore rubber or latex gloves when doing so. On March 29, 1989, thousands of ACTUP demonstrators returned to New York's City Hall to protest the city's AIDS policies. ACTUP's "Target City Hall" events featured protesters staging "die-ins," both to dramatize the stakes of the crisis and, in a show of passive resistance, to force police to move their bodies away from the scene. ACTUP's tactics were not confined to eastern cities: in June 1989, dozens of "gay-rights activists, AIDS patients, and healthcare workers" organized a die-in, recited names of county residents who had died of AIDS and drew chalk body outlines in a courtyard outside of the Civic Center in Santa Ana, California, to protest the Orange County Board of Supervisors' decision to reject a non-discrimination ordinance. Before a backdrop of protesters holding signs that read "Hate begets hate," "Selma '62, Santa Ana '89," and "Orange County: 457 cases of AIDS," Jeff LeTourneau—whom the *Los Angeles Times* identified as the co-chairman of the Orange County Visibility League (a gay-rights group)— told a reporter: "The days are over when gays and lesbians walk away with their heads down. We will fight back."[7]

The increasing radicalization of AIDS patients and their allies perhaps owed something to the scarcity of hopeful AIDS-related news in the closing years of the 1980s. Even the promise of AZT was tempered by concerns about the drug's price and toxicity. Then too, the culture clash occasioned by the homosexual identity of many AIDS patients was persistent and deep-seated. The Orange County protesters were met with equally impassioned critics—a news report quoted one counter demonstrator, the Rev. Louis P. Sheldon of the Traditional Values Coalition, as saying that "these people have chosen death with their behavior." In the Spring of 1987, a house in Queens that had been intended for a New York City–run program to provide foster care for six "boarder babies," who had been living in hospitals since they were born, was damaged by arson. The babies' parents typically were drug addicts and AIDS patients, and the city's foster care system, already overwhelmed, could not place the homeless infants. In May, officials in Harlem opened a home for 15 such babies who had been diagnosed with AIDS—most were expected to die before reaching their second birthday.[8]

On June 24, 1987, President Ronald Reagan signed Executive Order 12601, establishing the Presidential Commission on the Human Immunodeficiency Virus Epidemic. Presidential recognition of the seriousness of the outbreak, however, did little to quell the persistent fear with which many Americans continued to react to people with HIV. Earlier in June, the United States Senate had voted 96 to 0 to require the Immigration and Naturalization Service to test all immigrants for HIV. President Reagan had advocated for such a policy, as well as for regular HIV testing of prisoners, patients in drug treatment programs, and applicants for marriage licenses. Those affected by AIDS, in turn, continued to try to find ways to escape the isolation and discrimination they faced. Just two months after the creation of the Presidential Commission, Clifford and Louise Ray of Arcadia, Florida, won an injunction to force the De Soto County School Board to admit their three sons, ages eight to ten, into regular classrooms with non-infected children. Ricky, Robert, and Randy Ray had all tested positive for antibodies to the AIDS virus after treatments with tainted clotting factor for their hemophilia. As in Russiaville and Kokomo, Florida, parents organized against the boys: just as Western Schools had its Concerned Citizens, so De Soto County had its Citizens Against AIDS in Schools Committee. Committee members boycotted classes—parents kept half the student body home on the Ray boys' first day of school. Even the mayor of Arcadia withdrew his son from the school, and some callers phoned the Rays with death threats. On August 28, an arsonist burned the Rays' house down. The family moved to nearby Sarasota. U.S. Surgeon General C. Everett Koop honored that city in April 1989, for extending its hospitality to the Ray family.[9]

Variations of the scene repeated throughout the country that fall. In Waynesboro, Virginia, Shawn Decker, a boy with "mild" hemophilia who had been diagnosed with HIV earlier in 1987 and was subsequently expelled from sixth grade when the state health department notified his school, geared up for a fight to attend seventh grade. His mother, Pam Decker, arranged a meeting with the committee empowered to decide her son's fate that summer, bringing with her Shawn's nurse, doctor, and kindergarten teacher (the latter to attest to Shawn's character). The witnesses answered questions about risk factors and the transmission of HIV, and after a four-hour meeting, the committee recommended to the superintendent and school board that Shawn be allowed to attend school. In the end, Shawn was allowed to attend the seventh grade—but not until authorities had sent a flyer to every student in the school system (excluding the high school), informing them that an (unnamed) student was infected with the AIDS virus and explaining the connection between hemophilia and HIV. Shawn assumed everyone knew it was he—after all, he was not permitted to participate in physical education classes and was required to use a special bathroom stall. Electing not to speak of his status or to confirm anything, he missed more than 100 days of school in seventh grade—not because he was sick, but because he could not face his peers. Writing of her family to Jeanne White, his mother Pam explained: "We were the test case in Virginia—Shawn was expelled when he was diagnosed. We owe you and Ryan and Andrea a lot. They let Shawn in school after the Rays [sic] house was burned.... I call myself 'The Bitch' as I've had to fight the school and try to protect Shawn. The hardest thing is the hurt I sometimes see in his eyes."[10]

Some parents decided not to fight: the parents of a 12-year-old boy with hemophilia and AIDS, Dwayne Mowery of Lake City, Tennessee, withdrew him from school after two days of protests, picketing parents, and widespread absenteeism. After receiving threats, the family arranged for Dwayne to be taught at home. While some of his fellow students protested the treatment he received, Dwayne's opponents were by far the more vocal group. News reports indicated that 250 parents attending a school board meeting loudly cheered when the superintendent informed the crowd of the Mowerys' decision to keep Dwayne at home. In a 1988 interview with *USA Today* just before the release of the Presidential Commission's report on the HIV epidemic, commission chair James Watkins mentioned the Ray and Mowery families' ordeals as specific examples of the need for education: "We've seen a society too ready to reject, deny, condemn. I wouldn't have expected to see the three boys' home from Arcadia, [Florida], burned. I wouldn't have expected to see Dwayne Mowery from east Tennessee have his car stoned."[11]

As the Whites, the Rays, the Deckers, and the Mowerys grappled with intolerance and even outright violence in the late 1980s, people with AIDS continued to stage protests against stigma and discrimination. In August 1987, a decorated Viet Nam veteran, Leonard Matlovich, walked into the San Francisco International Airport wearing a t-shirt that read, "I'm a human with AIDS," strode up to the Northwest Airlines ticket counter, tried to buy a ticket, and was turned away because he lacked a note from his doctor certifying that he was not "contagious." The requirement of a physician's statement was actually an improvement over Northwest's earlier position, which had prohibited all people with AIDS from flying on its planes. Delta, USAir, and United also featured policies that had evolved from outright bans to allowing air travel with certain documentation during 1987, even though by this time, the circumstances under which the virus was transmitted were well-known.[12]

While ACTUP's shock troops engaged in confrontational direct action, and individual activists like Matlovich bravely called attention to corporate discrimination, San Francisco activist Cleve Jones and the NAMES Project favored a more poignant, but equally dramatic, type of publicity. Jones and his colleagues displayed the first 1,900 panels—two blocks' worth—of their NAMES Project quilt (the AIDS memorial quilt) at a march in Washington, D.C., on October 11, 1987. Within a year, the quilt had grown to more than 8,200 squares. By 1991, it would weigh 14 tons and stretch four miles in length—powerful and tangible evidence of the direct human loss caused by the epidemic. Relatives, lovers, parents, friends, and even complete strangers volunteered to sew quilt squares commemorating those who had died of AIDS. The colorful fabric squares often included text that ranged from the simple ("He loved dancing") to the complex ("I have decorated this banner to honor my brother. Our parents did not want his name used publicly. The omission of his name represents the fear of oppression that AIDS victims and their families feel"). The quilt told many different stories; a film about it and the stories embedded within it, *Common Threads: Stories from the Quilt*, won an Academy Award for best feature-length documentary in 1990.[13]

The AIDS memorial quilt gave a human face to the relentless drumbeat of casualty statistics. By January 1, 1988, the World Health Organization (WHO) reported 73,747 cases of AIDS in 129 countries; however, officials estimated that the actual number of cases was probably double that—closer to 150,000. The WHO estimated that between five and ten million people worldwide were infected with HIV, and predicted that by 1991, at least one million new cases of AIDS would develop in people who were currently HIV-positive. In an effort to curb the spread of the virus in the United States, Surgeon General C. Everett Koop prepared a six-page mailer on AIDS that would be sent to every household in America. "Understanding AIDS: A Message from the Surgeon General" was the largest print order to date in American history: 107 million copies, according to Koop's memoir. Months later, however, a Gallup poll would find that 51 percent of adults admitted to not having read the brochure.[14]

In October 1988, the *Washington Post* reported on a *New England Journal of Medicine* review of more than 50 public opinion surveys conducted between 1983 and 1988. Hostility toward people with AIDS remained strong. The lone sign of tolerance involved AIDS patients in schools: in a 1988 survey, only 18 percent of respondents believed children with AIDS should be prevented altogether from attending school, a marked improvement from a 1985 survey in which 39 percent had favored an outright ban.

Attitudes such as these had driven students like Shawn Decker and so many others underground: even though people with hemophilia (especially those who were children) could be considered "innocent" victims of HIV because of their nonsexual means of infection, they still found themselves on the receiving end of discrimination. Decker has written about how it felt to be an HIV-positive seventh grader in the late 1980s:

> The hardest part ... was the social ramifications. ... Some of my closest friends, whom I'd known for most of my life, weren't allowed to come over to my house to play anymore.... I did my best to keep my HIV status quiet, and never talked about it with friends.[15]

By 1989, medical experts estimated that 50 percent of the nation's 20,000 people with hemophilia were HIV-positive, constituting over four percent of all diagnosed AIDS cases. AIDS had overtaken both hemorrhaging and liver disease as the most common cause of death among people with hemophilia. Experts were also disturbed about the way in which Decker and many other hemophilia patients seemed to be coping with the ravages of HIV—by hiding. Their rate of participation in clinical trials for new antiviral treatments was extremely low, and their denial put them at risk of infecting their sexual partners. As Dr. Margaret V. Ragni put it in 1989, "hemophiliacs have long and successfully used denial to cope.... Combined with their ability to treat themselves at home, this denial has enabled people with hemophilia to get on with their lives, obtain jobs, start families and to avoid dealing with their chronic disease." That coping strategy, while it may have proved effective in the years before HIV, proved disastrous during a pandemic. AIDS represented not just a mortal threat to people with hemophilia—it was also a social threat. Even though they were not "responsible" for their infections, their infected status still connected them to the "guilty" high-risk groups of IV drug users and gay men.[16]

This associative stigma forced many people with hemophilia to try to "pass"—not just as uninfected, but even as not having hemophilia. Despite their life-or-death interest in the latest developments regarding antivirals, or discrimination, many put as much distance as possible between themselves and AIDS. The consequences of "passing" could be deadly, as Professor Dirk Scheerhorn observed in 1990: "passing, for example, may involve negligence in observing safety limitations, in seeking quick treatment, or in safe-sex practices. Passing may also involve refraining from involvement in social support networks or the unwillingness to attend and participate in meetings with other hemophiliacs"—isolating behaviors that threatened one's emotional health.[17]

For every Ryan White, Ricky Ray, or Dwayne Mowery—people with hemophilia who openly and publicly acknowledged their infections with

HIV—there were scores more Shawn Deckers who hid their illness and pretended that they were healthy, lest they be shunned. The stigma that society placed upon people with AIDS was nothing new. As anthropologists and other students of social behavior have long noted, humans instinctively identify illness as a threat to their existence, and a new disease—especially one which can remain latent for years once a person is infected and for which there is no cure—disrupts our ability to separate that which is pure and healthy from that which is impure and unhealthy. An AIDS patient like Ryan White symbolically blurred the lines between pollution and cleanliness: he appeared to be a child, but a lethal, invisible agent had overtaken his young body. His very presence in public spaces triggered primordial fears among people in his own community, reminded them of their own vulnerability to disease, and threatened to disrupt the social order. His neighbors stigmatized Ryan and his family not only because of his illness, however—they responded as well to his deviant behavior in defying authority and asserting his right to attend school, to circulate among healthy people. He went public, stayed vocal, and refused to let the stigma define or shame him.[18]

As the sociologist Erving Goffman explained in his seminal work on stigma, our ability to function in human society depends in part on our ability to read people—we constantly categorize the people we encounter, and we assess them, often on a subliminal level. Do they represent a threat? Are they like us, or are they different? Goffman reminds us that the ancient Greeks "originated the term *stigma* to refer to bodily signs designed to expose something unusual and bad about the moral status of the signifier." Such signs were not organic; rather, they were "cut or burnt into the body and advertised that the person was a slave, a criminal, or a traitor—a blemished person, ritually polluted, to be avoided, especially in public places." Because, in Goffman's parlance, stigmatized persons were "not quite human," the non-stigmatized—those with intact social identities—felt free to discriminate.[19]

While it has sometimes made sense to isolate the sick—especially in earlier centuries, when understandings of contagion were more rudimentary—people have over time tended to draw on that isolation to conflate the infectious condition of an illness with a group's entire identity. The Jews of medieval Venice, for example, were confined to that city's ghetto and condemned as corrupt in both body and morals when the influx of Jews fleeing the Spanish Inquisition coincided with the 1494 arrival of syphilis in the port city. The mere synchronicity of the two events (as opposed to concrete evidence that Jews, not sailors and prostitutes, were the vectors) provided sufficient justification, as Richard Sennett has shown, to confine and monitor an entire population of Others. Nayan Shah has written of similar behavior in San Francisco from 1900 to 1904, when an outbreak of bubonic plague caused the city's public health officials to quarantine all of Chinatown and to place its residents under surveillance. Patricia Fanning has documented how the 1918 influenza pandemic needlessly decimated entire immigrant families in Norwood, Massachusetts, because of the majority's insistence that the newcomers remain confined and separated from the community's medical facilities. Amid the crisis of war and the anxiety of the Red Scare, an epidemic quickly became a political emergency as well as a public health crisis.[20]

At their core, Ryan White's very loud opponents in Kokomo were similarly afraid—even though, in hindsight, their fears that one adolescent could defile an entire building were clearly and tragically irrational. Even judged by the standard medical knowledge of their time, their actions were misguided—they, and many others in America, confused an infectious disease—HIV—with a contagious disease, and treated Ryan and all people with AIDS accordingly. Their fears of toxicity and contamination seem doubly misdirected when we consider the fate of Continental Steel in the late 1980s, for its 183-acre campus harbored its own very real menace to the community's health.

Steel

Chris MacNeil, the *Kokomo Tribune* reporter who won awards for his work on the Ryan White story, had been a lifelong Kokomo resident while he worked at the paper. MacNeil grew up on Brandon Street, immediately behind the Continental Steel plant, which he recalls as providing a constant soundtrack of clanging and hammering through his childhood. The activity at Continental was ceaseless, with 18-wheel delivery trucks driving past his home 24 hours a day, seven days a week. At night, the sight of flying sparks lighting up the sky added beauty and life to both his neighborhood and the city. In its heyday, he says, Continental Steel was simply "the steel mill" for Kokomo residents. By the time the plant shut down, MacNeil had long since left Brandon Street, and he seldom returned. But on the night his mother died, as he drove two of his sisters home from the hospital, he turned to go through the old neighborhood, hoping to recall memories of better times. MacNeil was soon sorry he had made that turn. The house in which he and his sisters had grown up was gone—demolished. Many of the neighboring homes were in ill repair. The steel mill was boarded up, quiet; only a couple of abandoned delivery vehicles remained behind. MacNeil experienced yet another sense of loss.[21]

The demise of Continental Steel still stung the people of Kokomo

as late as the summer of 1987, when the *Kokomo Tribune* published a letter to the editor complaining of a taxpayer-funded "giveaway" to Mont-
gomery County, Indiana, for the construction of a new steel mill when the
massive Continental site sat just 60 miles away, idle and shuttered. Tech-
nically, Continental's fate still rested in the hands of the U.S. Bankruptcy
Court. In the spring of 1988, Bankruptcy Trustee Wayne Etter published a
notice to all former employees announcing a proposed settlement with the
U.S. Environmental Protection Agency (EPA), the Indiana Department of
Environmental Management (IDEM), the Pension Benefit Guaranty Corporation, and all former Continental employees to pay claims for wages,
medical benefits, unemployment benefits, and other wage-related matters.
The proposed settlement totaled $6.5 million; the estimated total value of
the 90-year-old company's estate was $11.3 million. The proposal was set
for hearings on April 5 and 12, 1988. Those employees who filed claims by
the June 8, 1988, deadline would ultimately receive just a fraction of what
they were owed and, as a story in the *Tribune* put it, the lingering questions
about what had gone wrong—and what the future might have looked like,
had Continental survived—would never be answered fully.[22]

The protracted bankruptcy proceedings, of course, only prolonged the
city's suffering—by the time Etter announced his proposed settlement, the
mill had been in bankruptcy court since November of 1985. All told, the
claims against Continental easily exceeded $200 million: demands for pay-
ment included $105 million from employee groups, $60 million from the
Pension Benefit Guaranty Corporation, and $18 million from the Internal
Revenue Service. The EPA and IDEM had also filed claims with the court
that gave some indication of the scope of Continental's liability for environmental damage: the government agencies estimated costs ranging between
$50,000 and $20 million to clean the plant's contaminated lagoons. Under
the terms of the agreement, shareholders would receive nothing—neither
would unsecured creditors. Thomas Sigler, Continental's last president,
would get $15,000 in cash and payment of up to $3,000 in medical claims.
The rest of the former employees—salaried and hourly, active and retired—
would split $5.5 million, with perhaps another $1 million to come. And
despite the enormity of their claims, the government agencies responsible
for cleaning up the environmental damage at the abandoned plant would
receive just $1.5 million in a special trust account, plus a $1 million administrative claim, in exchange for releasing any future owners of the site from
environmental liability.[23]

Just when it seemed that the settlement would provide some kind
of closure, one of Continental's major creditors filed an objection to the
agreement. Continuous Casting Corporation, which owned the mill's new
caster and had financed its purchase, wanted repayment of a $20 million

unsecured claim and a $42 million administrative claim. That objection and the resulting appeals delayed the settlement process for all creditors. Former employees, who had been jobless for years, would have to wait even longer before the court could authorize Etter to cut checks. The appeal process dragged on until the summer of 1989, and ex-steelworkers did not begin to receive their settlement checks (averaging $200 for each year they had worked) until November 1989. In the meantime, hard feelings lingered between those who laid the blame for the firm's dissolution upon steelworkers' unwillingness to agree to further concessions and those who accused the union of failing its loyal members.[24]

Division and bitterness were not the only legacy Continental Steel left behind. The community soon learned that not only the acid lagoons, but the entire Continental site was toxic and likely contaminating the surrounding air, soil, and groundwater. The sprawling campus sat on both the north and south sides of busy Markland Avenue on Kokomo's west side. The Markland Avenue Quarry, a former limestone quarry that had been part of Continental's operations since 1947, took up most of the space north of Markland, close by Chris MacNeil's old neighborhood. The mill had used the 23-acre quarry to dispose of its waste materials. When IDEM inspectors checked the site in the late 1980s, they found that the quarry contained hundreds of empty drums and tanks—those drums had once held oils and solvents. The surface soil of the quarry was contaminated with PCBs (polychlorinated biphenyls)—a known carcinogen.[25]

The 94-acre Main Plant, on the south side of Markland Avenue, included enormous abandoned buildings, some with footprints as large as 400,000 square feet. The empty buildings' basements flooded with ground water, and the structures themselves deteriorated over time. Inspectors discovered that the Main Plant held more than 700 drums full of oil and solvents, as well as aboveground and underground storage tanks and vats containing oil, chlorinated solvents, and acids. IDEM and the EPA also found 24 electrical transformers, 200 capacitors, electric arc furnace dust, and exposed asbestos at the Main Plant. The main campus, desolate and overgrown with weeds, included Wildcat Creek on its west side and Kokomo Creek on its south; both creeks drained the adjacent land and fed into the mighty Wabash River. The Kokomo Wastewater Treatment Facility sat just west of Wildcat Creek and east of Continental's 56-acre Acid Lagoon area, comprised of ten lagoons that held pickling and finishing liquors. Finally, the nine-acre Slag Processing Area, west of the acid lagoons, held calcium and iron oxides, aluminum, chromium, lead, manganese, magnesium and zinc oxides.[26]

All of these substances threatened the health of Kokomo residents. Authorities at IDEM and the EPA began the process of placing the

Continental Steel site on the EPA's National Priorities List in 1988, which eventually led to its official status as a Superfund site in late 1989. According to one report, the site posed risks to both human health and the environment, in part because it was home to "various chemical constituents above the acceptable cancer risk range," as well as other substances present in a concentration "above the non-cancer risk quotient." In other words, the place was truly poisonous.[27]

Whatever the city's hopes for redeveloping the abandoned area or luring a new steel maker to the facility, they quickly faded with the realization of just how badly Continental had harmed its neighborhood. As early as July 1988, one letter-writer to the *Tribune* had remarked about the inability of the settlement to provide adequate recompense for environmental damages: "I wonder if residents should be granted compensation for their rusted cars and home siding that was caused by emissions from Continental Steel Corp. Maybe we should also consider testing area residents for harmful contamination." Although the city re-zoned the Continental site as an urban enterprise zone in 1989, officials acknowledged that the uncertainty over the extent of the site's pollution presented a problem. "Everybody ... we have talked to has had a problem with the environmental situation," Greg Tiernan, the economic development director for Public Service Indiana (PSI) told the *Tribune*. PSI, a utility company, was interested in finding a new customer to replace the Continental operation and had been integral to the city's efforts to market the site to new industries. "There's a lot of concern there and I think that's scaring a lot of people and projects," Tiernan observed. Regardless of their lack of success, the redevelopment efforts themselves became a source of division within the community. Members of a group called Kokomo Against Pollution sent a letter to Governor Evan Bayh expressing their outrage. "It concerns us that efforts are being directed more to finding a new occupant for the closed facility than to finding a solution to the existing pollution problems and hazardous waste element," the group wrote in early 1990. By March 1990, the point was moot—after successive discoveries of new caches of contaminated materials, PSI gave up its efforts to find a new customer to occupy the massive property. A month later came the news that Wildcat Creek was contaminated with PCBs downstream of Kokomo, and that Continental was a prime suspect.[28]

As a boy, Chris MacNeil thought the huge piles of coal sitting across the parking lot right behind his house were pretty—he liked how the dark coal sparkled and glinted on sunny days. But thanks to that coal, billows of smoke constantly issued from the massive plant, and when he and his friends were taken to the doctor as children, they were usually simply diagnosed with having "breathed something from the steel mill." His own uncle, his friends' fathers, and other relatives who worked at the mill had all died from lung ailments, MacNeil recalled. While people had always connected working at Continental with poor health, no one truly appreciated the enormity of the mill's environmental damage until its closure. Like Marie Curie in Adrienne Rich's poem, "Power," the people of Kokomo had long denied that a source of the city's power could also be a source of its wounds. Unlike the metaphorical contamination of the Whites' home on Webster Street, the danger to the community presented by the Continental Steel campus on Markland Avenue was very real. No stigma had surrounded the steel works for the 90 years in which it provided jobs, security, and stability to Kokomo. Yet its poisoned legacy would remain long after those jobs had left. For their part, the Whites could not leave Howard County soon enough. They wondered whether their new neighbors in Cicero would view them as innocent newcomers or something more sinister.[29]

Ryan White

The Whites' new home at 1580 Overlook Circle in Cicero was a large Cape Cod in Shorewood Estates, near Morse Reservoir. The quiet subdivision of newer homes featured wide streets and large yards, with ample trees providing shade, privacy, and character. The pleasant environment was enhanced by the welcome that Jeanne, Ryan, and Andrea received. The Trump family of nearby Noblesville—complete strangers to the Whites—sent Ryan a card in 1987 that read, "Just wanted to tell you that we are thinking about you. Hope you and your mother enjoy many happy experiences in our community." The warm reception continued when the Whites' neighbors, Mary Baker and Betsy Stewart, rang the doorbell and introduced themselves. Jim Stewart, Betsy's husband, was active in the local Kiwanis chapter and, along with the State Board of Health, had helped to organize an educational program for those in the community who wanted more information about HIV. In contrast to the warmth of their new surroundings, however, one cold fact remained: Ryan was desperately ill during his first summer in his new home.[30]

Ryan fought extreme fatigue and constant chills, along with nausea, shortness of breath, a tight chest, and a runny nose. He was even hospitalized for a short time. Normally, such discomfort would not be newsworthy, but that summer, Jim Gaines, the editor of *People* magazine, had decided to publish a cover story on AIDS. The resulting August 3, 1987, issue featured the magazine's first non-celebrity cover since 1983. On that cover, next to text that read, "24 hours in the crisis that is BREAKING AMERICA'S HEART Every day is a challenge for people with AIDS and those who love them.

What follows is the story of one such day," a gaunt, stricken Ryan appeared, his head on his mother's bosom. In a departure from the usual magazine format, the cover story actually began on the cover with the words, "Ryan White is 15, and he is dying." When *People*'s editorial staff had decided to portray a 24-hour snapshot of the epidemic, Bill Shaw, the magazine's stringer in Indiana, had immediately thought of Ryan. As a result of his powerful writing and the poignant photos of Taro Yamasaki, what had previously been mostly a national news item went global. *People* was a staple at newsstands, airports, grocery checkout lanes, and doctors' offices. Shaw's article revealed to readers everywhere the stark reality that confronted the Whites that awful summer, as he described Ryan's constant shivering amid the oppressive Indiana heat, Ryan's fatigue, Ryan's bedtime prayers. Despite its focus on Ryan's present condition, the piece did briefly mention Ryan's past treatment in Kokomo: "His school kicked him out. Townspeople slashed the tires on the family car and pelted it with eggs; schoolmates taunted him; someone fired a bullet through the living-room window." Later, the article recalled the "grassroots hate campaign against him" and described how callers to a local radio talk show (presumably "Male Call") had called him names, as well as how fellow students had shunned Ryan once he was readmitted to school.[31]

The brief description was enough to cement this basic narrative in the national consciousness: Kokomo was intolerant and cruel toward a vulnerable, sweet, gravely ill young man, while Cicero was tolerant, quiet, comforting. In his new community, the worst treatment the reporters witnessed were the stares of restaurant patrons as Ryan quickly raced to the restroom to vomit, held his hands under the dryer for ten minutes, and then walked back to his table. The special issue of *People*, which featured the stories of several individuals living with, and dying of, AIDS, moved readers immensely. In the magazine's August 24, 1987, "Mail" section, emotional readers detailed their reactions to the AIDS issue, including Ryan's story. "As a resident of Kokomo, Ind., I have followed Ryan White's story from the beginning and was not aware of all the travesties committed against this innocent boy and his family," wrote Lynne A. Kasey. "I had often seen Ryan … and wanted to tell him how much I admired his courage…." William G. Eaton of Westminster, Maryland, expressed his outrage at the treatment Ryan had received: "I cannot understand the cruelty and heartlessness imposed upon the innocent youth Ryan White and his caring mother in Kokomo, Ind. Ryan says, 'I didn't want to die there.' Frankly, I wouldn't want to live there," Eaton wrote. *People* also printed Jeanne's response to Eaton's letter: "Kokomo is a good town…. Most of our problems were caused by the same people over and over. It was just a few bad apples who wouldn't leave us alone. I don't hold the whole town responsible." Her attempt to rehabilitate her hometown's image was futile, however—as long as the magazine lay on waiting room end tables, living room coffee tables, and kitchen counters, the narrative was alive.[32]

The *People* issue also inspired hundreds of readers to write directly to Ryan; in just three weeks after its publication, he received more than 200 letters. The cover story had vastly increased the visibility of HIV and AIDS and helped the disease along its path toward public acceptance—a path that had begun with the high-profile death of Rock Hudson and continued with the involvement of megawatt celebrities such as Elizabeth Taylor in amfAR fundraisers and other events. Ryan's association with the story added a very sympathetic dimension to the process and helped transform AIDS in the public's mind from something associated with Others—with gay sex and IV drug users—to something that could happen in their own families, or to the boy next door. Gradually, Ryan White helped to reverse the overwhelming stigma attached to HIV/AIDS. Instead of avoiding him and taunting him, many of his new classmates would seek him out and come to value his friendship. Whether because of his growing celebrity or just the fact that he was smart and engaging, Ryan found himself becoming popular.[33]

Ryan's new classmates mirrored the outpouring of support from across the country; as the first day of school drew closer, Jill Stewart, a senior and president of the student body at Hamilton Heights High School, visited Ryan at home. Another neighbor, Wendy Baker, who was a junior, followed suit, and she and Jill brought other students over, as well. Ryan's health improved in August as his first day of school approached. On August 28, *USA Today* ran a story on Ryan starting over at his new school; the headline read, "AIDS, school, and Ryan White/People friendlier in a new city." The piece quoted Jeanne's observation, "Here, we're just another family."[34]

When Ryan walked into Hamilton Heights High on August 31, not a single protester met him. In his memoir, Ryan described registering for school and meeting with Tony Cook and Steve Dillon, the principal and assistant principal of Hamilton Heights High School. He had started school two weeks later than his peers, at the request of Cook and Dillon, in order for the administrators to give the students and staff a "crash course" on AIDS. Cook and Dillon worked with personnel from the State Board of Health to develop the program, which extended into the community at large. Noting that the people in his district comprised a "pretty well-read, educated populace," Cook told a reporter that not one person had come to his office and "protest[ed] vehemently" about Ryan's attendance. For his part, Ryan (whose picture graced the front page of *USA Today* on September 1) told reporters that his first day "went really great—really. Everybody was real nice and friendly." "I was terribly nervous," he admitted.[35]

The rest of 1987 went well for Ryan and his family. They traveled to

California for an Athletes and Entertainers for Kids event in September that
marked the launch of a program, the Ryan White National Fund, designed
to send teams of celebrities and AIDS experts into schools to talk to children. The Whites, along with a new friend of Ryan's, Heather McNew, also
attended a cast party for the upcoming television movie about his life. And
in December, Governor Robert Orr declared December 18 "Ryan White
Day" and honored both Ryan and Jeanne with one of Indiana's highest honors, the Sagamore of the Wabash award, at a convocation held at the high
school and attended by more than 600 students and teachers. Orr then presented the school with the inaugural "Spirit of the Heartland" award for
welcoming Ryan. That same day, ABC News named the 16-year-old its "Person of the Week."[36]

People featured a more robust, upbeat Ryan in its May 30, 1988, cover
story, titled "Amazing Grace." Although—or perhaps because—the story
focused entirely on Ryan and his family, authors Jack Friedman and Bill
Shaw wrote unsparingly of Kokomo, observing that "if responding to AIDS
has become one of the litmus tests of human decency, many in Kokomo
failed it badly." Predictably, the magazine received many letters commenting on the cover story; the editors chose to publish five, four of which were
positive in tone and commended the article for its inspirational outlook.
One writer specifically mentioned the healing effect that "those wonderful townsfolk in Cicero" must have had on Ryan's health. The fifth letter,
from a Kokomo resident, scolded the magazine for its "sensationalism and
unprofessional conduct. You are condemning a community of 48,000 people indiscriminately for the acts of a very few," wrote Deborah L. McDaniel. As all of the letters made clear, a contentious geographical narrative
had steadily taken shape in the national discussion of Ryan White: Kokomo
was a bad place with judgmental people, and Cicero was a good place with
accepting people.[37]

Some *People* readers could not abide McDaniel's rationale. On July 11,
Katy Metzner of Charleston, South Carolina, argued "the problem was not
the 'few jerks' who harassed Ryan White. It was the 'majority of people' who
sat by and let it happen. That is Kokomo's shame." Kokomo would remain
in the news for some time, thanks to Ryan's increasingly high media profile.
In August, crews began filming *The Ryan White Story* in Statesville, North
Carolina. The Whites stayed there for about a month providing assistance
and even acting—Ryan played the part of Chad, a fellow patient at Riley
Children's Hospital. That same month, a *People* magazine television special commemorating its tenth year of publication (*People on TV*) featured a
story about Ryan that included news footage of the emotional and rancor-
ous Western School Corporation meetings. The rebroadcast of that video
some two years after the fact reminded viewers of the hostility the Whites

had endured in their previous community and provided a powerful contrast to the serene images of Ryan's new hometown.[38]

Interviewed for the *Kokomo Tribune* on September 21, David Rosselot, the attorney who had represented the concerned parents' group in the lawsuit to keep Ryan out of school, made public his nervousness about the upcoming made-for-TV movie of Ryan's life. "The media has picked up on this…. *People Magazine* and television shows made it look like the bad people of Kokomo ran Ryan White out of town. That just didn't happen," he told reporter Kate Conlon. In the same story, Western School Corporation superintendent J.O. Smith acknowledged having been interviewed for the film in 1987 but denied any concern about how the movie would tell the story. "I don't have any concerns about the movie," Smith remarked. The apprehension of residents who feared the worst about the TV movie must have deepened as the months went by and Ryan's visibility increased. In October, he was featured in "'I Have AIDS'—A Teenager's Story," a *3–2–1 Contact* Extra produced by Children's Television Workshop. The special aired as a preview of the series' seventh season and received national publicity. In late November, Ryan appeared on *The Phil Donahue Show* before an audience made up of New York and New Jersey junior high school students. Just as each appearance on national television served to fix the Kokomo-Cicero narrative into viewers' consciousness, each outing also caused hundreds of people to write to Ryan and his family. He became a national icon.[39]

From 1986 to 1990, Ryan received more than 2,000 letters from correspondents around the world. Most were positive in tone, and most of the writers were female. Many were out-and-out fan letters from high-school-aged girls, while others specifically mentioned his appearances in *People* and *Time* magazines or on *The Phil Donahue Show*. The volume of letters and cards spiked after each national media appearance, and even the people who wrote before the TV movie aired often referred to Ryan's treatment in Kokomo. One such writer, 21-year-old Ryan Atwell of Philadelphia, was moved to write to Ryan White after watching the *People* television special in 1988. Referring to the news footage of the concerned parents' meetings, Atwell wrote, "I was really hurt by the way the people of Kokomo at the school spoke about you. It was cruel and ignorant of them…. However, I did feel a great warmth for the reception of you by the people of Cicero." The people of Kokomo were very aware of the growing prevalence of sentiments like Atwell's. In December, the *Tribune* ran a story about the television movie's impending release, noting "it has already churned up old wounds from when [Ryan] lived at Kokomo." The piece quoted Jeanne White as maintaining that the finished product "doesn't portray them as bad as they really were. They were a lot worse than what the movie shows." Mayor Steve Daily, who declined to preview the movie, told the Associated Press that he was "sick to death of what this thing has done to the community."[40]

The narratives were thus well established by the time ABC aired its made-for-TV movie on Monday, January 16, 1989. As Mayor Daily's statement suggested, Kokomo residents were priming themselves to argue that *they* were the story's true victims—regular folks who found their community's reputation in tatters because of the news media. In her appearances at early screenings and benefit showings, Jeanne White repeated her contention that the movie had underplayed the prejudice that her family encountered in Kokomo. Ryan, too, emphasized the film's easy treatment of his former home: "The movie doesn't show the people of Kokomo to be as bad as they were. It was a lot worse than it is in the movie. Of course, you don't want to make anyone out to look downright awful." Current Kokomo mayor Robert Sargent told a magazine that he felt "terrible" about what happened to Ryan. "Two years later, Kokomo would have welcomed Ryan White." Sargent's assessment, that Ryan's opponents were merely uneducated and ill-informed about AIDS, hinted at another defense used by the pro–Kokomo forces: we should not blame people who acted out of ignorance and who were misinformed; rather, their lack of knowledge should make them less culpable in our eyes.[41]

More than 16 million people tuned into *The Ryan White Story* that Monday night. Reviews were mixed: *People*'s "Picks and Pans" review section panned the movie, which came in second place in that night's Nielsen ratings. The *New York Times* reviewer focused more on the story's content than on its quality:

> It is a story not only about ignorance but also about an almost total lack of enlightened community leadership in Kokomo. Residents are understandably concerned and frightened, but panic is allowed to take over. Petitions to keep Ryan out of school are signed not only by neighbors but also by the local police. A radio station broadcasts vicious bilge. The print and electronic press push for sensationalism. The Whites find a bullet hole in their living-room window. Ryan is systematically isolated and ostracized. It is not a pretty story. Worse, it is a story that didn't have to happen.

However the critics appraised the movie, average viewers were deeply affected by it. Mayor Sargent reported receiving angry telephone calls to his office from as far away as Arizona and New Hampshire: "They've been calling, giving us thunder," he told the *Tribune*. Locally, letters to the editor reflected feelings on all sides of the issue. The Campbell family from Muncie, Indiana, wrote to say that they would never relocate to such a place; Susan Sandberg from Lafayette, Indiana, opined that with the people of

Kokomo as "our representatives, Indiana looks like a state full of half-witted morons." Every writer from Kokomo, on the other hand, complained of the movie's one-sided depiction of the City of Firsts. "I do not understand why the people who were compassionate and tried to help the Whites were never mentioned," wrote Amy Royal, while Stacy Miller observed that "they only had bad things to say about Kokomo" and C. Main wondered why the movie didn't show "his mom taking [Ryan] out to roam the world" after he was barred from school.[42]

The reactions of those who had lived the story were equally mixed. Ron Colby told the *Tribune* that "if the purpose of the film was to portray Ryan, his family and his feelings, then I am sure it was accurate as they saw it.... The film captured the relentless pressure applied to all by the media." Western School Corporation officials J.O. Smith and Dan Carter refused to watch the movie at all: Smith told the paper that he had "things to do," while Carter was more cynical. "I know the meaning of the word 'fiction,'" he told the paper. The Whites' lawyer, Charles Vaughan, told *Tribune* reporter Dave Wiethop that while the movie was accurate, it was also "very good to Kokomo. It didn't bring up the 25–26 students who set up their own classroom in the school." David Rosselot was displeased, calling the drama "a subtle insult to the community as a whole simply because it left the impression that the community was anti–Ryan White when in the proper context it was not anti–Ryan White, but anti–AIDS in the classroom." Finally, Mitzie Johnson, one of the leaders of the concerned citizens group, panned the film: "I thought it would be a little more educational about AIDS. It was really kind of boring.... It got blown out of proportion and I kind of expected the movie to do that, too."[43]

Ryan received hundreds of letters after the TV movie aired. So did the cities of Cicero and Kokomo. Cicero officials forwarded some of them to Ryan with a letter that read in part, "the TV movie was excellent and we are very proud to have you here in Cicero." One of the letters addressed to Cicero simply said, "Bravo!" Gayle Schertenleib of Newman Lake, Washington, wrote "to personally thank the beautiful city of yours, for opening your mind and hearts to the Ryan White family.... I've never met anybody in my life that has had Aids [sic] but if I ever do, I'll be like you, and love, understand and do what I can for the person. Thank you again Cicero...." While Cicero basked in its good image, some Kokomo residents were so moved by the film's depiction of Ryan's mistreatment that they wrote to apologize. One such writer, Gary Morgan, shared that "I feel that people here in Kokomo were worse than ever imaginable. I am ashamed to admit that I even live here!" The Kokomo Chamber of Commerce and mayor's office also received letters from writers who expressed their disappointment at the treatment of Ryan depicted in the movie. An unsigned note from Madison, Wisconsin, read, "I can't believe how cruel and heartless the people of Kokomo have been to a sick child…. It will be a long time before people all over the United States will forgive Kokomo, Ind. Thank God for Cicero!"[44]

The number and tone of letters that the city of Kokomo received—at the *Tribune*, the Chamber of Commerce, and the mayor's office—prompted Mayor Sargent and City Attorney Ken Ferries to draft a 26-page response which they mailed to every correspondent. The lengthy missive refuted every single plot point in *The Ryan White Story* that Sargent, Ferries, and others considered factually inaccurate (such as the film's placement of Ryan's school in Kokomo, not Russiaville), and added positive anecdotes— omitted in the film—about the community's efforts to help the Whites. One recipient of the 26-page letter, though, remained unconvinced of Kokomo's innocence. Joan Strouse Shropshire of Indianapolis answered Ferries' reply to her letter with another letter of her own, quoting Edmund Burke: "The only thing necessary for the triumph of evil is for good men to do nothing," Shropshire wrote. "Most assuredly there are good men in Kokomo, Indiana," she added. "But just not quite enough of them when needed, perhaps?"[45]

Just as the community had ostracized Ryan White, now Kokomo was experiencing its own stigmatization. Like the *People* magazine readers, viewers of the television movie looked at Kokomo and decided they did not want to be like those people in that city. Kokomo offered them a way to define themselves in a positive manner, as "not that"—not intolerant, not cruel, not ignorant. Writers to Ryan White commented regularly on the cruelty he endured in Kokomo, and so many regularly used that exact word: cruelty. Just as Ryan had deviated from norms dictating how the sick "should" behave, the people of Kokomo had deviated from normative expectations of how a true community should behave when faced with a sick child, and by doing so, they confirmed the beliefs and hopes of many others that, surely, their *own* communities would not have treated Ryan in that way. Goffman's analysis of stigmatization is just as applicable to a city as it is to human beings. In the wake of the TV movie, we see in the vitriolic letters to the *Tribune* about the Whites' conduct, in the bitter complaints about the unfairness of selective reporting, and in the defensive 26-page letter sent in response to every critical letter the city received, nothing less than a reaction to stigmatization. According to Angelo A. Alonzo and Nancy R. Reynolds, a sociologist and nurse who wrote of HIV and stigma, "stigmatized groups" can develop "stigma theories and 'sad tales'" to "correct misinformation and its consequences in terms of fear, prejudice and discrimination." Statements such as "We didn't know enough about AIDS when Ryan White lived here," or complaints about an overly generalized depiction of the entire city as ignorant and biased, operate as "ideological defenses" or "strategies to avoid or minimize discrediting social attributions."[46]

Another argument that residents of Kokomo used to defend themselves against their city's depiction in the media was that Ryan White and his family were being "used" by powerful outside forces to further a larger agenda. John Wiles, former editor of the *Kokomo Tribune*, believed that "it became orchestrated and I think why it did was Ryan was used as the poster boy. And Reagan wasn't funding AIDS research because, again, it was looked at as a homosexual disease. And people saw this as an opportunity to get research money by showing that, you know, it affects other people too." Pointing to celebrities like Elton John and Michael Jackson, Wiles said, "look at their backgrounds, and you understand why. They were funding this. And then the movie came out and it was ridiculous." Wiles was not the only one who believed that Ryan's rise to prominence, and the accompanying impression of Kokomo as intolerant and Cicero as desirable, were part of a concerted effort to gain attention and funding for AIDS. David Whitman, a commentator writing in *U.S. News & World Report*, lent credence to such beliefs. "The truth is that children, and not just Ryan White, are often used by politicians, advocates and the media to make horrors publicly palatable." Homeless children, Whitman wrote, were profiled more often than homeless alcoholics and drug addicts, even though, he maintained, the former were much rarer than the latter. Race also entered the equation: political scientist Cathy Cohen has noted that although black and Latino children comprised the majority of pediatric AIDS patients, white children such as Ryan White and the Ray brothers dominated the evening news' coverage of children with AIDS between 1981 and 1993. If celebrities and the media had manipulated the Whites and victimized Kokomo in order to score political and social points, as Wiles maintained, it would not have been the first time that the innocent image of a child was put to such use. Nor would it be the last. In fact, when Congress enacted a large funding package to assist people with AIDS, it was named the Ryan White CARE Act. AIDS would thereafter be both bureaucratically and financially associated with a white youth who had contracted it blamelessly, via contaminated blood—not a child of color, and not a man who engaged in gay sex.[47]

Whatever the motivations of journalists, photographers, Hollywood scriptwriters, and celebrity fundraisers may have been, the people of Kokomo felt damaged by media portraits of their community. As Alonzo and Reynolds would have characterized it, the community told "sad tales." Many believed the city was the victim of the story, not its villain. "But it was an interesting time," Jeri Malone of the Howard County

Health Department reflected. "It was always ... in some ways uncomfortable because our community was a victim." Ken Ferries, the city attorney, believed that the outside world saw Kokomo as "this very backwards community of self-satisfied, sanctimonious burghers living in the middle of the soybean belt, and I think that's the image we have." Ferries believed that image would endure for a long time.[48]

After the television movie, Ryan's profile as a national speaker only increased. Because he often appeared alongside Jill Stewart, the class president who had helped to welcome him, his story was necessarily one of contrasts between then and now, between Kokomo and Cicero. Although Ryan continued to attend high-profile events like the Emmy Awards in September of 1989 (his *3–2–1 Contact* episode had been nominated for an award), his health was declining. Even as he recorded public service announcements about AIDS, he endured staph infections in his eyes and legs, an inoperable hernia and painful swelling, and hospitalizations. Dr. Kleiman cleared him to return to school in February of 1990, and he managed to attend a few events in California in March before returning to Riley Children's Hospital in Indianapolis with a severe respiratory infection in late March. By April 1, he was in critical condition and on life support.[49]

Elton John, who happened to be in Indianapolis for the Farm Aid IV concert, rushed to Ryan's bedside and stayed with Jeanne the entire time, except for when he performed "Candle in the Wind" at the concert and dedicated it to Ryan as 45,000 people sang along. Callers anxious to learn the latest on Ryan's status quickly overwhelmed the Riley Hospital switchboard. To handle the calls, Sprint installed a national hotline at Riley, with the number (800) 733-RYAN. Hospital officials reported receiving calls at the rate of one every seven seconds; others counted 5,000 a day. President George H.W. Bush, in the city for other reasons, planted a White House elm in downtown Indianapolis and dedicated it to Ryan. In Washington, D.C., as a Senate committee voted unanimously for a bill that would provide $1.2 billion over two years to fight AIDS, Senator Edward Kennedy (D-MA) said, "This one's for you, Ryan." And the people of Kokomo once again found themselves under the scrutiny of the national media as reporters reminded everyone of Ryan's story. The *Chicago Tribune* ran a story on April 5 headlined "Ryan White's Old Town Fights 'Rap,'" while *USA Today* chose "Even Kokomo is Grieving" for its headline. "I'm sad to hear it," David Rosselot told *USA Today* of his reaction to Ryan's grim condition.[50]

Ryan died on Palm Sunday, April 8, 1990, at the age of 18. The next day, Kokomo and Howard County officials lowered flags to half-staff at city and county buildings in Ryan's memory, as did Western School Corporation and Hamilton Heights High School officials. Underneath the symbolic honors, however, emotions simmered. Paula Adair, the teachers' association president when Ryan was barred from school at Western, told the *Kokomo Tribune* "there was never any hostility toward Ryan or his family by the school corporation" and called his death "devastating." Adair went on to blame the media for scapegoating Western "for the actions of a small group of people" and singled out *People* magazine for publishing articles she termed "exploitive." Hostile letters again poured into the city's mayoral, newspaper, and Chamber of Commerce offices. Pamela Palmer, of Honeoye Falls, New York, asked the people of Kokomo, "Are you happy now? The festering Philistinism displayed by our homophobic citizenry proves that your town is more deeply diseased than Ryan White ever was. May his specter sear your consciences forever, if indeed you possess consciences. Your neighbors in Cicero put you to shame." A sympathy card sent by Patricia Bartlett from North Bay, California, contained the note, "In reflection of your bigotry, hate, and ignorance/We wish you of Kokomo a speedy recovery."[51]

Western Middle School also received much angry mail immediately after Ryan died. Betty Mosteller of Endicott, New York, sent Western Middle School a greeting card: on the outside, it featured a picture of a medal and read, "You Deserve a Medal!" On the inside, Mosteller added her own sentiments: "Put this on your bulletin board. I certainly hope you all are very proud of yourselves for the way you treated Ryan White and the heartaches he and his family had to endure. Thank God, I don't live in your town. Maybe you can all kid yourselves that you did right—at least that way maybe you can sleep nights!" Dozens of other correspondents expressed similar disgust, outrage, and disappointment.[52]

Jeanne and Andrea White, meanwhile, received thousands of cards, notes, and letters. Even then, many of the condolences specifically mentioned Kokomo. Laura Cheng of Atlanta, Georgia, wrote of "a town [that] will forever be scorned." And Michael E. Sharkey of Sharpsville, Indiana, wrote of his remorse at not speaking out on behalf of Ryan when he had the chance:

> During Ryan's years in Kokomo, (after he became afflicted with AIDS) occasionally I would see him in town. One particular incident was when your family was having dinner at RAX. People were whispering and it was obvious. But on the outside it didn't bother Ryan. The whispers continued, but Ryan was still all smiles. I wish at that time I would of had the courage to stand up to those people. I wish I would of walked over to Ryan to shake his hand and tell him how proud I was to meet him. I'm very sorry I did not do this. I am embarrassed for the city of Kokomo. I feel the community was so cruel to your family. I apologize for our ignorance and hope that thanks to Ryan's work and dedication that no one will ever have to go through this discrimination again.

Sharkey's heartfelt letter was written on the same day that mourners jammed traffic in Carmel, Indiana, outside a funeral home where Ryan's body lay for viewing. The next day, April 11, CNN broadcast Ryan's funeral service live from Second Presbyterian Church in Indianapolis, where more than 1,500 people attended, including First Lady Barbara Bush. The nation had become transfixed by Ryan White's story—but that story was not finished yet.[53]

7

Blood, Steel
and Ryan White

Erasure and Visibility,
1990–2020

Americans would keep Ryan White in their collective gaze for months and even years following his death. His life story took on new meaning in the 1990s and 2000s, and ultimately signified courage, hope, and resilience to later generations. His mother Jeanne would become the chief architect of this legacy, and she endeavored to cast the events of the 1980s in as positive a light as possible, rarely mentioning Kokomo by name. She played an instrumental role in the permanent memorialization of her son at a major museum and lobbied in Congress for AIDS funding in his honor. But in Kokomo, the answers to the question "What next?" did not come as easily. With an empty, contaminated steel mill and acres of spoiled land on their hands, residents struggled with questions of erasure and memory. How best to deal with such an equivocal legacy?

In the events recounted in this chapter, the element of blood becomes associated with visibility, while the element of steel is linked with erasure. Just when gays began to hit their collective stride with respect to AIDS activism in the late 1980s, in the 1990s—in marked contrast to earlier decades—people with hemophilia also no longer hid their condition, went underground, or tried to "pass" as "normal." Instead, they emerged purposefully, to confront not only the NHF, but also blood shield laws, the federal government, and the blood products industry. At the same time, Jeanne White's efforts after Ryan's death immortalized her son and guaranteed he would always be visible on some level as a positive force for change, despite his former community's ambivalence about formally acknowledging his impact. And in Kokomo, as in other cities affected by deindustrialization and the environmental ruin often left in its wake, neighbors witnessed the systematic dismantling and literal erasure of the steel mill from the landscape.

Ryan's funeral—an event worthy of his international celebrity— would not be the last heart-wrenching tribute to his life. The cover of the April 23, 1990, issue of *People* magazine featured a full-color photo of Ryan in California, taken two weeks before his death, with an inset showing Jeanne and Elton John keeping a vigil at his bedside. Inside, Publisher Elizabeth P. Valk briefly recounted the magazine's relation- ship with the Whites and told readers about the powerful emotions that writer Bill Shaw and photographer Taro Yamasaki experienced as they documented the vigil at Riley Hospital. Shaw's cover story, titled "Can- dle in the Wind" after Elton John's song of the same name, promised readers the "moving, untold story of the final hours of Ryan White, the boy whose battle with AIDS touched America's heart." The article gen- erated a record number of letters to the editor—more than 800 cards, poems, and letters featuring "touching personal accounts of relatives or friends battling AIDS," according to the magazine's May 14, 1990, "Mail" section. The tone of the letters was overwhelmingly reverential. "Silently and carefully I read the story of Ryan White's passage from this world," wrote Angela Kristine Klindworth of Monticello, Minnesota. Of Jeanne, Jo Starr of Philadelphia wrote, "She has truly humbled me with her strength and guts. I guess I know where Ryan got his." Lauri Johnson of Garden Grove, California, shared, "Never have I been so emotionally shaken as by Bill Shaw's tender and dignified account of Ryan's last days of life." And Contessa Shade of North Hollywood, California, told the magazine: "In all the years I've been reading *People*, your article on Ryan White was by far the most important and meaningful story you have ever published."[1]

The magazine did publish one letter from a resident of Kokomo, Lau- ren Leep. Leep expressed her frustration at Kokomo's national reputation for intolerance, her pride in knowing her community had played a part in America's growing understanding of AIDS, and her admiration of Ryan. Leep also offered a positive spin on Ryan's time in Kokomo:

> While most in Kokomo don't ... excuse ... those who persecuted the Whites, we do ask that Americans remember the alarmist mentality that pervaded our country ... in 1985. Ironically, it was largely because of Ryan's ordeal in Kokomo that Americans stopped, took a deep breath and listened [to] the facts ... about AIDS.

Leep's interpretation provided a way for residents of Kokomo to admit their wrongdoing and save face at the same time, and it would echo throughout the ensuing decades. For Jeanne White, however, Kokomo was long gone.

Rather than dwelling on past events, she spent the weeks after Ryan's death looking ahead—to Washington, D.C., and Congress.[2]

Less than two weeks after Ryan's funeral, Jeanne White strode into the U.S. Capitol in a pair of white tennis shoes and fulfilled a promise she had made to Senators Edward Kennedy (D-MA) and Orrin Hatch (R-UT) as her son lay on his deathbed: she lobbied every Senator who would talk with her for passage of the $600 million bill (co-sponsored by Hatch and Kennedy) to provide funds for fighting AIDS. Half of the money would go to states for the care of people with AIDS, and the other half to the 13 cities hardest hit by the disease. Republican Senator Jesse Helms of North Carolina, one of the most virulently anti-gay lawmakers of the 1980s and 1990s, refused to meet with her—but most of his colleagues did, and 61 Senators agreed to co-sponsor the Ryan White CARE (Comprehensive AIDS Resource Emergency) Act. It took weeks of effort by activists to get enough votes to overcome Helms' stalling tactics. Finally, on May 15, 1990, the body voted to end the delay and schedule a vote on the merits. Helms objected, saying, "Little Ryan White was not an intravenous drug user, nor was he a promiscuous homosexual.... The tragedy of Ryan White is being exploited to promote a political agenda of the homosexual community." Jeanne, who had sat in the gallery and observed the voice vote on the Senate floor below her, later told a reporter that "Ryan didn't feel like that at all.... Ryan always felt that he did not blame anybody, so why should you[?]"[3]

In fact, Ryan's story had helped to turn the tide in favor of the legislation. Congressman John Lewis of Georgia and others specifically mentioned Ryan's influence. "In recent days, the life and death of Ryan White brought [AIDS] home to many, many people," Lewis told a reporter. Conservatives like Hatch and Indiana Republican Senator Dan Coats found Ryan's story to be useful political cover for their votes to fund the bill. Instead of supporting IV drug users and men who had sex with men, as Helms' rhetoric suggested, they were supporting "innocent" sufferers of AIDS like Ryan and voting for legislation to help overwhelmed hospitals treat the sick. The Senate approved the Ryan White CARE Act on August 5, and President George H.W. Bush signed the bill later that month.[4]

Ryan's story remained a fixture in public conversation well into the 1990s. The popular media did their part by showing reruns of the television movie, by covering posthumous honors awarded to Ryan, by including his death in year-end stories, and by running retrospectives on the anniversaries of his death. But the Whites were not the only family who had lost a loved one to contaminated Factor VIII, and those with hemophilia—and their families—who had been so silent in the 1980s would not stay underground in the 1990s. A newfound activism had awakened within that community, and along with it came demands for justice. By 1993, the process of holding the government and the blood products industry accountable for the widespread transmission of HIV to people with hemophilia had begun.

Blood

The DePrince family exemplified the growing activism and visibility of people with hemophilia. The biological parents of one son with the bleeding disorder known as Von Willebrand disease and another with hemophilia, they had adopted two more boys with hemophilia and were thus on the front lines of the AIDS epidemic in the 1980s and 1990s. Elaine DePrince did not hide her sons' condition—she herself also lived with Von Wille-brand disease—and she even went so far as to hold a blood drive in one son's name to accumulate credit toward the family's "clotting-factor costs" in the early 1980s. Neighbors were glad to help and eagerly participated in the drive—but, once the DePrince boys were diagnosed with HIV and AIDS, those neighbors turned on them. The DePrince family found their three-month-old puppy and their pet rabbits poisoned, the rabbit hutch damaged with an axe, their mail stolen, torn open, and then returned, their cars vandalized, and more. One former playmate's father shouted at little Cubby DePrince, "Go away, get out of here!" when he tried to ask his son out to play. Both Cubby and his brother Michael succumbed to AIDS, and the DePrinces, like so many other families, filed a lawsuit against the blood industry. The Whites had also pursued this tactic in the 1980s but had come up against the "blood shield laws" and saw their case tossed from court. Yet by the early 1990s, a sea change had occurred with respect to the way the courts viewed these cases.[5]

In July 1993, in response to congressional calls for investigation, U.S. Department of Health and Human Services Secretary Donna E. Sha-lala commissioned the prestigious Institute of Medicine (a division of the National Academy of Sciences) to investigate the widespread infection of hemophilia patients with HIV between 1982 and 1984. The study's time frame reflected scientists' belief that more than 50 percent of infections in those with severe hemophilia had occurred *before* 1985. Investigators would focus on what the blood products companies knew and when they knew it, as well as on what government officials knew, and when—and on whether both sectors had responded adequately to the threat to the nation's blood supply. Shalala also commissioned the investigators to make recommenda-tions based on their findings.[6]

In September of that same year, Jonathan Wadleigh and more than 20 other named plaintiffs (all either hemophilia patients with HIV or sur-viving family members of people with hemophilia who had died from

AIDS) filed a federal class action lawsuit against four large "fractionators," the industrial laboratories that separated blood plasma into clotting factor proteins—Rhone-Poulenc Rorer, Inc./Armour Pharmaceutical Co.; Miles, Inc. (which changed its name to Bayer in 1995); Baxter Healthcare Corporation; and Alpha Therapeutic Corporation—and against the National Hemophilia Foundation (NHF), resulting in *Wadleigh et al. v. Rhone-Poulenc Rorer et al.* The allegations were damning: in their complaint, plaintiffs accused the blood processors of knowing that viruses caused deadly diseases and that blood products were vectors for those viruses—witness the spread of hepatitis in the 1970s—and of negligently failing to take steps, such as heat treatment, that would have prevented the transmission of viruses. Had the firms used heat treatment (which was feasible in the late 1970s and was *de rigueur* in Germany) to kill the hepatitis virus, they argued, such measures would have also prevented HIV's spread in the blood products. The plaintiffs also alleged that the blood firms acted negligently once they became aware of HIV by continuing to pay donors for their plasma (a practice which they knew was likely to attract financially desperate individuals such as IV drug users), by failing to screen donors adequately, and by failing to warn people with hemophilia and their doctors about the true extent to which using Factor endangered their lives. As for the NHF, the plaintiffs accused that group of passing along the blood processors' assurances of safety to hemophilia patients and their families while under the influence of the same firms' significant monetary donations. The complaint formally charged the fractionators with negligence, strict product liability, breach of implied warranty, and conspiracy; the NHF faced charges of negligence and breach of fiduciary duty.[7]

As serious as those allegations were, what likely caused the blood products industry the most concern was the request from Wadleigh and his fellow plaintiffs to be certified as a class. The specter of mass-tort litigation—the plaintiffs estimated that easily half of the nation's 20,000 people with hemophilia were already infected with HIV and could potentially qualify for inclusion in a class action lawsuit if Wadleigh prevailed, along with the roughly 2,000 who had already died—might drive the companies out of the blood products business altogether. Indeed, at the time Wadleigh filed his suit in September, there were at least 300 other class action lawsuits pending in federal and state courts against the blood processors across the U.S.; the federal panel on multi-district litigation ordered the federal cases consolidated into the Northern District of Illinois, where Judge John F. Grady heard the pretrial motions. If Judge Grady allowed the plaintiffs to be certified as a class, the stakes would get very high very quickly. In 1994, Grady did certify the class, but only with respect to two questions: whether the blood processors had been negligent, and whether the NHF

had breached a fiduciary duty to its members. The blood companies immediately appealed to the Seventh Circuit Court of Appeals in Chicago, which
ordered the decertification of the class in 1995—in other words, there
would be hundreds of separate trials in federal courts—a victory of sorts
for the defendants, to be sure. But the blood products industry had seen
and heard enough during the nearly two years of arguments, motions, and
rulings to become motivated to find a way out of the legal thicket. In its
SEC Form 10-Q filing for the first quarter of 1996, Rhone-Poulenc disclosed
that it was named in some 450 pending lawsuits in the U.S., Canada, and
Ireland alone, related to Armour's blood products.[8]

Even in Indiana, the tide had turned against the blood products industry. In a state court lawsuit brought by the parents of a minor child who
had died of AIDS as a result of treatments with a tainted clotting factor,
the Indiana Court of Appeals found that the state's blood shield law did not
apply to the blood processors—the judges held that the clotting factor was a
product, not a service, and thus was subject to products liability laws. This
legal opinion signaled a dramatic change from the decision rendered by the
federal district court in 1985 against the Whites, wherein Charles Vaughan
had been stymied by the same blood shield law. Within the span of just
11 years—a relatively short time in jurisprudential terms—two courts had
read the same statute and come to very different conclusions. Rulings such
as these finally opened the courts to people with hemophilia and provided
them with a remedy for the events of the 1980s—and exposed the blood
processors to a threat that, just a decade earlier, had seemed inconceivable.
The blood shield laws, which protected corporate interests instead of individual health and lives, had been designed to insulate the blood products
industry from this very problem. This calculus had made economic sense
to lawmakers in the 1960s when legislatures around the country had passed
those laws, but in the decades afterward, when people with hemophilia
and transfusion recipients alike contracted hepatitis and then HIV, the ful-
crum had undeniably shifted. It could be argued that, in reading the blood
shield laws less sympathetically, courts in the 1990s had begun to weigh
individual pain and suffering more heavily than corporate viability when
balancing capital interests. As historian Keith Wailoo has noted in *Pain: A
Political History*, courts have often served as "the site of conflict and resolution" for questions of whose pain is more legitimate. In both Queens and
Kokomo/Russiaville in 1985–1986, when parents sued to stop students with
AIDS from attending school, and then later in the 1990s with the tort cases
against blood products manufacturers, the role of courts in both situations
involved, as Wailoo puts it, "how to measure distress and how to define the
right to relief." In our culture, Americans almost instinctively turn to courts
for legitimization, redress, and valuation of their grievances—regardless of

whether the courts are in fact a "good fit" for every social or personal problem. Legal scholars such as David Ray Papke have cast the trial as "the most important ritual of the legal faith"—that faith being our national belief in the rule of law that is "central to our ideology ... our sense of ourselves as a people ... our culture as a whole." The increasing willingness of people with hemophilia to "out" themselves as people with AIDS, combined with a cultural belief in the courts' inherent fairness, impelled them to choose lawsuits as their means of redress.[9]

In addition to financial concerns, the blood processors also had to consider penal consequences for their missteps. Blood company executives had only to look to France in the 1990s, where judges sent Drs. Michel Garretta and Jean-Pierre Allain of the National Blood Transfusion Center to prison for dispensing tainted clotting factor in the 1980s. Industry insiders also kept an eye on the dramatic events in Japan. In 1996, after trials in Osaka and Tokyo had dragged on for years, the country's new health minister, Naoto Kan, ordered the release of all government documents pertaining to the AIDS crisis, apologized in person to two hundred plaintiffs and their families, and accepted responsibility on behalf of the government. Kan's actions helped spur the blood processors to settle the Japanese lawsuits; the settlement was announced in a televised news conference, during which executives (including Wolfgang Plischke, president of Bayer, and Bob Hurley, president of Baxter's Japanese affiliate) made statements and bowed before the plaintiffs to convey their shame. Takehiko Kawano, the president of Green Cross, the largest supplier of clotting factor to Japan's hemophilia patients, displayed his abject contrition to a distraught mother of an AIDS victim by walking up to her, getting down on "his hands and knees, and bowing so deeply that his forehead touched the floor." Later in 1996, Dr. Takeshi Abe, vice-president of Teikyo University, renowned expert on hemophilia, and respected leader of Japan's blue-ribbon AIDS panel, went to jail for his own actions in 1983: he had helped delay his government's approval of Baxter's heat-treated, pasteurized clotting factor so that Green Cross could "catch up" with its own version, which did not happen until 1985. Abe's delay had resulted in the needless infection of more than 1,000 Japanese with HIV. Abe was joined in confinement by three executives of Green Cross, the company that had continued to sell its non-heat-treated, contaminated products on into 1987 rather than pulling them from distribution.[10]

Back in the United States, the Institute of Medicine released its report in 1995, as hundreds of lawsuits were still pending. The experts concluded that the events of the 1980s had "revealed an important weakness in the system—its ability to deal with a new threat that was characterized by substantial uncertainty." Aware that scientists knew much more in the mid–1990s than they had in the early 1980s, the authors took a considered tone: they grouped their conclusions under such measured headings as "Decision-making Under Uncertainty," "Bureaucratic Management of Potential Crises," and "Presumptive Regulatory and Public Health Triggers." But the report, titled *HIV and the Blood Supply: An Analysis of Crisis Decision-making*, contained no fewer than 14 solid recommendations for avoiding a repeat of the catastrophe—and its contents would doubtless have played a role in the litigation against the blood processors.[11]

The growing militancy of individual hemophilia patients and their families placed pressure on the blood products industry—and on the NHF. At the Foundation's annual meeting in October 1993—coincidentally taking place in Indianapolis, just a short drive from Cicero where Jeanne White still lived—the battle lines were drawn. According to writer Douglas Starr's account in *Blood: An Epic History of Medicine and Commerce*, the mood was adversarial; panels from the AIDS Memorial Quilt hung in breakout rooms, and representatives from the blood processors uncharacteristically stayed away. The Foundation had attempted to negotiate a compensation package for the patients and families affected by HIV, but those in attendance would have no part of that offer, because they found it "insultingly low." Children sat in hallways making posters; one read, "I was betrayed by the NHF." The audience at a "town meeting" about the proposed financial settlement proved unreceptive to the idea of compromise. One member announced a class action lawsuit, while others questioned the NHF's silence during the early years of the AIDS pandemic. An observer witnessed Jeanne White stand up and tell the audience that "she received no support from the Foundation—'no support at all' when the school district so ignorantly castigated her son."[12]

Even as late as 1995, financial assistance for AIDS patients was not guaranteed—lawsuits are slow, adversarial processes, and compensation could take years to arrive if the plaintiffs won, because the defendants would surely appeal. Congress had funded medical and social programs at least since the passage of the Ryan White CARE Act in 1990, but that process was usually subject to much debate—funding was never a foregone conclusion. Senator Jesse Helms led a drive, in late June 1995, to cut federal funds for AIDS programs, blaming the sufferers' "deliberate, disgusting, revolting conduct" for their infections. President Bill Clinton spoke out against the move to cut financing in a speech at Georgetown University on July 5, and at least one letter to the editor of the *New York Times* cited Ryan White in rebuttal to Helms's position: "Does the Senator not know that Ryan White contracted AIDS through a blood transfusion, as did Arthur Ashe?" wrote Jim Smith of Staten Island. Five years after his death, Ryan's was still the name many Americans automatically equated with the "innocent victims" of the disease. He was easily as much a celebrity as the professional tennis star Ashe, the only black man to win Wimbledon, the U.S. Open, and the Australian Open (Ashe had died in 1993).[13]

In 1995, Senator Mike DeWine (R-OH) and Representative Porter Goss (R-FL) introduced the Ricky Ray Hemophilia Relief Fund Act, which aimed to create a government trust fund to compensate people with HIV who had contracted the disease as a result of using contaminated clotting factor between July 1, 1982, and December 31, 1987. Under the legislation, each infected person (or a designated survivor) would receive a one-time "compassionate assistance" payment of $100,000. On November 12, 1998, President Bill Clinton signed the bill into law in a ceremony at the National Hemophilia Foundation's annual meeting in Orlando. With all of these considerations—pending federal legislation to compensate victims, hundreds of lawsuits, executives and doctors incarcerated in France and Japan, increasing rage on the part of those with hemophilia and their families—in play, the four defendants in *Wadleigh v. Rhone-Poulenc* tendered an offer in April 1996 to settle the claim of every single person with hemophilia who had become infected with HIV due to their products—as well as the claims of those who became infected by the users of the products. The defendants paid according to their market share: Bayer 45 percent, Alpha 15 percent, Rhone-Poulenc/Armour, 20 percent, and Baxter, 20 percent. Each infected person would receive $100,000; in cases such as Ryan's where patients had not survived, decedents' immediate family members received the settlement.[14]

The conclusion of the lawsuits did not necessarily provide satisfaction, however, for those family members. In her memoir, *Cry Bloody Murder*, Elaine DePrince recounted her efforts in 1995 and 1996 to lobby for the passage of a "Hemophilia Justice Act" in New Jersey, which would alter the statute of limitations for suits against blood products manufacturers, and remarked that blood shield statutes were still on the books in 47 states. (Indiana's law can still be found at Ind. Code 16–41–12–11.) Along with changes to the laws, DePrince, who penned her book in 1997, wanted "closure. Some entity must accept responsibility and apologize." Perhaps, however, in the wake of a painful social tragedy, what is needed is catharsis as well as closure. Our nation's legal apparatus—the enactment of laws and the mounting of trials—was designed more for certainty than for catharsis: when the settlement checks are written and cashed, the courts' job is done. But victims' and survivors' definitions of "justice" and "success" include an emotional reckoning, something courts cannot provide.[15]

Although AIDS patients (or their survivors) would see no further recompense, the federal government has continued to fund AIDS programs well into the twenty-first century via the Ryan White CARE Act. The law has helped all AIDS patients—not just those who had contracted the disease due to their hemophilia. In October 2009, President Barack Obama signed a reauthorization of the legislation and announced that the U.S. would lift its 22-year travel and immigration ban on people with HIV in early 2010. For people with hemophilia, the risk of infection with AIDS from clotting factor finally ended with heat treatment and pasteurization; since the 1990s, patients have had the additional option of using factor made from recombinant DNA, which is also safe. The government stopped making payments under the Ricky Ray Hemophilia Relief Fund Act in November 2003. On paper, the crisis for those affected by hemophilia and HIV was officially over in 2003; but the bitterness and mistrust would linger.[16]

Steel

Mistrust of government officials also hung in the air in Kokomo. In the summer of 1990, residents questioned the safety of the shuttered Continental Steel site. Workers from the EPA had recently concluded three weeks' worth of "investigation, sampling, and emergency response" at the campus, and had pronounced it safe. "Safe," in this context, meant that no *immediate* threats remained; authorities believed they had been able to contain or remove anything that was mobile. "Safe" did not mean, however, that the public should be on site. "As you are aware," EPA official Karen Martin commented to a reporter for the *Kokomo Tribune*, "there is much work left to be done by both EPA and IDEM, and the site is not considered safe for the public to enter and tour." Martin's assessment was correct. Workers from both the state and federal environmental agencies would be occupied for more than a decade handling what remained of the mill.[17]

Throughout the 1990s and into the 2000s, environmental workers operated under a continuous mist of water in order to reduce dust at the sprawling Continental cleanup site. They removed lead, PCBs, asbestos, and other contaminants by excavating and draining the underground chemical and fuel storage tanks, draining contaminated sediments, and burying some of the toxins in a landfill. They hauled other toxins off site, and filled, covered, and fenced off what remained. Between 1990 and 1994, the EPA removed 2,450 buried drums; 1,250 cubic yards of contaminated soil; 90 cubic yards of lead dust; 121 cubic yards of PCBs; 2,284 tons of solidified soil; more than 200 chemicals from an abandoned metallurgical laboratory, and a reported 65,647 gallons of No. 6 bunker oil. In 2006, IDEM removed twelve underground storage tanks and their wastes, as well as 676 cubic yards of buried material containing asbestos. Even as late as 2007, after millions of dollars and years' worth of effort, workers still found surprises: contractors dredging the Kokomo and Wildcat creeks that summer and fall found nearly *double* the contaminated material they had anticipated. (Authorities had expected to find 8,000 cubic yards; 30 cubic yards fills one dump truck.) In addition, at the Kokomo Creek site, workers encountered a completely new area full of crushed drums, something no one had anticipated. And from the quarry near Chris MacNeil's former home, workers had, by October 2008, removed 17,494 cubic yards (27,990 tons) of contaminated sediments. All of this was necessary because the EPA estimated that more than 1,600 people obtained their drinking water from private wells within just three miles of the site.[18]

The buildings on the Continental campus were dismantled beginning in 1999, but first to go was the iconic sign that faced Markland Avenue. The sign was removed as part of a ceremony documented by photographer Joel David Butler, whose haunting photos of the abandoned structure before its demolition in the 1990s have since been added to the Howard County Historical Society's web catalog. Some in Kokomo expressed resentment over the buildings' removal: government agencies had contracted with a New York firm to dismantle the structures, and so very few local citizens were employed as a result.[19]

While the agencies' goal was to ensure that no trace of the mill—or its pollutants—remained, the Howard County Historical Society wanted to create a strong archival record of Continental's presence. To that end, in 2009 Society volunteers spent nearly 4,000 hours taking oral histories from former Continental employees, both salaried and hourly workers. On the evening of October 20, 2009, 300 former employees gathered at a banquet at the Continental Ballroom, just west of the old mill's campus on Markland Avenue, to celebrate the project, watch a slideshow featuring photos and portions of the histories, and reminisce. All of the infighting and resentment between labor and management seemed to have vanished; all that remained was camaraderie and a shared sense of loss. Any rancor that remained was directed at Penn-Dixie and Jerome Castle, not at the union or management, and not at the community. "At its height the mill operated as an extended family. Before it fell apart there was a golden time when people worked as much for each other as for a paycheck," wrote a reporter for the *Kokomo Tribune* on the gathering. The article contained several sentimental anecdotes shared by the former workers, including one by L.E. Smith, whose father had been chief engineer at the mill for over three decades. "We lived about a mile from the plant," Smith recounted. "I remember, in the middle of the night sometimes my Dad would wake up and say, 'Something's wrong at the mill. It doesn't sound right.' And he'd get up, get dressed and go down there," Smith said. Just as a parent knows when a child's cry indicates something wrong, so Smith's father knew by the mill's sound when there was a malfunction. When Continental closed, Kokomo lost more than an economic mainstay; it lost a part of its community.[20]

Many cities shared Kokomo's problem: what to do with former factory sites in the wake of deindustrialization? Because of their toxic remains, the best many could hope for entailed a transition from Superfund site to brownfield—a place not quite habitable, but not completely desolate, either. The fate of the campus was partially settled in 2011, when the city announced plans for a 60-acre soccer complex on the site of the old acid lagoons near the Wildcat Creek. The Wildcat Creek Soccer Complex houses nearly 30 fields built on a two-foot-thick layer of clean soil the EPA deposited over the lagoons after workers excavated and graded the area. Because the "soil cap" cannot be disturbed, it would not be practical to build any permanent structure that required a foundation in that spot, so athletic fields fit well within the site's restrictions. The sports park sits adjacent to the Parks and Recreation Department's Wildcat Creek Walk of Excellence, a mixed-use trail that unites several city parks and ties together significant locations in the city's history. The Walk of Excellence in turn intersects with Kokomo's Industrial Heritage trail to the east, a rail-to-trail project that follows the path of a rail line that formerly supplied the city's largest manufacturers, including Continental Steel. The installation of a large solar farm in another vast stretch of empty space on the former Continental site attests to the city's ongoing efforts to restore some economic viability to the premises.[21]

The process of remaking the former Continental space will continue, even though environmental damage prevents the erection of permanent buildings onsite. At present, nothing tangible marks the space to hint at its former glory. Continental's history is invisible, its legacy ambiguous. But some 30 miles to the south, in Indianapolis, a very different situation exists with respect to Ryan White. There, thanks to his mother, a thoroughly memorialized, destigmatized narrative of Ryan's life and struggle to attend school awaits visitors to the Children's Museum of Indianapolis.

Ryan White

In the months immediately after Ryan's death, Jeanne White, on leave from her job at Delco, immersed herself in activism. In addition to her lobbying efforts on behalf of the Ryan White CARE Act, she accompanied *People* writer Bill Shaw to the White House Correspondents' Dinner in the spring of 1990. In June, she received a standing ovation at the National PTA Convention in Indianapolis. She then flew to Los Angeles to speak on AIDS education. When she was home, Jeanne drove Andrea to roller skating meets and worked on finishing Ryan's autobiography, begun while he was still alive.[22]

Throughout 1990 and into 1991, the repeated commemorations and invocations of Ryan and his legacy must have seemed relentless to the Whites. In September, officials presented the first Norman Vincent Peale Positive Thinker Awards to former President Ronald Reagan, to a Mississippi nun, Sister Anne Brooks, and to Ryan. The defacement of Ryan's Cicero gravesite that same month made news not only in Indianapolis and Kokomo, but also in *USA Today*. In Brooklyn, when parents threatened protests and school boycotts in response to an 11-year-old boy's disclosure that he had contracted HIV in a blood transfusion during a heart transplant, his mother commented, "It's like they are still back in the Ryan White era." As Jeanne and Andrea faced their first Christmas without Ryan, the Indianapolis Colts honored him with ceremonies at their December 22 game. *USA Today* remembered Ryan in its "Passages 1990" feature later that month, and *People* devoted four paragraphs to Ryan, his mother, and his sister in the magazine's annual "Sequels" section. The *Indianapolis Star* named Ryan its "Man of the Year" and Jeanne its "Woman of the Year." And in March 1991, Jeanne mustered the courage to join a typically confrontational ACTUP demonstration in front of the White House, calling on President Bush to help ensure that Congress fully funded the Ryan White CARE Act.[23]

Ryan's legacy was still very much in the public consciousness as talk-show host Phil Donahue commemorated the first anniversary of the teen's death, along with the Associated Press and *People* magazine. Jim Borgman, a cartoonist for the *Cincinnati Enquirer*, won a Pulitzer Prize in May for, among other works, a cartoon showing Ryan White on a cloud hugging an angel. The caption read, "A place where no one is afraid to hug." And *Ryan White: My Own Story*, an autobiography the teen had co-authored with Ann Marie Cunningham, rose to twelfth on the *New York Times'* bestseller list that same month. Closer to home, though, sales of the book were mixed. An Indiana distributor told the *Kokomo Tribune* that "two or three" local stores refused to sell the book at all, while another retailer "purposely turned all the books facing the wrong way when it received its shipment." Every tribute, every newspaper article, and every reading of his bestselling book furthered Ryan's public image as a courageous fighter who had withstood persecution, bigotry, and hate. Despite his near-canonization by the mass media, local antagonism toward this image did not abate. As late as July 1991, vandals continued to topple the nearly seven-foot-tall headstone at his grave in Cicero Cemetery. With every such desecration making national news, the familiar narrative repeated itself in shorthand form, usually with Ryan personifying the brave survivor,

Kokomo standing for cruelty and injustice, and Cicero representing tolerance and acceptance—despite the actions toward Ryan's grave.[24]

Throughout the 1990s, Ryan's memory remained prominent. In a special 1997 issue commemorating 20 years of publication, *Indianapolis Monthly* looked back at noteworthy people and stories. Ryan and Jeanne's names appeared with a caption, "Profiles in Courage," in an article reviewing the magazine's 20 most important stories. Its author, Susan Barker, wrote, "the Whites were all but excommunicated from Howard County." In October 1998, only a month before President Clinton signed the Ricky Ray Relief Fund Act, the *Chicago Tribune* published a long-form piece by Achy Obejas titled, "Ryan's Town Remembers." "In White's story," Obejas wrote, "Kokomo is always portrayed as a town without pity. But that, say its citizens, is a lie." Residents' statements to Obejas revealed the depth and immediacy of the community's outrage, even eight years after Ryan's death. Chad Gabbard, one of the named plaintiffs in the suit to enjoin Ryan from returning to classes at Western Middle School, was now 25. In his comments to the *Chicago Tribune*, he tried to convey both himself and Kokomo as victims of media bias: "[The media] listened to everything we said, then ignored it. I guess if we hadn't been these horrible people who wanted to keep this little kid down it wouldn't have been such a good story." But Gabbard also admitted that Ryan endured his fair share of mistreatment once he returned to Western, such as classmates giving him an extra wide berth in the hallways and calling him "fag." Gabbard maintained that this was normal junior high hazing, however. "These were the same people who picked on you for being overweight or wearing glasses," he told Obejas. The reporter, for her part, was impressed by how consistently Kokomo residents voiced that assertion: "in Kokomo, this line of reasoning is repeated over and over. Absolutely nobody [I] talked to for this story would say White received any but the most common teen harassment."[25]

Gabbard also alleged that Ryan had victimized *him*, "play[ing] on his fears of infection." "In art class one time, we had to draw an object from one angle, then move and draw it from another," he recounted to Obejas. "So when it came time to move, Ryan intentionally sat in my seat and just smiled at me, just to get me," Gabbard told her. Ron Colby, Ryan's former principal, also complained about unfairness. When Ryan told the President's Commission on AIDS that people at his new school, Hamilton Heights, treated him better, Colby had tried to correct the record, but the Commission refused to let him testify. Colby wanted it known that he had personally worked with the Hamilton Heights administration to educate them on universal precautions, spill kits, and the like. Colby also criticized the Whites themselves and resurrected old complaints about the blue-collar Whites crossing class lines. Saying the media had given the Whites a pass and overlooked all of Ryan's absences from school, Colby remarked, "Let's see, you call in and say your kid's too sick to come to school and then, hey, at 6 a.m. the next day, there's Ryan on a TV show in New York. Did people resent that? Yes." The last person featured in Obejas's story was Mitzie Johnson, who shared the bitterness of Gabbard and Colby—especially the resentment at the media's contrast of Kokomo and Cicero. "They [Cicero and Arcadia] had us as an example; we'd done all the homework for them on how not to do it," Johnson told the reporter. "We were far more educated than people ever knew," she insisted.[26]

People tracked down Gabbard and Johnson just a few months later for a story that ran in its March 15, 1999, issue. They sounded the same themes as they had with the *Chicago Tribune*, but this time for a national audience. Referring to the media's "Kokomo vs. Cicero" narrative, Mitzie Johnson told a reporter, "They made it sound like we were ignorant … but we [consulted] hospitals, the CDC, the AMA. We were opposed to the disease, not the people." Gabbard recalled a dearth of knowledge on AIDS. "I don't regret it, not a bit…. It took a lot of courage … the whole nation was against us," referring to the lawsuit to prevent Ryan from attending school. When *Indianapolis Monthly* published a special "Millennium Issue" in December 1999, and listed Ryan among its "Hoosier 50: A Chronicle of Indiana's Most Memorable Sons and Daughters"; when the *Kokomo Tribune* ran a story commemorating the tenth anniversary of Ryan's death in April 2000; when *People* published a "Sequel" item about Jeanne White closing down Ryan's foundation due to dwindling funds—each time, the people of Kokomo were cast as villains, and each time, that portrayal fueled their feelings of persecution.[27]

The community of Kokomo continued to see itself as the victim well into the twenty-first century. In September 2006, the *Kokomo Tribune* marked the twentieth anniversary of the dramatic Ryan White story with a set of lengthy articles. A headline proclaimed to readers that "Kokomo took a beating in the national news" in 1986, while the former managing editor John Wiles blamed the national media for Kokomo's negative image. Charlie Cropper, the former co-host of WWKI's "Male Call" with the late Dick Bronson, opined that Ryan was used by people "to further their own cause." In an article on Ryan's court battle published in March 2007, the *Tribune* noted that it was "still a sore subject locally." It was against this backdrop that, on November 10, 2007, the Children's Museum of Indianapolis enshrined Ryan White along Ruby Bridges and Anne Frank in a permanent exhibition called *The Power of Children: Making a Difference.*[28]

One of the nation's foremost museums, the venerable Children's Museum was founded in 1925. The world's largest children's museum houses diverse exhibits and programming—a haunted house every October, a

planetarium, a "dinosphere," and the occasional installation honoring Bar-
bie and Hot Wheels. The institution also mounts large traveling exhibitions, such as a display of the treasures of King Tut. A recent snapshot of its
vital statistics reflects both the scope and vibrancy of the museum's work: in
one year alone, the massive building contained 13 permanent and four temporary exhibit galleries, stored more than 130,000 artifacts and specimens,
and employed 300 full- and part-time staff members. The museum's annual
attendance regularly tops one million visitors. Even with its long history
of innovation, and all of the formidable resources at its disposal, the Children's Museum took years to develop *The Power of Children*, just as it took
Jeanne White years to let go of Ryan's belongings.[29]

Jeanne had married her Cicero neighbor, Roy Ginder, in August 1992.
She had kept her home, however, and left Ryan's room exactly as it was
when he went into the hospital in 1990. When Jeanne and Roy decided to
move to Florida in the late 1990s, Ryan's was the last room in the house to
be packed—and Jeanne could not face the task. Disposing of Ryan's cloth-
ing and personal effects, his posters, collections, and toys meant acknowledging the finality of her loss, and in a sense, she felt, losing him all over
again. When Jeanne decided to contact local museums to see whether they
were interested in Ryan's belongings, she had no definite idea about how
the items should be used—only that she did not want her son's property
reduced to a collection of celebrity keepsakes and 1980s memorabilia. She
felt that Ryan's legacy should stand for more than just a t-shirt he got in
California, a "Max Headroom" poster, or a photograph of him with Elton
John. So in January of 2001, Jeanne White called Andrea Hughes, Curator
of the American Collection at the Children's Museum. Jeanne wanted to
transfer Ryan's belongings to an institution that would accept all of them—
his entire room—and do something with the objects that would honor her
son. After traveling to Cicero and viewing Ryan's room in person, Hughes
and her colleagues knew they wanted it for their collection, although they
had no firm plans for its exhibition at the time. A month later, the museum
and Jeanne came to terms and the institution formally acquired the contents of Ryan's room. After accession, the museum staff measured the bedroom, which was in a large attic space above a two-and-a-half-car garage,
in order to faithfully recreate it at a later date. Before they packed the items,
Hughes and her co-workers interviewed Jeanne on video as she led them
through Ryan's room and discussed the importance of each object. They
loaded the furniture and boxes in a box truck and two minivans, drove to
the downtown Indianapolis museum, and began the months-long task of
processing all of the material.[30]

Before acquiring Ryan's things, the Children's Museum had previously mounted three temporary exhibitions on Anne Frank. The first two

consisted of a traditional, flat-panel format, but for the third, the museum had recreated the secret annex where the Franks had lived and hired an actress to portray Anne and read excerpts from her diary. According to Jennifer Pace-Robinson, the museum's Vice President for Experience Development and Family Learning, the third iteration showed the curators that an individual child's story made history more immediate and powerful for visitors. The museum staff had wanted to remake the facility's history exhibits anyway, Pace-Robinson recalled, because they were more than 20 years old by the time Jeanne transferred the contents of Ryan's room—and they wanted to continue the concept of having a historical figure address visitors. As they worked with Jeanne, the staff recognized similarities between Anne Frank and Ryan White: their stories were still present in popular memory; both had faced discrimination; and both had people in their lives who helped them through their difficulties—Miep Gies for Anne Frank, Dr. Kleiman for Ryan. Although the concept for the permanent installation developed relatively slowly, Pace-Robinson, Hughes, and their colleagues realized that a story from the civil rights movement of the 1960s would fit perfectly in this timeline—since Anne Frank's story occurred in the 1940s and Ryan's in the 1980s, and also because of the commonalities they shared. A senior museum official had a personal connection with Ruby Bridges, who in 1960 had been the first black child to attend an all-white elementary school and contacted her. After five more years, the museum had its final design.[31]

The exhibition promised to take people back in time and immerse them in each child's story; visitors would walk a "history path" in Anne's, Ruby's, and Ryan's shoes. Andrea Hughes and Jennifer Pace-Robinson assembled a panel of advisors—Holocaust experts, civil rights historians, public health experts—and designed an exhibition that combined factual historical information with personal accounts from each child in order to present history from the child's perspective. After all, Ruby Bridges had been only six years old when she integrated the William Frantz Public School in New Orleans, and thus could not have articulated the impact of historical figures like Dr. Martin Luther King, Jr., or historical forces such as slavery. Workers built each section to include not only traditional aspects such as objects with interpretive labels, but also to incorporate lighting and sound elements specific to each child's narrative, and to create a space for various actors to perform. After visitors encountered the actors, they would proceed along the pathway to find out what happened next—a way of discovering the legacies of Anne Frank, Ruby Bridges, and Ryan White.[32]

Since opening the permanent exhibition in late 2007, the Children's Museum has emphasized *The Power of Children*'s educational value. From its debut through May 2012 alone, more than 19,000 schoolchildren partook of *The Power of Children*'s guided learning experiences in person, while many others worked through Units of Study online. *The Power of Children: Making a Difference* occupies almost half of the museum's third floor. At its entrance, larger-than-life-sized photos of the three children—Frank, Bridges, and White—greet visitors and guide them to the "History Path." The path winds through the exhibition in chronological order, so a visitor must first travel through Anne's hiding place and Ruby's classroom before reaching Ryan's bedroom. This journey through space and time provides a historical context for Ryan's story: he was not the first child to encounter prejudice and discrimination. The story is scheduled to be updated to include a fourth hero in 2020: Malala Yousafzai, who won the Nobel Peace Prize at age 17, will be honored with a permanent spot in the exhibition for her own inspirational and courageous fight to attend school in defiance of the Taliban regime in Pakistan.[33]

When visitors arrive at the section on Ryan White, they learn about Ryan's hemophilia and then his infection with HIV. Graphic displays relate his efforts to return to classes at Western Middle School and the opposition he encountered. Ryan's room is located at the back of the space. Here, visitors view artifacts and listen to live actors portraying Ryan himself or his friends, Heather McNew and Jill Stewart.

Just outside of Ryan's room, a display depicts the legal battle over Ryan's school attendance. "Ryan won … and lost," a sign informs visitors, as sliding panels list the concessions Ryan made in order to attend Western: not participating in gym class, using plastic utensils, agreeing to a separate bathroom and water fountain. Another display shows a photo of Ryan by a school bus and quotes the teen: "Being back at school was almost as lonely as being at home." Visitors can also see a facsimile of Ryan's defaced locker; when they open the locker, they hear loudly whispered taunts, including: "Watch out!" "There he is!" "Don't let him touch you!" "He'll spit in your food!" "He shouldn't be here!" and "Keep away from him!" A sign at the top features a quote from Ryan. "I couldn't believe all the rumors going around about me." The text below reads, "Some people said he was biting kids and spitting on vegetables. Some restaurants threw his dishes away and people at church wouldn't shake his hand. At school, some kids would throw themselves against the wall and scream, 'Don't touch me' when he walked by." Middle and bottom signs read: "Have you ever stood up for someone … or had someone stand up for you? What was it like?"

For every negative element in the exhibition, curators have juxtaposed at least one positive element. For example, Ryan's statement about the loneliness of school stands beside a display of some of the cards and letters he received from around the world, along with photographs of Ryan with celebrities. And although the online teaching aid mentions that Ryan and his family lived in Kokomo, Indiana, the text omits any mention of the town of Russiaville, and the terms "Western Middle School" or "Western" appear rarely. Significantly, the place names of Kokomo and Russiaville appear nowhere within the exhibition itself, although at least one label mentions the *Kokomo Tribune*. Jeanne White wanted it that way. She recalled, "I [didn't] want to focus on Kokomo, because it could have happened anywhere. I mean, it might have even been worse somewhere else." Likewise, none of the actors' monologues mention Kokomo by name; however, the narrative freely mentions Hamilton Heights High School in Arcadia, and the town of Cicero. Typical of the exhibition's handling of the situation is a panel that speaks of Ryan's desire to move away and explains that the proceeds from the rights to the TV movie enabled the Whites to move. A viewer of the panel would not know that the Whites had lived in Kokomo but would know that they moved to Cicero once they had the funds. A succeeding panel, however, which focuses on Ryan's happiness and friendships after the move, mentions Hamilton Heights by name.[34]

Although it is possible to visit the exhibition and not realize that Russiaville and Kokomo were the communities where the Whites endured mistreatment, *The Power of Children: Making a Difference* has struck a nerve with some of the people who lived through the history that it depicts. Wanda Bowen Bilodeau and her brother Heath Bowen, Ryan's friends and former neighbors in Kokomo, went to the exhibition with Wanda's husband and children. A mother of three, Wanda was a regular visitor to the Children's Museum, but had not seen *The Power of Children* until she went with Heath and her family. The verisimilitude of Ryan's room took them both aback at first; Heath had to step outside and compose himself. An actor playing a janitor at Ryan's school talked about how (in Wanda's words) "Ryan used to have friends, but now that he's back at Western, he doesn't have *any* friends." Wanda and Heath objected to the all-or-nothing depiction of Ryan's life in Kokomo; *they* had been his friends, had they not? Heath and Ryan had slept over at each other's houses, and Heath had accompanied Ryan on trips to New York and met Elton John, Johnny Carson, and other celebrities with his friend. Now Heath and Wanda were faced with what they viewed as a total erasure of the friendship and support that their family had offered Ryan. "And not just us," Wanda recalled, "but a lot of people in Kokomo that truly were supportive of them in their own way, countless people that I'm sure I'm not aware of. But for anyone from Kokomo to go and see that, I just thought it was dishonest."[35]

The aim of *The Power of Children: Making a Difference* is not so much to relate historical stories as accurately as possible, however, as it is to inform children of their agency and to empower visitors of all ages to speak out against injustice and discrimination. This distinction drives the narrative that the Children's Museum has used to accompany the exhibition—Kokomo and Russiaville as places in and of themselves are not as important to the story as the events that occurred in those places. The material objects lend an authentic feel to each child's story and help communicate the child's relationship with the larger world. Viewed in that light, it is of no import whether the museum used Ryan's actual locker or constructed a facsimile. The written narrative for each portion of the exhibition is designed to provide a historical context for the three children's actions in order to illustrate why they were so remarkable. By necessity, some historical facts will be omitted. The actors' spoken pieces introduce drama, immediacy, and variety into the presentation. Again, whether they are actual, verbatim monologues from a documented or recorded speech or writing is not as important as the message the words convey. The Children's Museum's narrative of Ryan's story tries mightily to step around the place names of Russiaville and Kokomo, to avoid staining those communities with examples of the bad behavior of some of their residents. The exhibition recounts the cruelty and intolerance directed against the Whites only to the extent necessary to illustrate the social burdens of Ryan's disease. The isolation he experienced as a teen with AIDS could have accompanied any public health crisis, in any age, and in any place.

The Power of Children's curators had a variety of narratives from which to choose. Edward T. Linenthal, in his study of the memorialization of the Oklahoma City bombing, discussed Holocaust historian Lawrence Langer's concept of "preferred narratives"—interpretations that humans construct from tragic events of incomprehensible proportions, as a means to help us comprehend senseless destruction. While the details of humanity's awful deeds vary with each occurrence, whether it be the African slave trade, the Holocaust, the Oklahoma City or Boston Marathon bombings, or even the events of 9/11, any effort to officially remember those episodes necessarily involves decisions about what story to tell. According to Linenthal, the "progressive narrative" is one that finds positive elements in the story—acts of human decency and nobility amid chaos and suffering. The "redemptive narrative" elevates tragic events so that they take on a religious significance: acts so terrible they cause believers to question their faith in a divine God are revealed to be meaningful and, in hindsight, part of a larger plan. Finally, the "toxic narrative" makes no attempt to find meaning in suffering and hate. This approach finds no larger meaning in trauma, nor does it salvage lessons about the human spirit. The Power of Children uses the first strategy—a progressive narrative—to communicate an uplifting message to its juvenile audience. The installation publicly memorializes Ryan White in a meaningful, dignified, and honorable fashion. Ryan's story—and Kokomo, Russiaville, and Western's—in The Power *of Children* is meant to serve the purpose of inspiring museumgoers, not of vilifying communities. Each of those communities has dealt with Ryan's legacy in different ways.[36]

In Russiaville, a visitor to Western Middle School twenty years after Ryan's death would have to work hard to find any trace of his presence. In the mid–2010s, a walk down a busy hallway would end in a small room off of the library, where a stack of three-ring binders rested on shelves full of other materials. Inside those binders sat the school's collection of newspaper clippings, correspondence, CDC bulletins, and pamphlets related to Ryan White and AIDS. Though Swansea, Massachusetts, named a school after Mark Hoyle, there is no movement within the Western School Corporation to similarly commemorate Ryan's tenacity and heart. His story is nowhere to be found, his impact invisible. By comparison, the Hamilton Heights School Corporation in Arcadia, Indiana, applied for and received a state historical marker to commemorate its role in Ryan's story. The marker was erected in a special ceremony on August 30, 2019.[37]

In Kokomo, the legacy is not one of erasure but complexity. In 2010, the Howard County Historical Society embarked on a years-long, award-winning oral history project to record the memories of people like Mitzie Johnson, David Rosselot, Ron Colby, Dr. Alan Adler, and others. The Ryan White Oral History Project has ensured that the voices of those who were directly involved in the events will be accessible for generations, long after the principals in the story are gone. As the project's director, Allen Safianow, has noted, although each interviewee made "sincere efforts … to explore a difficult and often uncomfortable subject," each subject's individual recollection created not a complete picture, but one full of both contradiction and agreement, complicated and nuanced, like history itself. Taken as a whole, Safianow observed, the interview transcripts present "a community still seeking exoneration … from the harsher judgments of the outside world." It is true that oral history, as a means of investigating past events, has advantages and disadvantages. Interview subjects can be remarkably open in their first-person accounts, and sometimes bring along important documents, newspaper clippings, and personal photographs to augment their narratives and supplement their sometimes-frail memories. Safianow allows that some of the project's subjects might well have been biased, but rightly points out that "media accounts and even historical accounts are intrinsically incomplete and 'biased.'" The human memory is fallible, but nothing can replace the immediacy and the emotion that accompany a person's vivid recollections of important events. The oral histories provide that dynamic element. Finally, in 2014, the historical society selected Ryan White as one of six inductees into the Howard County Hall of Legends. Dave Broman, the executive director of the historical society, told the *Kokomo Tribune* that the selection committee emphasized leadership and service in its deliberations: "Howard County has always been proud of its sons and daughters and the things we've given the world. The people in the Hall of Legends represent that. They're a point of pride for the community."[38]

If the people of Kokomo are unhappy with *The Power of Children's* material representation of the historical events and actors, it is within their power to build upon the Historical Society's oral history project and Hall of Legends induction in a way that is more tangible and visible. After all, a visitor to the community could easily miss the Hall of Legends and the oral history project, whereas an exhibition like *The Power of Children* reaches hundreds of thousands of visitors annually. The community could borrow from Swansea and honor Ryan White's memory by naming a middle school after him, or by placing a plaque at the existing Western Middle School building in Russiaville. The city of Kokomo could name a street after Ryan, or—perhaps more fitting, given the teen's passion—dedicate a skateboarding park in his honor. Naming a street, or a school, or a park after Ryan White would mean taking a risk, though—the same risk taken by the curators at the Children's Museum. Which narrative to choose? The stakes are very high, because they involve the city's image, its constitutive narrative. While the narrative at the Children's Museum is flexible (the actors can change their scripts at any time, and curators can refabricate and mount new displays), a monument or public fixture carries more permanency in the form of words engraved in stone or cast in bronze, or names on maps. Memorializing Ryan White would inevitably rouse emotions and spark disagreement about what to say, where to say it, and how to say it: for example, should there be a moral to the story? Consensus will be impossible, because as Sanford Levinson put it in his discussion of Confederate memorials in the contemporary South, consensus about the meaning of monuments in the public realm "would require the existence of a singular public, whereas the reality of our society is its composition by various publics," and those different constituencies, with their individual life experiences, will never agree.[39]

The lack of public, visible memorials to Ryan White in Kokomo and Russiaville means the communities risk losing a chance to craft their own coherent and lasting narratives about past events. Driving through the streets of Kokomo today, a person would never know that the city had a resident in the international spotlight nearly three decades earlier, just as a visitor would not know there had once been a colossal steel mill on Markland Avenue. In stark contrast to that emptiness and silence, the Children's Museum's exhibition confers a legacy upon Ryan that is both heroic and meaningful to future generations.

A Community Divided

In Kokomo, Indiana, blood and steel combined with disease and economic disaster to divide a community along lines of class, gender, and health. Ryan White's determination to attend school, and his family's active support of that position, represented a rejection of his community's unspoken rules. Instead of passively accepting the school system's ban, Ryan broke the rules: he went public, stood apart from the crowd, and fought back. With a mother working the line at Delco, Ryan's family was solidly working-class, but the Whites did not remain at their social station. Instead, as Ryan defied Western School Corp. and broke with convention, he and his family traveled abroad and befriended celebrities on both the east and west coasts. From Hollywood to New York, from Rome to Disneyland, Ryan White was a household name in the 1980s. That very public behavior, and the notoriety that accompanied it, produced resentment in the Whites' community. Jeanne's coworkers watched helplessly as Continental Steel went under and layoffs rocked the auto industry. Yet Jeanne, one of their own, took her family on glamorous trips which were paid for by celebrities. As Jeanne White's hometown turned against her, the community also turned against itself. Members of the business class blamed workers' anemic productivity for Continental Steel's bankruptcy, while the workers blamed executives for poor decisions and bad managerial skills. The larger public, meanwhile, blamed both factions for leaving behind a financial and environmental mess, and for seeking "handouts."

The elements of blood and steel also divided the city along gender lines. "Steel," in this sense, refers to the tempered strength of both the Whites and their opponents. During the most direct conflict, when Ryan and the Concerned Parents were in and out of court, their positions hardened. As a divorced, single mother working in a male-dominated industry, Jeanne White made a rich target for those who lacked compassion. Time and again, Jeanne's critics focused on her status as Ryan's mother. They publicly criticized her parenting skills and wondered what kind of mother would send a child with a fatal disease out into the world. They asked why she let him decide whether to fight Western schools and why she supported his decision. They seriously considered making an official child welfare complaint regarding her fitness as a mother. During the time she lived in Kokomo, Jeanne White received a steady stream of mail containing invective, judgment, and abuse. Her opponents even called popular radio programs to speculate whether promiscuous behavior on her part had somehow led to Ryan's HIV. Steelworkers, no longer able to provide for their families, felt their own worthiness questioned as they became dependent upon charity and government programs for their economic survival.

And of course, blood and steel divided Kokomo along fault lines related to health. Ryan White's visibility in the public sphere flouted long-standing cultural taboos associated with the proper behavior of the sick. Although his HIV was not contagious, his opponents treated him as though he was capable of infecting them at will. Ironically, of the two elements which are the subjects of this book, the one that carried real toxicity to Kokomo was not blood, but steel—Continental Steel. The ups and downs of capitalism and disinvestment resulted in not only an economic disaster for those associated with Continental, but also an environmental disaster for the entire community. For generations, the people of Kokomo had turned a blind eye to what they suspected might be poisonous because of the prosperity and job security the mill offered. Once it closed, they learned the true extent of Continental's environmental degradation, and the true cost of that prosperity.

That Continental's economic woes occurred at the same time as Ryan White's opponents filed a lawsuit to prevent him from attending school compounded the damage to the community's social fabric. The media had created a simple "good/bad" narrative to explain the events surrounding Ryan White—an intolerant, regressive place discriminated against a sympathetic victim of AIDS—and that narrative built an image of Kokomo as unwelcoming and ignorant in the larger public mind. Even as the Whites experienced stigmatization at the hands of the Concerned Parents and their allies, the city of Kokomo felt the sting of national disapproval rub salt into the open wounds Continental left behind. Restoring the city's image took resilience, and that in turn involved erasure: a physical erasure effected by the decontamination of the Continental Steel site, and a psychic erasure wrought by forgetting Ryan White. Although the Howard County Historical Society's efforts to memorialize Ryan were meaningful, they have not been especially visible. Thanks to his mother, however, Ryan White's memory has both a permanent meaning and a permanent home—far from Kokomo, far from his home.

Chapter Notes

Preface

1. "Mom, I Want to Go to School," Transcript of audio recording of Jeanne White Ginder, The HIV/AIDS Program: Who Was Ryan White? U.S. Department of Health and Human Services, Health Resources and Services Administration, http://hab.hrsa.gov/abouthab/ryanwhite.html, accessed October 26, 2014.

2. Britt, a gay San Francisco city supervisor, was quoted in Manuel Castells, *The City and the Grassroots: A Cross-Cultural Theory of Urban Social Movements* (Berkeley: University of California Press, 1983), at 138. Julie Abraham elaborates on how gays and cities helped define each other in her cultural history *Metropolitan Lovers: The Homosexuality of Cities* (Minneapolis: University of Minnesota Press, 2009); she discusses the Britt quote on p. 264.

3. Sean Strub, *Body Counts: A Memoir of Politics, Sex, AIDS, and Survival* (New York: Scribner, 2014); Shawn Decker, *My Pet Virus: The True Story of a Rebel Without a Cure* (New York: Penguin, 2006); Jay Hoyle, *Mark: How a Boy's Courage in Facing AIDS Inspired a Town and the Town's Compassion Lit Up a Nation* (South Bend, IN: Langford Books, 1988); Elton John, *Love Is the Cure: On Life, Loss, and the End of AIDS* (New York: Little, Brown, 2012); Kate Scannell, *Death of the Good Doctor: Lessons from the Heart of the AIDS Epidemic* (San Francisco: Cleis, 1999); Cleve Jones and Jeff Dawson, *Stitching a Revolution: The Making of an Activist* (New York: HarperCollins, 2000, 2001); C. Everett Koop, *Koop: The Memoirs of America's Family Doctor* (New York: Random House, 1991).

4. Randy Shilts, *And the Band Played On: Politics, People, and the AIDS Epidemic* (New York: St. Martin's, 1987, 2007); David Black, *The Plague Years: A Chronicle of AIDS, the Epidemic of Our Times* (London: Picador/Pan Books, 1985, 1986).

5. David L. Kirp, Steven Epstein, Marlene Strong Franks, Jonathan Simon, Douglas Conaway, and John Lewis, *Learning by Heart: AIDS and Schoolchildren in America's Communities* (New Brunswick, NJ: Rutgers University Press, 1989).

6. Mirko D. Grmek, *History of AIDS: Emergence and Origin of a Modern Pandemic*, trans. Russell C. Maulitz and Jacalyn Duffin (Princeton: Princeton University Press, 1990); Jacques Pepin, *The Origins of AIDS* (Cambridge: Cambridge University Press, 2011).

7. Charles E. Rosenberg, *Explaining Epidemics and Other Studies in the History of Medicine* (Cambridge: Cambridge University Press, 1992); Allan M. Brandt, *No Magic Bullet: A Social History of Venereal Disease in the United States Since 1880* (New York: Oxford University Press, 1987); and Victoria A. Harden, *AIDS at 30: A History* (Washington, D.C.: Potomac Books, 2012).

8. Susan Resnik, *Blood Saga: Hemophilia, AIDS, and the Survival of a Community* (Berkeley: University of California Press, 1999); Douglas Starr: *Blood: An Epic History of Medicine and Commerce* (New York: Alfred A. Knopf, 1998); and Stephen Pemberton, *The Bleeding Disease: Hemophilia and the Unintended Consequences of Medical Progress* (Baltimore: Johns Hopkins University Press, 2011).

9. Eric A. Feldman and Ronald Bayer, eds., *Blood Feuds: AIDS, Blood, and the*

Politics of Medical Disaster (New York: Oxford University Press, 1999).

10. John Griggs, ed., *AIDS: Public Policy Dimensions* (New York: United Hospital Fund of New York, 1987); Elizabeth Fee and Daniel M. Fox, eds., *AIDS: The Burdens of History* (Berkeley: University of California Press, 1988); Douglas A. Feldman, ed., *Culture and AIDS* (New York: Praeger, 1990); Elizabeth Fee and Daniel M. Fox, eds., *AIDS: The Making of a Chronic Disease* (Berkeley: University of California Press, 1992); Phil Tiemeyer, *Plane Queer: Labor, Sexuality, and AIDS in the History of Male Flight Attendants* (Berkeley: University of California Press, 2013), 144–146; and Richard A. McKay, *Patient Zero and the Making of the AIDS Epidemic* (Chicago: University of Chicago Press, 2017).

11. Cathy J. Cohen, *The Boundaries of Blackness: AIDS and the Breakdown of Black Politics* (Chicago: University of Chicago Press, 1999); Jennifer Brier, *Infectious Ideas: U.S. Political Responses to the AIDS Crisis* (Chapel Hill: University of North Carolina Press, 2009); Michael P. Brown, *RePlacing Citizenship: AIDS Activism and Radical Democracy*, Mappings: Society/Theory/Space Series (New York: Guilford Press, 1997); Deborah B. Gould, *Moving Politics: Emotion and ACTUP's Fight Against AIDS* (Chicago: University of Chicago Press, 2009); and Steven Epstein, *Impure Science: AIDS, Activism, and the Politics of Knowledge*, Medicine and Science Series (Berkeley: University of California Press, 1996).

12. Cindy Patton, *Inventing AIDS* (New York: Routledge, 1990); Lee Edelman, *No Future: Queer Theory and the Death Drive* (Durham: Duke University Press, 2004); and Catherine Waldby, *AIDS and the Body Politic: Biomedicine and Sexual Difference*, Writing Corporealities Series (London: Routledge, 1996).

13. Robert A. Beauregard, *Voices of Decline: The Postwar Fate of U.S. Cities*, second ed. (New York: Routledge, 2003); Thomas J. Sugrue, *The Origins of the Urban Crisis: Race and Inequality in Postwar Detroit* (Princeton: Princeton University Press, 1996, 2005), 127–128; Jefferson Cowie, *Capital Moves: RCA's Seventy-Year Quest for Cheap Labor* (New York: The New Press, 1999, 2001), 34; David Harvey, *A Brief History of Neoliberalism* (Oxford: Oxford University Press, 2005), 45.

14. Barry Bluestone and Bennett Harrison, *The Deindustrialization of America: Plant Closings, Community Abandonment, and the Dismantling of Basic Industry* (New York: Basic Books, 1982), 6; Steven P. Dandaneau, *A Town Abandoned: Flint, Michigan, Confronts Deindustrialization* (Albany: State University of New York Press, 1996), xiii.

15. Nelson Lichtenstein, *State of the Union: A Century of American Labor*, rev. ed. (Princeton: Princeton University Press, 2013); Steve Babson, *The Unfinished Struggle: Turning Points in American Labor, 1877-Present* (Lanham, MD: Rowman & Littlefield, 1999), 146–159.

16. Steven High, *Industrial Sunset: The Making of North America's Rust Belt, 1969-1984* (Toronto: University of Toronto Press, 2003), 96; Steven High and David W. Lewis, *Corporate Wasteland: The Landscape and Memory of Deindustrialization* (Ithaca, NY: ILR Press, 2007); Sherry Lee Linkon and John Russo, *Steeltown U.S.A.: Work and Memory in Youngstown* (Lawrence: University of Kansas Press, 2002); and Dale Maharidge and Michael Williamson, *Journey to Nowhere: The Saga of the New Underclass* (New York: Hyperion, 1985, 1996).

17. Jefferson Cowie and Joseph Heathcott, eds., *Beyond the Ruins: The Meanings of Deindustrialization* (Ithaca, NY: ILR Press, 2003), and Ruth Milkman, *Farewell to the Factory: Auto Workers in the Late Twentieth Century* (Berkeley: University of California Press, 1997).

18. Richard C. Longworth, *Caught in the Middle: America's Heartland in the Age of Globalism* (New York: Bloomsbury, 2008, 2009), 5, 265; Jon C. Teaford, *Cities of the Heartland: The Rise and Fall of the Industrial Midwest* (Bloomington: Indiana University Press, 1993, 1994), ix–xii.

19. Robert S. Lynd and Helen Merrell Lynd, *Middletown: A Study in Modern American Culture* (New York: Harcourt, Brace, 1929, 1956), 22.

20. Abe Aamidor and Ted Avanoff, *At the Crossroads: Middle America and the Battle to Save the Car Industry* (Toronto: ECW Press, 2010), 10; Thomas Bender, *Community and Social Change in America* (Baltimore: Johns Hopkins University Press, 1978), 148–149; and Robert N. Bellah, Richard Madsen, William M. Sullivan, Ann Swidler, and Steven M. Tipton, *Habits of the Heart: Individualism and Commitment in*

American Life (Berkeley: University of California Press, 1985, 2008), 251.

Chapter 1

1. Worcester Polytechnic Institute, "Profiles in Innovation: Stainless Steel, Invented by Elwood Haynes, Class of 1881," http://www.wpi.edu/about/history/steel.html, accessed January 8, 2013.
2. Booth Tarkington, *The Works of Booth Tarkington*, vol. XXIII: *The World Does Move* (Garden City, NY: Doubleday, Doran & Co., 1928, 1932), 119.
3. Continental Steel Corporation, *Getting Acquainted with Steel and Continental* (Kokomo, IN: Continental Steel Corporation, 1947), no page number (promotional pamphlet); "Steel Firm Has Been Growing with Kokomo for 79 Years," *Kokomo Tribune*, October 19, 1975; Vincent P. De Santis, *The Shaping of Modern America: 1877–1920*, third ed. (Wheeling, IL: Harlan Davidson, 2000), 2, 60–61.
4. Charlie Sparks, ed., *Kokomo: City of Firsts* (Kokomo, IN: Kokomo Development Corp., 1982), 1; James A. Glass, "The Gas Boom in East Central Indiana," *Indiana Magazine of History* 96, no. 4 (Dec. 2000), 321–322; 326; 332.
5. Sparks, *Kokomo: City of Firsts*, 2; "Haynes Heritage—80 Years Plus of Innovative Metallurgy," www.haynesintl.com/Heritage.htm, accessed December 19, 2012.
6. Glass, "The Gas Boom in East Central Indiana," *Indiana Magazine of History*, 331–332, emphasis added. Continental Steel Corporation, *Getting Acquainted with Steel and Continental*; "Steel Firm Has Been Growing with Kokomo for 79 Years," *Kokomo Tribune*, October 19, 1975.
7. Continental Steel Corporation, *Getting Acquainted with Steel and Continental*; "Fine Office Quarters: The Official and Clerical Force at the Steel Mill Are Housed in Desirable Rooms," *Kokomo Daily Tribune*, July 27, 1918; "Steel Firm Has Been Growing with Kokomo for 79 Years," *Kokomo Tribune*, October 19, 1975.
8. Continental Steel Corporation, *Getting Acquainted with Steel and Continental*; "Steel Firm Has Been Growing with Kokomo for 79 Years," *Kokomo Tribune*, October 19, 1975; William Scheuerman, *The Steel Crisis: The Economics and Politics*

of a Declining Industry (New York: Praeger, 1986), 52.
9. "Steel Firm Has Been Growing with Kokomo for 79 Years," *Kokomo Tribune*, October 19, 1975.
10. Steve Daily, interview by Judy Lausch, January 23, 2009, transcript, Continental Steel Corporation, Howard County Historical Society, Kokomo, IN; "Nothin' Like 1950s Lunch Counters," *Kokomo Perspective*, http://kokomoperspective.com/generations/nothin-like-s-lunch-counters/-article_49bee847-eb0d-52ba-b29d-f251e4573eb5.html, accessed February 22, 2015.
11. Scheuerman, *The Steel Crisis: The Economics and Politics of a Declining Industry*, 73–74.
12. "Jerry's Castle," *Forbes*, June 15, 1976, 21–22.
13. *Ibid*.
14. "Jerry's Castle," *Forbes*, 21–22; "Continental, Penn-Dixie Merger Approved," *Kokomo Tribune*, April 18, 1973.
15. Joel Kotkin, "A Commitment Forged in Steel," *Inc.*, June 1983, 93; "Former Penn-Dixie Head Indicted," *Kokomo Tribune*, October 11, 1978; "Ex-Penn Dixie Chief Sentenced to 15 Months in Prison," *ibid.*, October 24, 1979.
16. Scheuerman, *The Steel Crisis: The Economics and Politics of a Declining Industry*, 138–143; 160, 164–165; 169.
17. Kotkin, "A Commitment Forged in Steel," *Inc.*, 83, 88; "Jerry's Castle," *Forbes*, 23; "Steel Firm Has Been Growing with Kokomo for 79 Years," *Kokomo Tribune*, October 19, 1975; Pasquale Rocchio, "Penn-Dixie Files to Reorganize," *ibid.*, April 7, 1980; Scheuerman, *The Steel Crisis: The Economics and Politics of a Declining Industry*, 189.
18. James H. Madison, *Indiana Through Tradition and Change: A History of the Hoosier State and Its People, 1920–1945* (Indianapolis: Indiana Historical Society, 1982), 309–312.
19. *Ibid.*, 320–323.
20. G. I. C. Ingram, "The History of Haemophilia," *Journal of Clinical Pathology* 29 (1976), 469; Susan Resnik, *Blood Saga: Hemophilia, AIDS, and the Survival of a Community* (Berkeley: University of California Press, 1999), 5–7.
21. Resnik, *Blood Saga: Hemophilia, AIDS, and the Survival of a Community*, 15–19 (emphasis in original); National

Hemophilia Foundation, "History of Bleeding Disorders," https://www.hemophilia.org/Bleeding-Disorders/History-of-Bleeding-Disorders, accessed August 28, 2012.

22. David L. Kirp, et al., *Learning by Heart: AIDS and Schoolchildren in America's Communities* (New Brunswick, NJ: Rutgers University Press, 1989), 29; Resnik, *Blood Saga: Hemophilia, AIDS, and the Survival of a Community*, 17–18; 20; National Institutes of Health, NIH History, "The NIH Almanac: Chronology of Events," http://nih.gov/about/almanac/historical/chronology_of_events.htm#nineteenthirty, accessed February 21, 2015; Kathleen M. Berry, "A Multibillion-Dollar Business in a Nonprofit World," *New York Times*, July 7, 1991; Douglas Starr, *Blood: An Epic History of Medicine and Commerce* (New York: Alfred A. Knopf, 1998), 174; Keith Wailoo, *Dying in the City of the Blues: Sickle Cell Anemia and the Politics of Race* (Chapel Hill: University of North Carolina Press), 126; Keith Wailoo, *Pain: A Political History* (Baltimore: Johns Hopkins University Press, 2014), 45.

23. Resnik, *Blood Saga: Hemophilia, AIDS, and the Survival of a Community*, 31, 32; Baxter, Company Profile, "History," http://www.baxter.com/about_baxter/company_profile/history.html, viewed November 29, 2012.

24. Resnik, *Blood Saga: Hemophilia, AIDS, and the Survival of a Community*, 31, 32.

25. *Ibid.*, 32. Marc A. Franklin, in "Tort Liability for Hepatitis: An Analysis and a Proposal," *Stanford Law Review* 24 (1971–1972), 443–444, quoted a contemporary (1970) estimate from the National Research Council of "30,000 cases of serious overt illness annually ... associated with transfusions, of which some 1,500 to 3,000 are fatal.... 'the ratio of sub-clinical hepatitis cases associated with transfusion to cases of the overt disease may be as high as 5:1.'" For a lengthy discussion of the involvement of prisoners as donors and lax governmental oversight, see Sophia Chase, "The Bloody Truth: Examining America's Blood Industry and its Tort Liability Through the Arkansas Prison Scandal," *William & Mary Business Law Review* 3, no. 2 (2012), 597–644. The blood services industry in the United States is easily worth billions of dollars. Kathleen M. Berry, "A Multibillion-Dollar Business

in a Nonprofit World," *New York Times*, July 7, 1991. Chase compares the 1998 value of a barrel of crude oil—$13—with the value of a barrel of whole blood—over $20,000. "If the blood were separated, or fractionated, into its derivative products, the value of the same quantity in 1998 rises to more than $67,000, while the barrel of oil, including all of *its* derivatives, was worth $42." Chase, "The Bloody Truth," at 607–608 (emphasis in original); 610, note 95.

26. Resnik, *Blood Saga*, 22; 37–38; 40–42. Interestingly, Resnik notes that a concurrent development was necessary: the technology to produce plastic bags. Starr, *Blood: An Epic History of Medicine and Commerce*, 101–106.

27. Starr, *Blood: An Epic History of Medicine and Commerce*, 224; Resnik, *Blood Saga*, 47–50; Stephen Pemberton, *The Bleeding Disease: Hemophilia and the Unintended Consequences of Medical Progress* (Baltimore: Johns Hopkins University Press, 2011). Pemberton discusses the pull of normality in depth at 116–117.

28. Pemberton, *The Bleeding Disease: Hemophilia and the Unintended Consequences of Medical Progress*, xi; Resnik, *Blood Saga*, 53; Starr, *Blood: An Epic History*, 224–225.

29. Glenn F. Pierce, Jeanne M. Lusher, Alan P. Brownstein, Jonathan C. Goldsmith, and Craig M. Kessler, "The Use of Purified Clotting Factor Concentrates in Hemophilia: Influence of Viral Safety, Cost, and Supply on Therapy," *JAMA* 261, no. 23, June 16, 1989, 3434; Kirp et al., *Learning by Heart: AIDS and Schoolchildren in America's Communities*, 30; Titmuss, *The Gift Relationship: From Human Blood to Social Policy*, 25–27. Lawrence K. Altman, "Use of Commercial Blood Donors Increases with Shortage in U.S.," *New York Times*, September 5, 1970. Starr, *Blood: An Epic History*, 256–257. "Transfusion Blood Soon Must Indicate Volunteer Donors," *New York Times*, January 14, 1978; United Press International, "Blood to Identify Donor as 'Paid' or 'Volunteer,'" *ibid.*. May 16, 1978.

30. Resnik calls this period the "Golden Era." See chapter 7, generally, in her *Blood Saga*, for compelling anecdotes about life before and after "cryo," and before and after "Factor." She discusses the regional disparities in the quality of treatment (which would endure throughout the 1970s) in the early part of that chapter. Robert

E. Johnson, Dale N. Lawrence, Bruce L. Evatt, Dennis J. Bregman, Lawrence D. Zyla, James W. Curran, Louis M. Aledort, M. Elaine Eyster, Alan P. Brownstein, and Charles J. Carman, "Acquired Immune Deficiency Syndrome Among Patients Attending Hemophilia Treatment Centers and Mortality Experience of Hemophiliacs in the United States," *American Journal of Epidemiology* 121, no. 6 (1985), 801. Marsha F. Goldsmith, "Hemophilia, Beaten on One Front, Is Beset on Others," *JAMA* 256, no. 23 (Dec. 19, 1986), 3200.

31. Resnik, *Blood Saga*, 109. Johnson et al., "Acquired Immunodeficiency Syndrome Among Patients Attending Hemophilia Treatment Centers and Mortality Experience of Hemophiliacs in the United States," 799. Dr. Bruce Evatt, quoted in "Protecting the Hemophiliacs," *Saturday Evening Post* 260, no. 2, March 1988, 100–101.

32. Jeanne White and Susan Dworkin, *Weeding Out the Tears: A Mother's Story of Love, Loss, and Renewal* (New York: Avon Books, 1997), 32; Jeanne White Ginder, interview with author, October 25, 2012, Children's Museum of Indianapolis, Indianapolis, IN. *1936–1996 Delco Electronics 60th Anniversary Video*, "Generations of GM," history.gmheritagecenter.com/wiki/index.php/1936–1996_Delco_Electronics_60th_Anniversary_Video, viewed January 15, 2013. The name "Delco" was actually an acronym for a General Motors conglomerate, the Dayton Engineering Laboratories Company. See Joseph W. Barnes, "Rochester and the Automobile Industry," *Rochester History* 43, nos. 2 and 3 (April and July 1981), 35. GM moved Delco to its Delphi Automotive Systems in 1997 and renamed the new entity "Delphi Delco Electronics Systems." In 1999, GM let go of Delphi Automotive Systems, allowing it to become a separate, publicly traded company, Delphi Corp. Delphi Corp. declared bankruptcy and filed for a Chapter 11 reorganization in 2005. "Delphi's History in Kokomo," *Kokomo Tribune*, October 10, 2006. Just as Delphi was preparing to emerge from bankruptcy, in 2009, GM (which was itself on the verge of filing under Chapter 11) acquired a huge stake in Delphi again; GM would sell it back to Delphi two years later, for $3.8 billion. Delphi has been privately held since it emerged from its own restructuring. Nick Bunkley, "G.M. Sells Delphi Stake for $3.8 Billion," *New York Times*, March 31, 2011.

33. White and Dworkin, *Weeding Out the Tears: A Mother's Story of Love, Loss, and Renewal*, 36–37; Jeanne White Ginder, interview with author, October 25, 2012, Children's Museum of Indianapolis, Indianapolis, IN.

34. White and Dworkin, *Weeding Out the Tears: A Mother's Story of Love, Loss, and Renewal*, 21–23; 27–32; White Ginder, interview.

35. White and Dworkin, *Weeding Out the Tears: A Mother's Story of Love, Loss, and Renewal*, 37–40; Ryan White and Ann Marie Cunningham, *Ryan White: My Own Story* (New York: Signet, 1992), 14–15.

36. White and Dworkin, *Weeding Out the Tears*, 41; "Drive Starts," *Kokomo Tribune*, March 17, 1973, p. 2.

37. White and Dworkin, *Weeding Out the Tears*, 42–43, 50–51.

38. *Ibid.*, 51–54. Wayne White died only one month after retiring from Delco, in 1999. White Ginder, interview and e-mail message to author, January 28, 2013.

39. White and Dworkin, *Weeding Out the Tears*, 54–58; White and Cunningham, *Ryan White: My Own Story*, 32–38.

Chapter 2

1. The campaign ad, titled "Prouder, Stronger, Better," was specifically designed to resonate with voters on an emotional level. "The Living Room Candidate-Commercials-1984-Prouder, Stronger, Better," www.livingroomcandidate.org/commercials/1984/prouder-stronger-better," accessed August 25, 2016.

2. Jeanne White and Susan Dworkin, *Weeding Out the Tears: A Mother's Story of Love, Loss, and Renewal* (New York: Avon Books, 1997), 58–59; Ryan White and Ann Marie Cunningham, *Ryan White: My Own Story* (New York: Signet, 1992), 38–39. Wanda Bilodeau, interview by Allen Safianow, June 7, 2011, transcript, Ryan White Project, Howard County Historical Society, Kokomo, IN. Ford passed away in 2017. George Myers, "Ryan White's Stepdad, Unheralded Father Figure, Remembered by Family After Passing," *Kokomo Tribune*, May 30, 2017.

3. U.S. Department of Commerce, Bureau of the Census, *1980 Census of Population and Housing, Census Tracts, Kokomo, Ind., Standard Metropolitan Statistical*

Area (Washington, D.C.: U.S. Department of Commerce, Bureau of the Census, 1983), Table P-2, "General Characteristics of White Persons: 1980," and Table P-3, "General Characteristics of Black Persons: 1980." Ongoing Ku Klux Klan activity may have played a part in the reluctance of minorities to settle in this area. The *Kokomo Tribune* ran a story about a Klan march around the courthouse in downtown Kokomo, planned for April 26, 1980. John Stowell and Linda Miller, "Anti-Klan Coalition Seeks Parade Permit," *Kokomo Tribune*, April 17, 1980.

4. Glen R. Boise, *A Land Use Plan for the City of Kokomo, Indiana* (Kokomo: Kokomo-Howard County Plan Commission, 1976), 10.

5. White and Cunningham, *Ryan White: My Own Story*, 41–49. Wanda Bilodeau, interview transcript, Ryan White Project, Howard County Historical Society, Kokomo, IN.

6. White and Cunningham, *Ryan White: My Own Story*, 48–49; White and Dworkin, *Weeding Out the Tears*, 59–61. Lauren B. Leveton, Harold C. Sox, Jr., and Michael A. Stoto, eds., *HIV and the Blood Supply: An Analysis of Crisis Decisionmaking* (Washington, D.C.: National Academy Press, 1995), 61–64, citing "Current Trends Update: Acquired Immunodeficiency Syndrome (AIDS)—United States," *MMWR* 33, no. 47 (Nov. 30, 1984), 661–664.

7. The manufacturers had already withdrawn their untreated products by the time the FDA finally issued the order. Leveton et al., *HIV and the Blood Supply: An Analysis of Crisis Decisionmaking*, 155. Gilbert M. Gaul, "Judge Allows Use of AIDS Memo in Hemophiliacs' Suit," *Philadelphia Inquirer*, May 16, 1990; White and Dworkin, *Weeding Out the Tears*, 68.

8. Lawrence K. Altman, "Rare Cancer Seen in 41 Homosexuals," *New York Times*, July 3, 1981. See also the August 29, 1981, article headlined "2 Fatal Diseases Focus of Inquiry: Rare Cancer and Pneumonia in Homosexual Men Studied." James W. Curran and Harold W. Jaffe, "AIDS: The Early Years and CDC's Response," *MMWR* 60, Supplement (Oct. 7, 2011), 64. The two criteria in the original case definition were: "biopsy-proven" Kaposi's sarcoma in people under 60 years old or "biopsy- or culture-proven life-threatening or fatal" opportunistic infections; and "no known

underlying illness (e.g. cancer or immune deficiency disease) or history of immunosuppressive therapy."

9. Jacques Pepin, *The Origins of AIDS* (New York: Cambridge University Press, 2011), 233–234; Phil Tiemeyer, *Plane Queer: Labor, Sexuality, and AIDS in the History of Male Flight Attendants* (Berkeley: University of California Press, 2013), 144–146.

10. Curran and Jaffe, "AIDS: The Early Years and CDC's Response," *MMWR* 60, Supplement (Oct. 7, 2011), 65. See also "A Cluster of Kaposi's Sarcoma and Pneumocystis carinii Pneumonia among Homosexual Male Residents of Los Angeles and Orange Counties, California," *MMWR* 31, no. 23 (June 18, 1982), 305–307; Robert M. Swenson, "Plagues, History, and AIDS," *American Scholar* 57, no. 2 (Spring 1988), 188–189.

11. "Current Trends Update on Acquired Immune Deficiency Syndrome (AIDS)—United States," *MMWR* 31, no. 37 (Sep. 24, 1982), 507–508; 513–514. The CDC had formally established the term "Acquired Immune Deficiency Syndrome" (AIDS) and identified four risk factors over the summer of 1982. The risk factors were male homosexuality, intravenous drug use, Haitian ethnicity, and hemophilia A. "Epidemiologic Notes and Reports *Pneumocystis carinii* Pneumonia Among Persons with Hemophilia A," *MMWR* 31, no. 27 (July 16, 1982), 365–367.

12. Susan Resnik, *Blood Saga: Hemophilia, AIDS, and the Survival of a Community* (Berkeley: University of California Press, 1999), 115, 118.

13. Johnson et al., "Acquired Immune Deficiency Syndrome Among Patients Attending Hemophilia Treatment Centers and Mortality Experience of Hemophiliacs in the United States," *American Journal of Epidemiology* 121, no. 6 (June 1985), 797–798; Resnik, 119–121. In 1976, the CDC, fearing an epidemic outbreak of swine flu, advocated for a widespread inoculation program. Not only did the epidemic not occur, the vaccine itself sickened a number of people with a rare illness that caused paralysis called Guillain-Barré syndrome. Then, when a different strain of influenza threatened, the public was not receptive to the idea of flu vaccinations. The Secretary of the U.S. Department of Health, Education, and Welfare, Joseph A. Califano, Jr., asked

the director of the CDC at the time, Dr. David Sencer, to resign in the wake of the affair, which had seriously undermined the public's faith in the CDC. "Califano Moves to Remove Doctor Who Guided Swine Flu Program," *New York Times*, February 8, 1977. Leveton et al., *HIV and the Blood Supply: An Analysis of Crisis Decisionmaking*, 20.

14. Resnik, *Blood Saga: Hemophilia, AIDS, and the Survival of a Community*, 124; "Update on Acquired Immune Deficiency Syndrome (AIDS) among Patients with Hemophilia A," *MMWR* 31, no. 48 (Dec. 10, 1982), 644–646; 652.

15. "Epidemiologic Notes and Reports Possible Transfusion-Associated Acquired Immune Deficiency Syndrome (AIDS)— California," *MMWR* 31, no. 48 (Dec. 10, 1982), 652–654; Katie Leishman, "San Francisco: A Crisis in Public Health," *The Atlantic* 256, no. 4 (Oct. 1985), 31; Resnik, *Blood Saga*, 125.

16. *Ibid.*, 126–127. Randy Shilts, in his account of the early years of the AIDS pandemic, offers a much more detailed description of the January 4, 1983 meeting. See Randy Shilts, *And the Band Played On: Politics, People, and the AIDS Epidemic* (New York: St. Martin's, 1987; 20th anniv. ed., 2007), 220–224.

17. Leveton et al., *HIV and the Blood Supply: An Analysis of Crisis Decisionmaking*, 70–73, 78, 154–155; "Current Trends Prevention of Acquired Immune Deficiency Syndrome (AIDS): Report of Inter-Agency Recommendations," *MMWR* 32, no. 8 (March 4, 1983): 101–103. The CDC would prove that heat treatments were fatal to the AIDS virus in October of 1984.

18. Leveton et al., *HIV and the Blood Supply: An Analysis of Crisis Decisionmaking*, 74–75; 147; 155; 174–178; 196, 169.

19. Pasquale Rocchio, "Local Auto Plants Say More Layoffs"; Associated Press, "Economic Indicators Point to Long-Predicted Recession"; and Associated Press, "State to Begin Talks with Chrysler," *Kokomo Tribune*, April 17, 1980.

20. Pasquale Rocchio, "Local Auto Plants Say More Layoffs"; Associated Press, "Economic Indicators Point to Long-Predicted Recession"; and Associated Press, "State to Begin Talks with Chrysler," *Kokomo Tribune*, April 17, 1980; Dale Maharidge and Michael S. Williamson, *Someplace Like America: Tales from the New*

Great Depression (Berkeley: University of California Press, 2011), 31.

21. Pasquale Rocchio, "Local Auto Plants Say More Layoffs"; Associated Press, "Economic Indicators Point to Long-Predicted Recession"; and Associated Press, "State to Begin Talks with Chrysler," *Kokomo Tribune*, April 17, 1980. Pasquale Rocchio, "Penn-Dixie Mill Gets First OK," *ibid.*, December 12, 1980.

22. Pasquale Rocchio, "Continental Steel May Return Here," *Kokomo Tribune*, January 20, 1981; "Penn-Dixie Hearing Reset June 18," *ibid.*, June 3, 1981.

23. Sue Tidler, "Penn-Dixie Workers Told to Face Facts," *Kokomo Tribune*, June 21, 1981.

24. John Stowell, "Penn-Dixie Tax Debt Growing at $800,000 Rate," *Kokomo Tribune*, October 28, 1981.

25. Pasquale Rocchio, "Penn-Dixie's Troubles Near End?" *Kokomo Tribune*, January 9, 1982; John P. Hoerr, *And the Wolf Finally Came: The Decline of the American Steel Industry* (Pittsburgh: University of Pittsburgh Press, 1988), 63–64; William Scheuerman, *The Steel Crisis: The Economics and Politics of a Declining Industry*, 190–191; United Steelworkers Local 2-369, "Past/Current International Presidents," http://www.usw12-369.org/?ID=22, viewed February 4, 2013.

26. Hoerr, *And the Wolf Finally Came*, 64–67.

27. Pasquale Rocchio, "Local Chamber Finds Easy Does It," *Kokomo Tribune*, October 6, 1982; Associated Press, "Agreement Is Reached on Steel Plant Wastes," *New York Times*, February 25, 1983.

28. Kotkin, "A Commitment Forged in Steel," *Inc.* (June 1983), 84, 88, 93; "Together We're Building a Brighter Future with Kokomo," *Kokomo Tribune*, April 17, 1983; Mary Ann McNulty, "Continental's New Rod Mill Goes on Display," *ibid.*, May 31, 1984; John Dempsey, "Chrysler Idles Plants," *ibid.*, December 18, 2008.

29. Mary Ann McNulty, "Continental Waste Case Dismissed," *Kokomo Tribune*, August 22, 1984.

30. Linda Miller, "Continental Steel Fires Up for a New Life," *Kokomo Tribune*, March 25, 1984; Mary Ann McNulty, "Continental's New Rod Mill Goes on Display," *ibid.*, May 31, 1984.

31. United States Environmental Protection Agency, Region 5 Cleanup Sites,

"Continental Steel," http://www.epa.gov/region5/cleanup/continental/index.htm, accessed February 4, 2013.

32. "Billet Caster Looks Like a 'Go,'" *Kokomo Tribune*, November 2, 1984.

33. White and Dworkin, *Weeding Out the Tears*, 61–64; Donald Fields, interview by Judy Lausch, June 6, 2011, transcript, Ryan White Project, Howard County Historical Society, Kokomo, IN.

34. Jeanne White Ginder, interview with author, October 25, 2012, Children's Museum of Indianapolis, Indianapolis, IN; White and Dworkin, *Weeding Out the Tears*, 69–70.

35. White and Dworkin, *Weeding Out the Tears*, 73–74; White and Cunningham, *Ryan White: My Own Story*, 66–68; Wanda Bilodeau, interview by Allen Safianow, June 7, 2011, transcript, Ryan White Project, Howard County Historical Society, Kokomo, IN. Det. Sgt. Roger Smith, Howard County Sheriff's Department, Criminal Investigations Division, January 20, 1989, Ken Ferries papers, Ryan White Project, Howard County Historical Society, Kokomo, IN.

36. White and Dworkin, *Weeding Out the Tears*, 74; White and Cunningham, *Ryan White: My Own Story*, 69–71; Jeanne White Ginder, interview with author, October 25, 2012, Children's Museum of Indianapolis, Indianapolis, IN.

Chapter 3

1. Jeanne White and Susan Dworkin, *Weeding Out the Tears: A Mother's Story of Love, Loss, and Renewal* (New York: Avon Books, 1997), 78; Christopher M. MacNeil, "AIDS Case Confirmed," *Kokomo Tribune*, January 10, 1985.

2. Jeanne White Ginder, interview with author, October 25, 2012, Children's Museum of Indianapolis, Indianapolis, IN.

3. Steve Marschand, "Local Youth Faces AIDS," *Kokomo Tribune*, March 3, 1985.

4. Donald P. Francis, "Commentary: Deadly AIDS policy failure by the highest levels of the U.S. government: A personal look back 30 years later for lessons to respond better to future epidemics," *Journal of Public Health Policy* 33, no. 3 (2012), 294–295; Susan Resnik, *Blood Saga: Hemophilia, AIDS, and the Survival of a*

Community (Berkeley: University of California Press, 1999), 136. The controversial question of who "discovered" the virus that causes AIDS pitted American scientist Robert Gallo against his French counterpart, Luc Montagnier. The question was settled diplomatically in March 1987, with a written agreement between HHS and the Pasteur Institute signed by Ronald Reagan and Jacques Chirac. Even the virus's name, HIV, was the subject of mediation by the Human Retrovirus Subcommittee of the International Committee on the Taxonomy of Viruses in 1986. Ultimately, Chermann and Barré-Sinoussi would be awarded the Nobel Prize in 2008 in recognition of their work to isolate HIV. For two good, in-depth, scholarly discussions of this controversy, see Mirko D. Grmek, *History of AIDS: Emergence and Origin of a Modern Pandemic*, trans. Russell C. Maulitz and Jacalyn Duffin (Princeton, NJ: Princeton University Press, 1990), esp. chapters 6 and 7; and, Steven Epstein, *Impure Science: AIDS, Activism, and the Politics of Knowledge* (Berkeley: University of California Press, 1996), esp. pp. 66–88. "ELISA," an acronym for enzyme-linked immune assay, is a common laboratory test for antibodies in blood. "ELISA: MedlinePlus Medical Encyclopedia," U.S. National Library of Medicine, U.S. Department of Health and Human Services, National Institutes of Health, http://www.nlm.nih.gov/medlineplus/ency/article/003332.htm, accessed February 6, 2013. Because the ELISA test could result in a false positive for HIV, positive ELISA tests are always followed by Western blot tests. "ELISA/Western blot tests for HIV," U.S. National Library of Medicine, National Institutes of Health, http://www.nim.nih.gov/medlineplus/ency/article/003538.htm, accessed July 13, 2014; Christopher M. MacNeil, "AIDS Test Has Health Officials Worried," *Kokomo Tribune*, March 3, 1985.

5. Kim Painter, "A Checkered History of Tragedy, Despair and Hope," *USA Today*, June 4, 1991; David Black, *The Plague Years: A Chronicle of AIDS, the Epidemic of Our Time* (London: Picador/Pan Books, 1985, 1986), 14–15.

6. "AIDS Epidemic: The Price of Promiscuity," *Human Events* 43, no. 25 (June 18, 1983), 5.

7. Ronald S. Godwin, "AIDS: A Moral and Political Time Bomb," *Moral Majority Report*, July 1983, 2. Italics in original.

8. *Life*, July 1985, 12, 19. After a lengthy study of an unusually concentrated AIDS outbreak in Belle Glade, Florida, the CDC concluded in October 1986 that mosquitoes were not to blame; instead, the virus was transmitted via sexual activity and IV drug use. *Aids Policy & Law* 1, no. 19, Oct. 8, 1986, 2.

9. *Newsweek*, August 12, 1985, 27. In early July, Rock Hudson and his publicist had given reporters various reasons for his appearance, including flu and liver disease, but soon after, news reports emerged that he had AIDS. Kim Painter, "A Checkered History of Tragedy, Despair and Hope," *USA Today*, June 4, 1991. Hudson died of AIDS on October 2, 1985. Burt A. Folkart, "Rock Hudson Is Dead at 59; His AIDS Moved the World," *Los Angeles Times*, October 2, 1985.

10. Kim Painter, "A Checkered History of Tragedy, Despair and Hope," *USA Today*, June 4, 1991; Francis, "Commentary: Deadly AIDS Policy Failure," *Journal of Public Health Policy*, 298; Ronald Sullivan, "Parishioners Block Archdiocese's AIDS Shelter," *New York Times*, August 31, 1985; Associated Press, "Blood Center's Officials Waving Red Flag," *Kokomo Tribune*, September 19, 1985; Judy Foreman, "Mass. Neurosurgeon Suggests Quarantine for AIDS Carriers," *Boston Globe*, November 21, 1985. At the time that Mark made his statements, the 87-acre island in Buzzards Bay served as a wildlife sanctuary.

11. Kelly Kaiser, "Brochure Touts Continental Steel," *Kokomo Tribune*, January 27, 1985.

12. "Continental Ups Sales Revenues," *Kokomo Tribune*, April 5, 1985.

13. "Shuffle Ejects Sigler," *Kokomo Tribune*, July 5, 1985; Kotkin, "A Commitment Forged in Steel," *Inc.*, 86.

14. "8 Continental Steel Directors Resign," *Kokomo Tribune*, September 24, 1985.

15. Pickle liquor is a corrosive mixture of acids that steelmakers use to remove iron oxide scale from steel; they soak the steel in a bath of the liquor. Manufacturers began pickling steel in this manner in 1891 and disposing of the used pickle liquor involves dangerous work. G. A. Howell, "Waste Pickle Liquor Disposal," *Sewage and Industrial Wastes* 29, no. 11 (Nov. 1957), 1278. "NPL Site Narrative for Continental Steel Corp.," http://www.epa.gov/superfund/ sites/npl/nar1164.htm, accessed February 13, 2013.

16. Kelly Lasecki, "Steel Firm Names Head," *Kokomo Tribune*, November 21, 1985; "Continental Idles 200," *ibid.*, November 22, 1985.

17. Kelly Lasecki, "Continental Seeks Relief in Court," *Kokomo Tribune*, November 26, 1985.

18. Kelly Lasecki, "Continental Seeks Relief in Court," *Kokomo Tribune*, November 26, 1985; "Continental Steel Reaches an Accord with Two Utilities," *ibid.*, December 7, 1985; Kelly Lasecki, "Continental OKs Upfront Utility Paying," *ibid.*, December 10, 1985.

19. Cory SerVaas, "The Happier Days for Ryan White," *Saturday Evening Post* 260, no. 2 (March 1988), 54.

20. Jeanne White Ginder, interview with author, October 25, 2012, Children's Museum of Indianapolis, Indianapolis, IN.

21. Ryan White and Ann Marie Cunningham, *Ryan White: My Own Story* (New York: Signet, 1992), 92–95; italics in original.

22. Adler served as the county's health officer for nearly 30 years while he maintained his practice as a family physician. Ken de la Bastide, "Adler Resigning as County Health Officer," *Kokomo Tribune*, November 5, 2006; Dr. Alan Adler, interview by Judy Lausch, March 23, 2009, transcript, Ryan White Project, Howard County Historical Society, Kokomo, IN. In the 1980s, during a separate interview, Adler cited diarrhea alone as sufficient reason to exclude Ryan for the spring. See David L. Kirp et al., *Learning by Heart: AIDS and Schoolchildren in America's Communities* (New Brunswick, NJ: Rutgers University Press, 1989), 34.

23. Ron Colby, interview by Diane Knight and Allen Safianow, May 24, 2011, transcript; Daniel W. Carter, interview by Allen Safianow, February 9, 2011, transcript, Ryan White Project, Howard County Historical Society, Kokomo, IN; State Board of Health Office Memorandum, T. S. Danielson, Jr., M.D., M.P.H., February 6, 1985, Folder 1, State Board of Health, Commissioners File, Commissioner's Correspondence, GRADM-3, A9639, Box 2, 21-Q-4, Indiana State Archives, Commission on Public Records.

24. *Forbes*, Woodrow Myers Profile, http://www.forbes.com/profile/

woodrow-myers/, accessed February 20, 2013 (profile no longer available); Ken Kusmer, "Indiana's Controversial Health Chief: He's Ready to Shake Things Up," *Los Angeles Times*, August 17, 1986. Minutes of the March 13, 1985, meeting of the Executive Board of the Indiana State Board of Health, State Board of Health, Executive Board Minutes & Reports, GRADM-1, A8766, Box 1, 20-N-4, Indiana State Archives, Commission on Public Records. After many years out of the public eye, during which he became a wealthy venture capitalist, Myers announced that he would run for the Democratic nomination for governor of Indiana in 2020. Chris Sikich, "'I'm Running for Governor,'" *Indianapolis Star*, July 19, 2019.

25. Minutes of the July 10, 1985 meeting of the Executive Board of the Indiana State Board of Health, State Board of Health, Executive Board Minutes & Reports, GRADM-1, A8766, Box 1, 20-N-4, Indiana State Archives, Commission on Public Records.

26. Christopher M. MacNeil, "School Bars Door to Youth with AIDS," *Kokomo Tribune*, July 31, 1985; Judith Michaelson, "Rock Hudson Has AIDS: Diagnosis Made Over Year Ago," *Los Angeles Times*, July 26, 1985; Kirp et al., *Learning by Heart: AIDS and Schoolchildren in America's Communities*, 37; White and Dworkin, *Weeding Out the Tears*, 83. Italics in original.

27. Kirp et al., *Learning by Heart: AIDS and Schoolchildren in America's Communities*, 36–37; Mark Nichols, "Young AIDS Victim Barred from School," *Indianapolis Star*, July 31, 1985.

28. Charles E. Rosenberg, "What Is an Epidemic? AIDS in Historical Perspective," in *Explaining Epidemics and Other Studies in the History of Medicine* (New York: Cambridge University Press, 1992), 282; James Oleske et al., "Immune Deficiency Syndrome in Children," *JAMA* 249, no. 17 (May 6, 1983), 2345; Anthony S. Fauci, "The Acquired Immune Deficiency Syndrome: The Ever-Broadening Clinical Spectrum," *JAMA* 249, no. 17 (May 6, 1983), 2375–2376. A scientific study on the question of whether AIDS was transmissible by casual contact was already well underway in 1985, and the results were published in the *New England Journal of Medicine* in early 1986. This should have settled the matter. See Gerald H. Friedland et al., "Lack

of Transmission of HTLV–III/LAV Infection to Household Contacts of Patients with AIDS or AIDS-Related Complex with Oral Candidiasis," *New England Journal of Medicine* 314, no. 6 (Feb. 6, 1986), 344–349.

29. Carter interview transcript, Ryan White Project, Howard County Historical Society, Kokomo, IN; White and Dworkin, *Weeding Out the Tears: A Mother's Story of Love, Loss, and Renewal*, 82; Jeanne White Ginder, interview with author, October 25, 2012, Children's Museum of Indianapolis, Indianapolis, IN.

30. "Case in the Spotlight," *Kokomo Tribune*, August 1, 1985; Associated Press, "School in Indiana Bars Boy with AIDS," *Los Angeles Times*, July 31, 1985. Datelined "Kokomo, Ind.," the article mentioned Western Middle School but never specified the school's location in Russiaville. Jeanne White Ginder, interview with author, October 25, 2012, Children's Museum of Indianapolis, Indianapolis, IN; Carter interview transcript, Ryan White Project, Howard County Historical Society, Kokomo, IN. Denise Kalette, Mark Spearman, and Steven Findlay, "New Testing Would Save Other Kids," *USA Today*, August 1, 1985.

31. Mark Nichols, "Young AIDS Victim Barred from School," *Indianapolis Star*, July 31, 1985; Jeri Malone, interview by Judy Lausch, February 9, 2011, transcript, Ryan White Project, Howard County Historical Society, Kokomo, IN. "Guidelines for Children with AIDS/ARC Attending School, Indiana State Board of Health—July 1985," MSC 339, Jeri Malone Collection, 2011.042, Box 33, Folder 3, Howard County Historical Society.

32. Christopher MacNeil and Ann Nolan, "Guide Leaves Voids," *Kokomo Tribune*, August 1, 1985; "Guidelines for Children with AIDS/ARC Attending School, Indiana State Board of Health—July 1985," MSC 339, Jeri Malone Collection, 2011.042, Box 33, Folder 3, Howard County Historical Society.

33. Correspondence from A. J. Adler to All Kokomo-Howard County School Corporations, August 2, 1985, MSC 339, Jeri Malone Collection, 2011.042, Box 33, Folder 2, Howard County Historical Society; Editorial, "Every Right," *Kokomo Tribune*, August 2, 1985.

34. Mark Nichols, "Interested ICLU Sees Ryan's Case as One of Discrimination," *Indianapolis Star*, August 4, 1985.

Christopher M. MacNeil, "AIDS Verdict Up to Schools," *Kokomo Tribune*, August 2, 1985; Christopher M. MacNeil, "Ryan's Case May Go to Court," *ibid.*, August 3, 1985; Christopher M. MacNeil, "ICLU Offers Services to Whites," *ibid.*, August 6, 1985.

35. Christopher M. MacNeil, "ICLU Offers Services to Whites," *Kokomo Tribune*, August 6, 1985; Carter and Colby interview transcripts, Ryan White Project, Howard County Historical Society, Kokomo, IN. Myers did personally respond to Carter's questions: in a letter dated October 9, 1985, he enclosed an eight-page list of Western's 30 questions, complete with answers, titled "Questions and Answers About Children with AIDS in Schools." State Board of Health, Woodrow Myers Correspondence, Letter C 1986, Commissioners Files GRADM-3, A9644, Box 1, 21-Q-6, Indiana State Archives, Commission on Public Records.

36. Christopher M. MacNeil, "Some Support Gels for Western Schools," *Kokomo Tribune*, August 7, 1985. "Do You Agree with Western's Rule Barring an AIDS Pupil?" KT Streettalk, *ibid.*, August 12, 1985. The day after the "Streettalk" piece ran, the paper published three letters to the editor supporting the school.

37. Christopher M. MacNeil, "AIDS Suit Filed," *Kokomo Tribune*, August 8, 1985.

38. "Parents, Teachers Would Claim Damages," and Kay Bacon, "Worried Parents Attend Meeting," *Kokomo Tribune*, August 13, 1985; "AIDS Message Reaction Calm," and Christopher M. MacNeil, "Kokomo Attorney Offers Assistance," *ibid.*, August 30, 1985.

39. Kay Bacon, "Worried Parents Attend Meeting," *Kokomo Tribune*, August 13, 1985.

40. Claudia Wallis et al., "AIDS: A Growing Threat," *Time*, Aug. 12, 1985, 45; David Gelman et al., "The Social Fallout from an Epidemic," *Newsweek*, Aug. 12, 1985, 28.

41. Christopher M. MacNeil, "Teachers Support Smith's Decision," *Kokomo Tribune*, August 16, 1985.

42. "Ryan's Lawsuit Stalls," *Kokomo Tribune*, August 16, 1985. *Ryan White b/n/f Jeanne White v. Western School Corporation et al.*, IP 85-1192-C, S. D. Ind., 1985, U.S. Dist. Lexis 16540 (written opinion dated August 23, 1985). The Rehabilitation Act of 1973, Public Law 93–112, was the federal anti-discrimination law for people with disabilities (referred to at the time of enactment as "qualified handicapped individuals"). See Wendy E. Parmet and Daniel J. Jackson, "No Longer Disabled: The Legal Impact of the New Social Construction of HIV," *American Journal of Law and Medicine* 23, no. 1 (1997), 12. Congress passed the Education for All Handicapped Children Act, Public Law 94–142, in 1975. The Act requires that schools provide special education and related services to all children, regardless of the severity of their disability. See Judith S. Palfrey et al., "Schoolchildren with HIV Infection: A Survey of the Nation's Largest School Districts," *Journal of School Health* 64, no. 1 (Jan. 1994), 22.

43. Mark Nichols, "Young AIDS Victim Barred from School," *Indianapolis Star*, July 31, 1985; Christopher M. MacNeil, "'Baloney,' Lawyer Says After AIDS Decision," *Kokomo Tribune*, December 1, 1985. Jeanne White Ginder, interview with author, October 25, 2012, Children's Museum of Indianapolis, Indianapolis, IN. Ind. Code 16-8-7-2, 1982 edition. The following articles illustrate the evolution of courts' and legislatures' thinking with respect to liability for transfusion-related diseases: Marc A. Franklin, "Tort Liability for Hepatitis: An Analysis and a Proposal," *Stanford Law Review* 24 (1971–1972): 439–480; Michael J. Miller, "Strict Liability, Negligence, and the Standard of Care for Transfusion-Transmitted Disease," *Arizona Law Review* 36 (1994): 473–513; George W. Conk, "Is There a Design Defect in the *Restatement (Third) of Torts: Products Liability?*" *Yale Law Journal* 109 (1999–2000): 1087–1133; Andres Rueda, "Rethinking Blood Shield Statutes in View of the Hepatitis C Pandemic and Other Emerging Threats to the Blood Supply," *Journal of Health Law* 34, no. 3 (Summer, 2001): 419–458; and Sophia Chase, "The Bloody Truth: Examining America's Blood Industry and its Tort Liability Through the Arkansas Prison Plasma Scandal," *William & Mary Business Law Review* 3, no. 2 (2012): 597–644. Currently, people with hemophilia A can choose between plasma-derived Factor VIII and recombinant Factor VIII; the latter has unlimited production capacity and is not vulnerable to contamination from an infected plasma donor. As of 2010, though, advances in viral

inactivation methods and in screening for viruses have resulted in no confirmed cases of blood-transfusion-associated transmission of either the hepatitis viruses or HIV since 1996—or since 1990, depending on which source one consults. See Massimo Franchini, "Plasma-derived versus recombinant Factor VIII concentrates for the treatment of haemophilia A: recombinant is better," *Blood Transfusion* 8, no. 4 (2010), 292, and Pier Mannuccio Mannucci, "Plasma-derived versus recombinant factor VIII concentrates for the treatment of haemophilia A: plasma-derived is better," *Blood Transfusion* 8, no. 4 (2010), 288. The reason there is a debate about the relative efficacy of plasma-derived vs. recombinant Factor VIII is because some patients with severe hemophilia A (about 20–30 percent) actually develop inhibitors that make Factor VIII ineffective. See Franchini, *infra*, at 292. When scientists successfully cloned the human Factor VIII gene in 1984, they were then able to begin development of the recombinant product. Jeanne M. Lusher, "Hemophilia: From Plasma to Recombinant Factors," American Society of Hematology, http://www.hematology.org/publications/50-years-in-hematology/4737.aspx, accessed February 28, 2013.

44. Christopher M. MacNeil, "'Baloney,' Lawyer Says After AIDS Decision," *Kokomo Tribune*, December 1, 1985. White and Cunningham, *Ryan White: My Own Story*, 106–109; Richard A. McKay, *Patient Zero and the Making of the AIDS Epidemic* (Chicago: University of Chicago Press), 357; Wanda Bowen Bilodeau, BBC World Service, *Witness* Archive 2011, "Witness: Ryan White," podcast audio, December 1, 2011, http://downloads.bbc.co.uk/podcasts/worldservice/witness/witness_20111201-0900a.mp3.

45. Bev Ashcraft, interview by Judy Lausch, January 27, 2011, transcript, Ryan White Project, Howard County Historical Society, Kokomo, Indiana.

46. The Indiana health department's guidelines were approved by the State Department of Education, which sent a copy of them to the superintendents of every school district in the state. Minutes of the September 11, 1985, meeting of the Executive Board of the Indiana State Board of Health, State Board of Health, Executive Board Minutes & Reports, GRADM-1, A8766, Box 1, 20-N-4, Indiana State Archives, Commission on Public Records. Children with AIDS were reported in 23 different states, the District of Columbia, and Puerto Rico; 75 percent of them lived in New York, California, Florida, and New Jersey. "Current Trends Education and Foster Care of Children Infected with Human T-Lymphotropic Virus Type III/Lymphadenopathy-Associated Virus," *MMWR* 34, no. 34 (Aug. 30, 1985): 517–21.

47. Dorothy Nelkin and Stephen Hilgartner, "Disputed Dimensions of Risk: A Public School Controversy Over AIDS," *The Milbank Quarterly* 64, Supplement 1, AIDS: The Public Context of an Epidemic (1986), 138–139.

48. "AFRAIDS," *The New Republic* 193, Oct. 14, 1985, 7; Erik Eckholm, "Fears on AIDS Termed Largely Without Cause," *New York Times*, September 13, 1985.

49. C. Everett Koop, *Koop: The Memoirs of America's Family Doctor* (New York: Random House, 1991), 194–196.

50. Transcript of the President's News Conference, September 17, 1985, Ronald Reagan Presidential Library, National Archives and Records Administration, http://www.reagan.utexas.edu/archives/speeches/1985/91785c.htm, accessed August 14, 2012.

51. Peter Baldwin, "Beyond Weak and Strong: Rethinking the State in Comparative Policy History," *Journal of Policy History* 17, no. 1 (2005), 21. For a spirited critique of the Reagan administration's handling of the early years of the AIDS epidemic, see retrovirologist and former CDC researcher Don Francis's article in the *Journal of Public Health Policy*. Donald P. Francis, "Commentary: Deadly AIDS Policy Failure by the Highest Levels of the U.S. Government: A Personal Look Back 30 Years Later for Lessons to Respond Better to Future Epidemics," *Journal of Public Health Policy* 33, no. 3 (2012): 290–300.

52. Transcript of the President's News Conference, September 17, 1985, Ronald Reagan Presidential Library, National Archives and Records Administration, http://www.reagan.utexas.edu/archives/speeches/1985/91785c.htm, accessed August 14, 2012.

53. Jay Hoyle, *Mark: How a Boy's Courage in Facing AIDS Inspired a Town and the Town's Compassion Lit Up a Nation* (South Bend, IN: Langford Books, 1988), 8, 26–28.

Dudley Clendinen, "'Epidemic of Fear' in U.S.," *New York Times*, September 8, 1985.

54. Ethan Bronner, "Emotions Run High at Meeting on AIDS," *Boston Globe*, September 12, 1985; Hoyle, *Mark: How a Boy's Courage in Facing AIDS Inspired a Town and the Town's Compassion Lit Up a Nation*, 57. Jay Hoyle's memoir contains a complete transcript of this meeting in chapter 3, at 42–101.

55. "Parents to Plan Next Step in AIDS Case," *Times* (London), September 18, 1985; "Pupils Return as AIDS Boy's Parents Call for Greater Understanding," *ibid.*, September 20, 1985. White and Dworkin, *Weeding Out the Tears: A Mother's Story of Love, Loss, and Renewal*, 150. Resnik discussed the fact that once people with hemophilia saw what transpired with Ryan White (and later, Ricky Ray and his family in Florida), they frequently withdrew from their larger communities and hid their status. Resnik, *Blood Saga: Hemophilia, AIDS, and the Survival of a Community*, 142, 153.

56. Joyce Purnick, "Pupils with AIDS a Risk, Koch Says," *New York Times*, September 2, 1985.

57. Robert G. Sullivan, "*District 27 v. Board of Education*," in John Griggs, ed., *AIDS: Public Policy Dimensions* (New York: United Hospital Fund of New York, 1987), 70; Joyce Purnick, "Pupils with AIDS a Risk, Koch Says," *New York Times*, September 2, 1985. In fact, a New York City school had sent the city's health department its first letter requesting information on handling a student with AIDS as early as the spring of 1983, although there was not yet an official policy from the health agency. See Frederick A. O. Schwarz, Jr., and Frederick P. Schaffer, "AIDS in the Classroom," *Hofstra Law Review* 14, no. 1 (Fall 1985), 163.

58. Carter interview transcript, Ryan White Project, Howard County Historical Society, Kokomo, IN. Christopher M. MacNeil, "National Moratorium Sought on AIDS Children in Schools," *Kokomo Tribune*, September 10, 1985; Jennifer Brier, "'Save Our Kids, Keep AIDS Out': Anti-AIDS Activism and the Legacy of Community Control in Queens, New York," *Journal of Social History* 39, no. 4 (Summer 2006), 967–968; Dudley Clendinen, "'Epidemic of Fear' in U.S.," *New York Times*, September 8, 1985.

59. Larry Rohter, "New York City Schools Open with Dual Goal," *New York Times*, September 9, 1985; Nelkin and Hilgartner, "Disputed Dimensions of Risk," *Milbank Quarterly*, 120–121; Brier, "'Save Our Kids, Keep AIDS Out': Anti-AIDS Activism and the Legacy of Community Control in Queens, New York," 965. United Press International, "5 N. Y. School Workers Said to Have AIDS," *Boston Globe*, September 12, 1985; Jeffrey Schmalz, "Panel of Doctors Picked to Screen AIDS Students," *New York Times*, September 25, 1985. The case is reported at *District 27 Community School Board v. Board of Education*, 130 Misc. 2d 398, 502 N.Y.S.2d 325 (Sup. Ct. 1986).

60. "Phone Hookup Links Ryan White with His School," *Kokomo Tribune*, August 21, 1985; John Schorg, "Ryan White Back in School by Telephone," *ibid.*, August 26, 1985; "AT & T to Get Bugs Out of Hook-Up," *ibid.*, August 27, 1985; Christopher M. MacNeil, "Via Phone: Ryan Can Even Hear a Pin Drop—Almost," *ibid.*, August 29, 1985. United Press International, "AIDS Victim Starts School Over Telephone," *New York Times*, August 27, 1985. Principal Colby told reporters that the school had received offers of equipment from firms in Chicago, New York, and Washington, among others.

61. "Compound Being Tried," *Kokomo Tribune*, August 30, 1985; Christopher M. MacNeil, "Ryan's Hospital Stay May End," *ibid.*, September 6, 1985; "Ryan White Continuing to Battle Fever, Cough," *ibid.*, September 18, 1985. "AIDS Student in Hospital," *USA Today*, September 5, 1985; "AIDS Victim 'Just Like Any Boy His Age,'" *ibid.*, September 18, 1985. Associated Press, "Indiana Hospital Says AIDS Boy Is Improving," *New York Times*, September 5, 1985. "Ryan White's Condition Good," *Indianapolis Star*, September 29, 1985. The national newspapers featured detailed stories about Ryan's condition, with *USA Today* including his photograph. For coverage of the administrative review: Associated Press, "Conference Set in Ryan's Case," *Kokomo Tribune*, September 17, 1985; Christopher M. MacNeil, "Ryan's Hope for School Continues," *ibid.*, September 19, 1985; Christopher M. MacNeil, "AIDS Conference Concludes on Silent Note," *ibid.*, September 20, 1985; and Christopher M. MacNeil, "Recommendation Not Surprising," *ibid.*, October 2, 1985. For Principal

Colby's findings, see the case conference report, Exhibit D, "Brief for Defendants, Ryan White by next of friend [sic] Jeanne White and Jeanne White," filed March 7, 1985, *Scott Bogart, b/n/f/ Daniel R. Bogart et al. v. Ryan White, b/n/f Jeanne White and Jeanne White*, Howard County Circuit Court cause no. 49192.

62. Colby interview transcript, Ashcraft interview transcript, Ryan White Project, Howard County Historical Society, Kokomo, IN. The kits, housed in small beige file cabinets emblazoned with a red cross, contained written instructions on cleaning up body fluids, rubber gloves, a bleach solution, and Voban (a sawdust-like vomit absorbent).

63. Christopher M. MacNeil, "School Doors Still Closed for Local AIDS Victim, 13," *Kokomo Tribune*, October 4, 1985; "White's Lawyer Files Appeal," *ibid.*, October 10, 1985; "Goodfellows Opens Fund for Ryan," *ibid.*, October 11, 1985; "White's Condition Slowly Improving," *ibid.*, October 15, 1985; Christopher M. MacNeil, "Goodfellows Helping Ryan White," *ibid.*, October 19, 1985; "Youth's Condition Reported as Good," *ibid.*, October 22, 1985. Ryan had been readmitted to the hospital September 25; see Christopher M. MacNeil, "Schools Head Would Bar AIDS Prone," *Kokomo Tribune*, November 1, 1985. Joseph P. Fried, "Lawyer in Queens Suit Says City Did Not Follow U.S. AIDS Policy," *New York Times*, October 13, 1985; Erik Eckholm, "Doctors Unit Urges Schools to Admit AIDS Victims," *ibid.*, October 24, 1985.

64. Christopher M. MacNeil, "Tempers Flare at AIDS Hearing," *Kokomo Tribune*, November 2, 1985.

65. New Jersey singer Alex Tiensivu donated $1,500, the proceeds from sales of his tapes of "Ryan's Song," to Goodfellows in October. Christopher M. MacNeil, "Receipts of Song Enrich White Fund," *Kokomo Tribune*, October 25, 1985. For Ryan's release from the hospital, see "Ryan Out of Hospital," *ibid.*, November 10, 1985. In November, country singer Jimmy Dee held a concert at Kokomo High School to raise funds for Ryan; also on the bill were comedian Elmer Fudpucker, singer Rich Mount, the Southbound Express Band, singer Marty Martell, and local talent Dorval Smith. "Ryan's Show Set for Saturday," *ibid.*, November 15, 1985. "Japanese TV

Crew Does Piece on Ryan," *ibid.*, November 22, 1985. "No Comment from School," and Christopher M. MacNeil, "Pleasure is Hard for Ryan White's Mother to Subdue," *ibid.*, November 26, 1985. For Madinger Angelone's ruling, see "Findings of Fact, Conclusions of Law, and Order," Exhibit E, "Brief for Defendants, Ryan White by next of friend [sic] Jeanne White and Jeanne White," filed March 7, 1985, *Scott Bogart, b/n/f/ Daniel R. Bogart et al. v. Ryan White, b/n/f Jeanne White and Jeanne White*, Howard County Circuit Court cause no. 49192. United Press International, "'Great' Present for AIDS Boy," *New York Times*, November 27, 1985.

66. Christopher M. MacNeil, "School Boards Grappling with AIDS Issue," *Kokomo Tribune*, November 24, 1985; Christopher M. MacNeil, "Avoid Boycott, Parents are Told," and "Smith, Colby Relax Position on Guidelines," *ibid.*, December 5, 1985.

67. "AIDS Case a Drain to School Finances," and Dawne Slater, "Western Agenda is Media Event," *Kokomo Tribune*, December 18, 1985.

68. Alex Tiensivu, letter to the editor, *Kokomo Tribune*, December 22, 1985; John Langone, "Special Report: AIDS," *Discover* 6 (December 1985), 49.

69. Christopher M. MacNeil, "Christmas Comes Early for Ryan," *Kokomo Tribune*, December 20, 1985.

Chapter 4

1. "Reporter, Tribune Earn Award," *Kokomo Tribune*, November 15, 1985. "1985: Kokomo's Ryan White was in Spotlight," *ibid.*, December 29, 1985. Christopher M. MacNeil, "Western's Appeal of Order on White is Open to Public," *ibid.*, Jan.1, 1986. John Wiles, interview by Judy Lausch, July 14, 2008, transcript, Ryan White Project, Howard County Historical Society, Kokomo, IN.

2. "Current Trends Update: Acquired Immunodeficiency Syndrome—United States," *MMWR* 35, no. 2 (Jan. 17, 1986): 17–21; Sam Stall, "Living with AIDS," *Indianapolis Monthly* 9, no. 5 (Jan. 1986), 35.

3. *AIDS Policy & Law* 1, no. 4 (Mar. 12, 1986), 3.

4. The New York Assembly passed a bill banning discrimination in housing on

the basis of sexual orientation in June 1985. "Bill to Extend Co-op Conversion Laws Goes to Cuomo," *New York Times*, June 26, 1985; "Texas Quarantine Plan Withdrawn by Official," *AIDS Policy & Law* 1, no. 1 (Jan. 29, 1986), 5.

5. Richard J. Meislin, "AIDS Said to Increase Bias Against Homosexuals," *New York Times*, January 21, 1986. John T. McQuiston, "City Finds Rise in Complaints of Bias Against Homosexuals," *ibid.*, March 8, 1986. "Anti-Gay Violence, Bias in New York Said Sharply Higher, Linked to AIDS," *AIDS Policy & Law* 1, no. 4 (Mar. 12, 1986), 1.

6. William J. Broad, "Thousands Watch A Rain of Debris," *New York Times*, January 29, 1986. Marlene Aig, "Tylenol: Police Find No Motive in Deaths," *Kokomo Tribune*, February 23, 1986.

7. Seymour Martin Lipset and William Schneider, *The Confidence Gap: Business, Labor, and Government in the Public Mind*, rev. ed. (Baltimore: Johns Hopkins University Press, 1987), 48–49. Leon Eisenberg, "The Genesis of Fear: AIDS and the Public's Response to Science," *Law, Medicine & Health Care* 14, no. 5–6 (Dec. 1986), 246–247.

8. Friedland et al., "Lack of Transmission of HTLV–III/LAV Infection to Household Contacts of Patients with AIDS or AIDS-Related Complex with Oral Candidiasis," *New England Journal of Medicine* 314, no. 6 (Feb. 6, 1986), 344–349. William F. Buckley, Jr., "Crucial Steps in Combating the AIDS Epidemic: Identify All the Carriers," *New York Times*, March 18, 1986; Alan M. Dershowitz, "Emphasize Scientific Information," *ibid.*, March 18, 1986. See also Eisenberg, "The Genesis of Fear: AIDS and the Public's Response to Science," at 243, for a critique of this aspect of Dershowitz's piece.

9. Keith Wailoo, "Stigma, Race, and Disease in 20th Century America," *The Lancet* 367 (Feb. 11, 2006), 533, quoting Linus Pauling, "Reflections on the New Biology: Foreword," *UCLA Law Review* 15, no. 2 (1967–1968), 269.

10. Michael D. Quam, "The Sick Role, Stigma, and Pollution: The Case of AIDS," in Douglas A. Feldman, ed., *Culture and AIDS* (New York: Praeger, 1990), 29–31.

11. Micheline Maynard, "Chrysler: A Short History," *New York Times*, April 30, 2009. Accessed online August 25, 2016.

http://www.nytimes.com/2009/05/01/business/01history.html?_r=0.

12. Associated Press, "Jobless Rate Eases Down," and Kelly Lasecki, "Firm's Offer Looks at Lopping," *Kokomo Tribune*, January 8, 1986.

13. Kelly Lasecki, "Steelworkers Threaten to Strike," and "Continental Wants Funds Back," *ibid.*, January 23, 1986.

14. James R. Asher, letter to the editor, *Kokomo Tribune*, February 5, 1986.

15. "Thinks Firm Can Work," and Kelly Lasecki, "Adviser Says Closing Would Solve Cash Flow," *ibid.*, February 13, 1986.

16. Kelly Lasecki, "Adviser Says Closing Would Solve Cash Flow," *Kokomo Tribune*, February 13, 1986; Kelly Lasecki, "Continental's Kokomo Plant is Shut Down," *ibid.*, February 17, 1986.

17. Kelly Lasecki, "Continental's Kokomo Plant is Shut Down," *Kokomo Tribune*, February 17, 1986.

18. Kelly Lasecki, "Jobless Facing Grim Reality," *ibid.*, February 18, 1986; Kelly Lasecki, "Trustee Picked at Steel Firm," *ibid.*, February 20, 1986.

19. "Steel Imports Level Is High," and Robert Haberfield, letter to the editor, *Kokomo Tribune*, February 20, 1986.

20. Lipset and Schneider, *The Confidence Gap: Business, Labor, and Government in the Public Mind*, 57, 203.

21. Kelly Lasecki, "Any Continental Sale Feasible," *Kokomo Tribune*, February 21, 1986.

22. "Steel Firm Here Accepts Sellout," *Kokomo Tribune*, February 25, 1986; Kelly Lasecki, "Workers Still Have Contract, Benefits," *ibid.*, February 26, 1986.

23. Christopher M. MacNeil, "Western Patrons Seek Funds for AIDS Case," *Kokomo Tribune*, January 12, 1986. David Rosselot, interview by Diane Knight and Allen Safianow, October 11, 2011, transcript, Ryan White Project, Howard County Historical Society, Kokomo, IN.

24. "White Hearing Has Been Shifted," *Kokomo Tribune*, January 17, 1986; Cynthia Tiensivu, letter to the editor, *ibid.*, January 28, 1986.

25. Paula Kincaid to Ronald Colby, undated, Western Middle School Library, Russiaville, IN.

26. Ryan White and Ann Marie Cunningham, *Ryan White: My Own Story* (New York: Signet, 1992), 123–124. "Passports in Hand, Whites Leave Today," *Kokomo*

Tribune, February 1, 1986. Associated Press, "Romans Lend Ryan an Ear," *ibid.*, February 4, 1986. "Home from Rome," and Christopher M. MacNeil, "Whites Keeping the Media Busy," *ibid.*, February 6, 1986.

27. "Nobody Claims Victory, Defeat," and Christopher M. MacNeil, "School Must Use Health Guidelines," *Kokomo Tribune*, February 7, 1986. "Final Findings of Fact, Conclusions of Law, and Order," Indiana Board of Special Education Appeals, Exhibit F, "Brief for Defendants, Ryan White by next of Friend [sic] Jeanne White and Jeanne White," *Bogart et al. v. White et al.*, No. 49192 (Howard Cir. Ct., Ind., filed March 7, 1986).

28. Final Findings of Fact, Conclusions of Law, and Order," Indiana Board of Special Education Appeals, Exhibit F, "Brief for Defendants, Ryan White by next of Friend [sic] Jeanne White and Jeanne White," *Bogart et al. v. White et al.*, No. 49192 (Howard Cir. Ct., Ind., filed March 7, 1986).

29. Christopher M. MacNeil, "Official Comment Nil in AIDS Ruling," *Kokomo Tribune*, February 7, 1986; Christopher M. MacNeil, "Lawyer Says Ruling Omits Rights of Others," *ibid.*, February 9, 1986.

30. Becky Graves, letter to the editor, *ibid.*, February 9, 1986.

31. Christopher M. MacNeil, "White Decision Comes Thursday," *Kokomo Tribune*, February 11, 1986. "Western Offers Guidelines," and Christopher M. MacNeil, "Western Officials Dismayed," *ibid.*, February 12, 1986.

32. *AIDS Policy & Law* 1, no. 3 (Feb. 26, 1986), 7; Dorothy Nelkin and Stephen Hilgartner, "Disputed Dimensions of Risk: A Public School Controversy Over AIDS," *The Milbank Quarterly* 64, Supplement 1, AIDS: The Public Context of an Epidemic (1986), 136–137.

33. *District 27 Community School Board v. Board of Education*, 130 Misc. 2d 398, 502 N.Y.S.2d 325 (Sup. Ct. 1986), at 335. See also Frederick A. O. Schwarz, Jr., and Frederick P. Schaffer, "AIDS in the Classroom," *Hofstra Law Review* 14, no. 1 (Fall 1985), at 176, for an in-depth discussion of this aspect of the case. Jennifer Brier, "'Save Our Kids, Keep AIDS Out'; Anti-AIDS Activism and the Legacy of Community Control in Queens, New York," *Journal of Social History* 39, no. 4 (Summer 2006), at 979–980.

34. Christopher M. MacNeil, "Ryan's Schooling is Medically OK," *Kokomo Tribune*, February 13, 1986. Ind. Code 16-1-9-7, -8, 1985 edition.

35. Associated Press, "Indiana School Told to Readmit 12-Year-Old Student With AIDS," *New York Times*, February 14, 1986. Christopher M. MacNeil, "Ryan's Schooling is Medically OK," *Kokomo Tribune*, February 13, 1986. Christopher M. MacNeil, "Ryan Poses No Threat" and "Mom's Happy Ryan's Going Back," *ibid.*, February 14, 1986.

36. Christopher M. MacNeil, "Western Plans No Further Action" and "Mom's Happy Ryan's Going Back," *ibid.*, February 14, 1986.

37. Gerald Vasconcellos to Ronald Colby, February 13, 1986, Western Middle School Library, Russiaville, IN; "Journalists Barred Friday at Western," and Christopher M. MacNeil and Dawne Slater, "State Health Chief to Resign? No Way," *Kokomo Tribune*, February 19, 1986.

38. Christopher M. MacNeil and Dawne Slater, "State Health Chief to Resign? No Way," *Kokomo Tribune*, February 19, 1986.

39. Associated Press, "Ryan Travels to New York Monday," *Kokomo Tribune*, February 16, 1986. "Journalists Barred Friday at Western," *ibid.*, February 19, 1986. White and Cunningham, *Ryan White: My Own Story*, 124–125. United Press International, "AIDS Victim 'Nervous' About Return to School," *New York Times*, February 18, 1986.

40. *Bogart et al. v. Howard County Board of Health et al.*, No. 49192 (Howard Cir. Ct., Ind. Feb. 19, 1986).

41. Transcript of proceedings, *Bogart et al. v. Howard County Board of Health et al.*, No. 49192 (Howard Cir. Ct., Ind. Feb. 19, 1986). Kay Bacon, "Court Rejects Ban on Ryan," *Kokomo Tribune*, February 19, 1986. Christopher M. MacNeil, "School Reaction Has Ryan's Mother, Officials Worried," *ibid.*, February 20, 1986.

42. Jacqueline K. and Jeffery L. Fetz, Jr., letter to the editor, *ibid.*, February 19, 1986.

43. Tammy Collier, letter to the editor, *ibid.*, February 20, 1986.

44. James Barron, "AIDS Sufferer's Return to Classes Is Cut Short," *New York Times*, February 22, 1986.

45. Christopher M. MacNeil, "100 Parents Plan Boycott at Western," *Kokomo Tribune*, February 20, 1986. Christopher M. MacNeil, "Citizens Will Take It to Court," *ibid.*, February 21, 1986.

46. *Bogart et al. v. Howard County Board of Health et al.*, No. 49192 (Howard Cir. Ct., Ind. Feb. 20, 1986). Kay Bacon, "Western Transfers Minimal, Queries Greater" and "Transfer Process Relatively Simple," *Kokomo Tribune*, February 21, 1986.

47. "AIDS Boy Back to School," and Cheryl Mattox Berry, "AIDS Victim's Return to Class Resisted," *USA Today*, February 21, 1986.

48. Christopher M. MacNeil, "Western Absentees Above 40%," *Kokomo Tribune*, February 21, 1986. "Absentee Rate is Back to Normal at Western School," *ibid.*, February 24, 1986. Donald A. Ozogar to Ronald Colby, February 21, 1986, Western Middle School Library, Russiaville, IN.

49. Susie White to Ronald Colby, February 23, 1986; Linda Cauble to Ronald Colby, February 24, 1986; Shirley Crites and Michael Crites to Ronald Colby, February 24, 1986, Western Middle School Library, Russiaville, IN.

50. Wanda Bowen Bilodeau, BBC World Service, *Witness* Archive 2011, "Witness: Ryan White," podcast audio, December 1, 2011, http://downloads.bbc.co.uk/podcasts/worldservice/witness/witness_20111201-0900a.mp3. Mark Nichols, "New Ruling Cuts Short Ryan's School Return," *Indianapolis Star*, February 22, 1986; *New York Times*, February 22, 1986, p. 6.

51. Colby interview transcript, Ryan White Project, Howard County Historical Society, Kokomo, IN. Christopher M. MacNeil, "All's Well as Ryan Goes Back to Western Classroom," *Kokomo Tribune*, February 21, 1986; "First Day Termed 'Success,'" *ibid.*, February 22, 1986.

52. Transcript of proceedings, *Bogart et al. v. White et al.*, No. 49192 (Howard Cir. Ct., Ind. Feb. 21, 1986).

53. Donald Fields, interview by Judy Lausch, June 6, 2011, transcript, Ryan White Project, Howard County Historical Society, Kokomo, IN. Transcript of proceedings, *Bogart et al. v. White et al.*, No. 49192 (Howard Cir. Ct., Ind. Feb. 21, 1986).

54. Transcript of proceedings, *Bogart et al. v. White et al.*, No. 49192 (Howard Cir. Ct., Ind. Feb. 21, 1986).

55. *Ibid.*

56. Ind. Code 16–1–9–7 and -9, 1985 edition. Transcript of proceedings, *Bogart et al. v. White et al.*, No. 49192 (Howard Cir.

Ct., Ind. Feb. 21, 1986). Indiana Constitution, Article 8, online at http://www.in.gov/history/2863.htm. "Many Hear Decision," *Kokomo Tribune*, February 22, 1986. "R. Alan Brubaker: Judge with a Secret," *Indianapolis Monthly* 18, no. 6 (Jan. 1995), 68; Transcript of proceedings, probable cause hearing, *State of Indiana v. R. Alan Brubaker*, No. 06D019407CF39 (Boone Sup. Ct. 1, Ind. July 19, 1994); "Across the USA: News from Every State," *USA Today*, October 28, 1994.

57. Colby interview transcript; David Rosselot, interview by Diane Knight and Allen Safianow, October 13, 2011, transcript, Ryan White Project, Howard County Historical Society, Kokomo, IN.

58. "Many Hear Decision," *Kokomo Tribune*, February 22, 1986. Christopher M. MacNeil, "Jeanne White Won't Give Up the Fight," *ibid.*, February 23, 1986.

59. James Barron, "AIDS Sufferer's Return to Classes Is Cut Short," *New York Times*, February 22, 1986. Editorial, "AIDS in Queens and Kokomo," *ibid.*, February 27, 1986.

Chapter 5

1. "Incumbent Wins in Indiana," *New York Times*, May 7, 1986. Kevin Roderick, "AIDS Measure Qualifies for Fall Election," *Los Angeles Times*, June 25, 1986. Kevin Roderick, "Questions on Prop. 64: Clearing the Confusion," *ibid.*, October 29, 1986.

2. Associated Press, "AIDS Spread by Air, Mosquitoes, LaRouche Says," *Los Angeles Times*, July 13, 1986. "Rally to Protest Proposition 64," *ibid.*, September 11, 1986. David L. Kirp, "Uncommon Decency: Pacific Bell Responds to AIDS," *Harvard Business Review* 67, no. 3 (May-June 1989), 148–149.

3. Kevin Roderick, "Toxics Measure Passes; AIDS Initiative Fails," *Los Angeles Times*, November 5, 1986. Kevin Roderick, "Prop. 64 Records Seized in State's LaRouche Probe," *ibid.*, November 20, 1986. On November 19, California authorities obtained a warrant to search La Rouche's state offices for evidence of illegal acts in furtherance of a criminal conspiracy behind Proposition 64, including forging signatures on petitions to get the measure on the ballot, and using out-of-state residents to circulate the petitions.

4. Robert Pear, "Rights Laws Offer Only Limited Help on AIDS, U.S. Rules," *New York Times*, June 23, 1986. Erik Eckholm, "Ruling on AIDS Provoking Dismay," *ibid.*, June 27, 1986. Wendy E. Parmet and Daniel J. Jackson, "No Longer Disabled: The Legal Impact of the New Social Construction of HIV," *American Journal of Law and Medicine* 23, no. 1 (1997), 14–16. In 1988, the Office of Legal Counsel changed its official position on this issue and advised that people who were HIV-positive but asymptomatic were handicapped and would be protected by the Rehabilitation Act of 1973.

5. Tamar Lewin, "Business and the Law: AIDS and Job Discrimination," *New York Times*, April 15, 1986. Wayne King, "Doctors Cite Stigma of AIDS in Declining to Report Cases," *ibid.*, May 27, 1986.

6. "Sanitation Workers Refuse to Work with Colleague," *AIDS Policy & Law* 1, no. 12 (July 2, 1986), 7. "Task Force Advises Against Firing, Mandatory Testing," *ibid.*, at 5. "New Guidelines Issued by NEA on Teachers, Students with AIDS," *AIDS Policy & Law* 1, no. 13 (July 16, 1986), 1, 4.

7. *Bowers v. Hardwick*, 478 U.S. 186 (1986). Larry Rohter, "Friend and Foe See Homosexual Defeat," *New York Times*, July 1, 1986. The decision was overturned in 2003 in *Lawrence v. Texas*, 539 U.S. 558 (2003). Goldsmith, "Hemophilia, Beaten on One Front, Is Beset on Others," *JAMA* 256, no. 23 (Dec. 19, 1986), 3200.

8. Kelly Lasecki, "Continental Trustee Preparing for Sale" and "Ex-Workers at Steel Firm are Worried Over Benefits," *ibid.*, February 27, 1986; "Trustee Files to Reject Pension," "Continental Salaried to Meet Sunday," and "Women's Support Meeting Set," *ibid.*, March 1, 1986.

9. "PBGC Provides Security," and Mary Ellen Podmolik, "Pension Plan to be Honored," *Kokomo Tribune*, March 2, 1986; Linda Miller, "Funds are Sought for Those Laid Off," *ibid.*, March 3, 1986; Kelly Lasecki, "Attorney Sees Sales Chance Encouraging" and "Steel Firm Interested in Continental Here?" *ibid.*, March 4, 1986.

10. Kelly Lasecki, "Continental Answers Won't be Easy," *ibid.*, March 18, 1986.

11. Barb Haberfield, letter to the editor, *Kokomo Tribune*, April 16, 1986; "Continental Steel, Region 5 Cleanup Sites, U.S. EPA," http://www.epa.gov/region5/cleanup/continental/index.htm, accessed July 29, 2012.

12. Mrs. Larry Causey, letter to the editor, *Kokomo Tribune*, June 29, 1986.

13. "Steel Skills No Use Elsewhere, Lt. Gov. John Mutz Remarks," and "Continental Financial Assist Reported Available at State," *ibid.*, August 8, 1986.

14. "Sheffield Buys Joliet," *Oklahoman*, http://newsok.com/article/2158296, Archive ID: 279964, accessed February 12, 2013; "Pension Pickets," *Kokomo Tribune*, September 24, 1986; John Schorg, "Kokomo Business Succumbs After 90 Years," *ibid.*, January 3, 1987; Mary Ellen Podmolik, "Fence Plant to Reopen?" *ibid.*, November 7, 1986.

15. Mary Ellen Podmolik, "City Looks to Different Approach," *ibid.*, December 24, 1986.

16. Sherry Lee Linkon and John Russo, *Steeltown U.S.A.: Work and Memory in Youngstown* (Lawrence: University Press of Kansas, 2002), 2–4. For the concept of a "constitutive narrative," Linkon and Russo cite the work of Robert N. Bellah et al.'s study of the meaning of community in American life, *Habits of the Heart: Individualism and Commitment in American Life* (Berkeley: University of California Press, 1985, 1996).

17. Kay Bacon, "Bond Hearing Tuesday," *Kokomo Tribune*, February 24, 1986; Kay Bacon, "Ryan's Foes Must Post a $12,000 Bond," *ibid.*, February 26, 1986.

18. "Parents Waste No Time Seeking Bond Funds," *Kokomo Tribune*, February 26, 1986; Thales Kaster, letter to editor; Margery Gilcrest-Hesse, letter to editor; Elsie Ward, letter to editor; Jeff L. Hayward, letter to editor, *ibid.*, February 27, 1986.

19. Christopher M. MacNeil, "Talk Show Irks Ryan's Mother," *ibid.*, February 28, 1986.

20. Jeanne White Ginder, interview with author, October 25, 2012, Children's Museum of Indianapolis, Indianapolis, IN. "Auction is Set to Aid Fight," *Kokomo Tribune*, February 28, 1986.

21. "Auction Is Set to Aid Fight," *Kokomo Tribune*, February 28, 1986; Kay Bacon, "AIDS Victim Opponents Reach Bond Money Goal," *ibid.*, March 3, 1986.

22. White and Cunningham, *Ryan White: My Own Story*, 112. For Ryan's description of the auction, see pp. 137–138. Steve Bell, "Look Back in Anger,"

Indianapolis Monthly 9, no. 11 (July 1986), 57. Ken Ford, "'Male Call' Has What It Takes," *Kokomo Tribune*, February 17, 1984. "WWKI Presents the Popular 'Mike' Show: 'Male Call for the Ladies,'" *Our Town* 2, no. 1 (Spring, 1980), 3. "History," WWKI-We Care, http://www.wecareonline.com/files/history.html, accessed October 1, 2012.

23. Bell, "Look Back in Anger," *Indianapolis Monthly*, 57.

24. *Ibid.* at 57–58, 104.

25. Kay Bacon, "AIDS Victim Opponents Reach Bond Money Goal," *Kokomo Tribune*, March 3, 1986; Kelly Lasecki, "Attorney Sees Sales Chance Encouraging," *ibid.*, March 4, 1986. Rogers Worthington, "Kokomo Bristles Over Publicity on AIDS Boy's Plight," *Chicago Tribune*, March 4, 1986.

26. "Wet T-Shirt, Briefs Contest to Help Continental's Jobless," and Josh Schorg, "Jobless May Be in for a Wait," *Kokomo Tribune*, March 5, 1986. Elmer and Emma Jean Gunnell, letter to the editor, and Mrs. Pendu Miller, letter to the editor, *ibid.*, March 6, 1986.

27. David A. Parrish and H. D. Waterman, letters to the editor, *ibid.*, March 6, 1986.

28. Carla Leffert and Ron DeGraaff, letters to the editor, *ibid.*, March 6, 1986.

29. Homer and Gail Trammell, letter to the editor, *ibid.*, March 5, 1986. Smith to Colby, March 19, 1986, Western Middle School Library, Russiaville, IN.

30. Anonymous correspondence, March 1986, Western Middle School Library, Russiaville, IN.

31. Fritz to Colby, March 8, 1986, Western Middle School Library, Russiaville, IN.

32. "Rosselot to Run," *Kokomo Tribune*, March 7, 1986. "Donations Accepted for Workers," and Bob Garrison, "Continental Widow Trying to Get Insurance," *ibid.*, March 9, 1986.

33. Christopher M. MacNeil, "AIDS: Town Spared Turmoil" and "He's Just Another Kid," *Kokomo Tribune*, March 9, 1986.

34. Thomas Hale, letter to the editor, *Kokomo Tribune*, March 13, 1986. Christopher M. MacNeil, "Ryan Fund to Help Other Kids," *ibid.*, March 11, 1986. Christopher M. MacNeil, "Methodists Offer Support to AIDS Victims" and "Ministers to Discuss Resolution," *ibid.*, March 16, 1986. Christopher M. MacNeil, "Local Ministers Approve AIDS Research Fund Drive," *ibid.*, March 19, 1986. United Press International, "Teen-Age AIDS Victim Learns Science at Home," *New York Times*, March 11, 1986. Frances Sempsel Hardin, interview by Diane Knight, April 26, 2011, transcript, Ryan White Project, Howard County Historical Society, Kokomo, IN.

35. Kay Bacon, "Ryan's Case to be Moved," *Kokomo Tribune*, March 13, 1986. "White Case Moves to Clinton County," *ibid.*, March 20, 1986. Kay Smith, letter to the editor, *ibid.*, March 20, 1986. Minutes of the Court, *Bogart et al. v. White et al.*, No. 49192 (Howard Cir. Ct., Ind., March 18, 1986).

36. Christopher M. MacNeil, "Local Ministers Approve AIDS Research Fund Drive," *Kokomo Tribune*, March 19, 1986. Christopher M. MacNeil, "White Says Benefit Could be Starting Point," *ibid.*, March 23, 1986.

37. Christopher M. MacNeil, "Ryan to Join National Fund Drive," *Kokomo Tribune*, March 26, 1986.

38. White and Cunningham, *Ryan White: My Own Story*, 134–135; Jeanne White Ginder, interview with author, October 25, 2012, Children's Museum of Indianapolis, Indianapolis, IN.

39. "Judge Sets April 9 Hearing for Ryan," *Kokomo Tribune*, April 5, 1986. Fran Richardson, "ICLU Filing Brief for AIDS Victim," *ibid.*, April 8, 1986. "Judge Rules Against Motion to Dismiss Injunction Suit," *ibid.*, April 10, 1986. "Brief of the Indiana Civil Liberties Union Amicus Curiae Submitted for the Hearing of April 9, 1986," *Bogart et al. v. White et al.*, No. 86–144 (Clinton Cir. Ct., Ind., April 8, 1986).

40. Sylvia Payne, letter to the editor, *Kokomo Tribune*, April 4, 1986.

41. Miriam E. Stewart and David Kaufman, letters to the editor, *Fort Wayne Journal Gazette*, March 22 or 24, 1986.

42. "Findings of Fact and Order," *Bogart et al. v. White et al.*, No. 86–144 (Clinton Cir. Ct., Ind., April 10, 1986). Kay Bacon, "Ryan's Back in Class," *Kokomo Tribune*, April 10, 1986. David Rosselot interview transcript, Ryan White Project, Howard County Historical Society, Kokomo, IN.

43. United Press International, "Indiana Judge Allows AIDS Victim Back in School," *New York Times*, April 11, 1986.

44. Kay Bacon, "Reports About Ryan Take Little Time to Travel," *Kokomo*

Tribune, April 11, 1986. White and Cunningham, *Ryan White: My Own Story*, 141–142.

45. Kay Bacon, "Parents Facing Liability Risks" and "Western Records Fewer Absences," *Kokomo Tribune*, April 11, 1986. Mary Kaull, "Teen AIDS Victim Returns to School; Lawyers to Appeal," *USA Today*, April 11, 1986. The *New York Times* did mention that fact in an article it ran when Ryan died, however, on April 9, 1990: Dirk Johnson, "Ryan White Dies of AIDS at 18: His Struggle Helped Pierce Myths," *New York Times*, April 9, 1990.

46. Sr. Julia Delaney to Ronald Colby, April 11, 1986, Western Middle School Library, Russiaville, IN.

47. Bob Garrison, "AIDS Campaign Suggested Here," *Kokomo Tribune*, April 13, 1986. Noel and Dianna Vandevender et al., letter to the editor, *ibid.*, April 15, 1986.

48. United Press International, "AIDS Victim Ryan White Decides Against Taking Bus to School," *Fort Wayne Journal Gazette*, April 15, 1986.

49. "Parents Are Invited to Home Study Meeting," *Kokomo Tribune*, April 17, 1986. Nikole Hannah-Jones, "It Was Never About Busing," *New York Times*, July 12, 2019. Associated Press, "Special Classes Start Tuesday," *Kokomo Tribune,* April 19, 1986.

50. United Press International, "Special School Planned to Avoid AIDS Victim," *New York Times*, April 20, 1986.

51. Mitzie Johnson, interview by Diane Knight, June 30, 2011, transcript, Ryan White Project, Howard County Historical Society, Kokomo, IN.

52. Arletta Reith, interview by Allen Safianow, February 16, 2011, transcript, Ryan White Project, Howard County Historical Society, Kokomo, IN.

53. Associated Press, "Louganis Keeps U.S. Diving Title," *New York Times*, April 21, 1986. Associated Press, "Mettle Earns Ryan a Medal," *Kokomo Tribune*, April 21, 1986. Christopher M. MacNeil, "Ryan Skips School 5 Days for AIDS Benefit," *ibid.*, April 23, 1986.

54. Michael Gross, "Fashion Industry Turns Out in Force for AIDS Benefit," *New York Times*, April 30, 1986. Associated Press, "Fashion, Glitter Party for AIDS/Back to Court for Ryan," *Kokomo Tribune*, April 30, 1986. Associated Press, "White in NYC for Benefit," *Fort Wayne News Sentinel*, April 30, 1986.

55. Kay Bacon, "Ryan Will Remain, Judge Rules," and Christopher M. MacNeil, "Ryan's Trip to New York 'Great,'" *Kokomo Tribune*, May 1, 1986.

56. Bell, "Look Back in Anger," *Indianapolis Monthly*, 57. White and Cunningham, *Ryan White: My Own Story*, 144. *Bogart et al. v. White et al.*, No. 86–144 (Clinton Cir. Ct., Ind., July 22, 1986). Associated Press, "Parents Drop Effort To Bar AIDS Student," *New York Times*, July 19, 1986. Associated Press and Bob Garrison, "Parents End Battle Against Ryan," *Kokomo Tribune*, July 19, 1986. *Ryan White b/n/f Jeanne White v. Western School Corporation et al.*, IP 85–1192-C (S. D. Ind., November 24, December 1, 1986).

57. Christopher M. MacNeil, "Ryan's Trip to New York 'Great,'" *Kokomo Tribune*, May 1, 1986. Christopher M. MacNeil, "Local AIDS Patient Ineligible for Experimental Treatment," *ibid.*, December 7, 1986. Bell, "Look Back in Anger," *Indianapolis Monthly*, 56–58. John Wiles, interview by Judy Lausch, July 14, 2008, transcript, Howard County Historical Society, Kokomo, IN.

58. Kay Bacon, "School Year Starts for Ryan White," *Kokomo Tribune*, August 23, 1986.

59. "Excited AIDS Victim Back in School: Some Concerned," *Los Angeles Times*, August 25, 1986. "AIDS Victim Starts 8th Grade After Opponents Drop Battle," *ibid.*, August 26, 1986. Associated Press, "14-Year-Old Boy with AIDS Attends School After 2 Years," *New York Times*, August 26, 1986. AP News Archive, September 5, 1986, http://www.apnewsarchive.com/1986/Group-That-Fought-AIDS-Victim-Ryan-White-Will-Announce-National-Organization/id-c0a3c751f6bac6968a89c1443b0e6d4a. accessed May 21, 2013.

60. Jeanne White and Susan Dworkin, *Weeding Out the Tears: A Mother's Story of Love, Loss and Renewal* (New York: Avon Books, 1997), 87–89. William Narwold, interview by Allen Safianow, May 4, 2011, transcript, Ryan White Project, Howard County Historical Society, Kokomo, IN.

61. Ken de la Bastide, "BBC Special Focusing on White," *Kokomo Tribune*, December 1, 2011. Wanda Bowen Bilodeau, BBC World Service, *Witness Archive 2011*, "Witness: Ryan White," podcast audio, December 1, 2011, http://downloads.bbc.co.uk/podcasts/

worldservice/witness/witness_20111201-0900a.mp3. Wanda Bilodeau, interview by Allen Safianow, June 7, 2011, transcript; and Chantel Kebrdle, interview by Allen Safianow, November 5, 2010, transcript, Ryan White Project, Howard County Historical Society, Kokomo, IN.

62. James C. Scott, *Domination and the Arts of Resistance: Hidden Transcripts* (New Haven: Yale University Press, 1990), 4–5, 14.

63. Jay Hoyle, *Mark: How a Boy's Courage in Facing AIDS Inspired a Town and the Town's Compassion Lit Up a Nation* (South Bend, IN: Langford Books, 1988), 207, 206–217; 227, 239, 243, 247. "Ryan White, 14, Back in Hospital," *Kokomo Tribune*, September 17, 1986. "Ryan White to be Released Soon," *ibid.*, September 18, 1986. "AIDS Victim Out of Riley Hospital," *ibid.*, September 21, 1986.

64. "That's What Friends Are For" won a Grammy in 1986 for Best Pop Performance by a Duo or Group with Vocal; Warwick, along with Elton John, Gladys Knight, and Stevie Wonder, took home statuettes. The royalties from the song were donated to amfAR. http://www.grammy.com/nominees/search?artist=Dionne+Warwick+and+Friends&field_nominee_work_value=That%27s+What+Friends+are+for&year=All&genre=All, accessed May 23, 2013. Hoyle, *Mark: How a Boy's Courage in Facing AIDS Inspired a Town and the Town's Compassion Lit Up a Nation*, 130–137; 157–158; 172–173; 151–153; 187–188.

65. Hoyle, *Mark: How a Boy's Courage in Facing AIDS Inspired a Town and the Town's Compassion Lit Up a Nation*, 149–150, 184, 250–51, 264, 272–274, 276, 279; http://hoyle.swanseaschools.org, accessed May 23, 2013.

66. Randy Lewis, "Pop Review: Elton John Stirs Up Memories," *Los Angeles Times*, October 6, 1986. White and Cunningham, *Ryan White: My Own Story*, 165–166. Associated Press, "Media Credited in Return to School of Teen with AIDS," *Indianapolis Star*, October 12, 1986.

67. White and Cunningham, *Ryan White: My Own Story*, 147–153. "FDA Clears Wider Testing Of AZT, a New AIDS Drug," *Wall Street Journal*, October 1, 1986. Associated Press, "Teen-Age AIDS Victim Ryan White in Hospital," *Los Angeles Times*, November 9, 1986. Associated Press, "Teen with AIDS to Return to School," *ibid.*,

November 18, 1986. "Ryan White in Hospital," *Indianapolis Star*, November 9, 1986. "Ryan White Home After Hospital Stay," *ibid.*, November 16, 1986. "Ryan White's Legal Battle Selected as Year's Top Story," *ibid.*, December 28, 1986. Associated Press, "AIDS Victim Gets Tests," *New York Times*, November 9, 1986.

68. Bob Garrison, "Whites Speak at AIDS Conference," *Kokomo Tribune*, February 8, 1987. "Mandatory Tests Won't Stop AIDS, Officials Say," *Indianapolis Star*, February 7, 1987. George Stuteville, "Victim's Mother Says AIDS Will Touch All in Some Way," *ibid.*, February 8, 1987.

69. "Kokomo Police Department, Initial Case Report," MSC 336, Ken Ferries Collection, 2011.012.0007, Police Reports, White Family, Box 33, Folder 7, Howard County Historical Society. Jeanne White Ginder, interview with author, October 25, 2012, Children's Museum of Indianapolis, Indianapolis, IN. "Kokomo Singing New Tune," and Associated Press, "Klan Marches in Delphi," *Kokomo Tribune*, March 15, 1987.

70. Fran Richardson, "It Was Smooth Sailing for Ryan," *ibid.*, August 31, 1987. Jeanne White Ginder, interview with author, October 25, 2012, Children's Museum of Indianapolis, Indianapolis, IN.

Chapter 6

1. Jeanne White and Susan Dworkin, *Weeding Out the Tears: A Mother's Story of Love, Loss, and Renewal* (New York: Avon Books, 1997), 114–115. Jeanne White Ginder, interview with author, October 25, 2012, Children's Museum of Indianapolis, Indianapolis, IN.

2. *Ibid.* at 105.

3. "Whites Moving to Area," *Heights Herald*, May 7, 1987, Ken Ferries Collection, Howard County Historical Society.

4. "School Board OKs Plan to Evoke Law," *Heights Herald*, May 14, 1987, 1–2. Ken Ferries Collection, Howard County Historical Society.

5. Kim Painter, "A Checked History of Tragedy, Despair and Hope," *USA Today*, June 4, 1991. "An AIDS Drug, at a Cost," *New York Times*, March 25, 1987.

6. Bradford Martin, *The Other Eighties: A Secret History of America in the Age of Reagan* (New York: Hill and Wang, 2011), 171–173. "An AIDS Drug, at a Cost," *New*

York Times, March 25, 1987. Bruce Lambert, "3,000 Assailing Policy on AIDS Ring City Hall: 200 Arrested as Koch Is Criticized Over Funds," *ibid.*, March 29, 1989.

7. Susan Okie, "AIDS Coalition Targets FDA for Demonstration," *Washington Post*, October 11, 1988. Paul Duggan, "1,000 Swarm FDA's Rockville Office To Demand Approval of AIDS Drugs," *ibid.*, October 12, 1988. Martin, *The Other Eighties: A Secret History of America in the Age of Reagan*, 174–177. Thomas Becher, "'Die-In' Staged to Protest Supervisors' Vote on AIDS Law," *Los Angeles Times*, June 21, 1989.

8. Thomas Becher, "'Die-In' Staged to Protest Supervisors' Vote on AIDS Law," *Los Angeles Times*, June 21, 1989. Joyce Purnick, "Arson Damages Disputed Foster Home in Queens," *New York Times*, April 22, 1987. Jane Gross, "Babies to Have AIDS Center in Harlem," *ibid.*, May 8, 1987. Esther Iverem, "Rise Seen in 'Boarder Babies,' But More Are Finding Homes," *ibid.*, May 31, 1987.

9. Text of Executive Order 12601, Presidential Commission on the Human Immunodeficiency Virus Epidemic, June 24, 1987, Ronald Reagan Presidential Library, National Archives and Records Administration, http://www.reagan.utexas.edu/archives/speeches/1987/062487c.htm, accessed September 5, 2016; Jonathan Fuerbringer, "Senate Votes to Require Test of Aliens for AIDS Virus," *New York Times*, June 3, 1987; Associated Press, "Callers Threaten to Kill Brothers," *Kokomo Tribune*, August 24, 1987. Associated Press, "Hoosier Teen to be in TV Film About AIDS Fears," *ibid.*, June 27, 1988. "Family in AIDS Case Quits Florida Town After House Burns," *New York Times*, August 30, 1987. White and Dworkin, *Weeding Out the Tears: A Mother's Story of Love, Loss, and Renewal*, 152. David L. Kirp et al., *Learning by Heart: AIDS and Schoolchildren in America's Communities* (New Brunswick: Rutgers University Press, 1989), 1. Associated Press, "Honor for Battling AIDS Fear," *New York Times*, April 12, 1989.

10. Shawn Decker, *My Pet Virus: The True Story of a Rebel Without a Cure* (New York: Penguin, 2006), 5, 42, 44–52. Pam Decker to Jeanne White, January 26, 1989, Ryan White Collection, E—Todd Cummings Dissertation Sources, Children's Museum of Indianapolis, Indianapolis, Indiana.

11. Associated Press, "Students Weep Over Boy's Leaving School," *Kokomo Tribune*, September 11, 1987. Kevin T. McGee, "AIDS Panel Chief Speaks; His Emphasis: Education," *USA Today*, June 23, 1988. "AIDS-Infected Boy to be Taught at Home in Wake of Threats," Associated Press, September 10, 1987, http://www.apnewsarchive.com/1987/AIDS-Infected-Boy-To-Be-Taught-At-Home-In-Wake-of-Threats/id-2706dda8e5ae7d0d0bf657f4b10f630d, accessed February 21, 2015.

12. Allyn Stone and Jeff Pelline, "Airlines' Confusing Policy for AIDS Passengers," *San Francisco Chronicle*, August 15, 1987.

13. Kim Painter, "A Checkered History of Tragedy, Despair and Hope," *USA Today*, June 4, 1991. Kim Painter, "AIDS Quilt: A Labor of Love for 25 Years," *ibid.*, June 22, 2012. Cleve Jones and Jeff Dawson, *Stitching a Revolution: The Making of an Activist* (New York: Harper Collins, 2000, 2001), 1, 166–167; http://www.oscars.org/oscars/ceremonies/1990, accessed February 21, 2015.

14. The Global AIDS Situation: WHO Update, January, 1988," *American Journal of Public Health* 78, no. 4 (April, 1988), 410. Koop, *Koop: The Memoirs of America's Family Doctor* (New York: Random House, 1991), 235. Susan Okie, "Much Hostility Seen Toward AIDS Carriers," *Washington Post*, October 13, 1988.

15. Susan Okie, "Much Hostility Seen Toward AIDS Carriers," *Washington Post*, October 13, 1988. Even in the later poll, one-third of parents said they would consider withdrawing their children from school if another child in the class had AIDS. Shawn Decker, "A Boy, a Virus, and the Education of a Community," *The Times Gone By*, January 15, 2014. http://www.waynesboroheritagefoundation.com/boy-virus-education-community, accessed January 20, 2014.

16. Margaret V. Ragni, "Medical Aspects of Hemophilia and AIDS," *FOCUS: A Guide to AIDS Research* 4, no. 5 (April 1989), 1–2. Dirk Scheerhorn, "Hemophilia in the Days of AIDS: Communicative Tensions Surrounding 'Associated Stigmas,'" *Communication Research* 17, no. 6 (Dec. 1990), 845.

17. *Ibid.*, 846.

18. Mary Douglas, *Purity and Danger: An Analysis of Concept of Pollution and Taboo* (London: Routledge, 1966,

2002), 140. Angelo A. Alonzo and Nancy R. Reynolds, "Stigma, HIV and AIDS: An Exploration and Elaboration of a Stigma Trajectory," *Social Science & Medicine* 41, no. 3 (1995), 305.

19. Erving Goffman, *Stigma: Notes on the Management of Spoiled Identity* (New York: Simon & Schuster, 1963, 1986), 1–2, 5.

20. Richard Sennett, *Flesh and Stone: The Body and the City in Western Civilization* (New York: W.W. Norton, 1994, 1996), 223. Nayan Shah, *Contagious Divides: Epidemics and Race in San Francisco's Chinatown* (Berkeley: University of California Press, 2001), 120–125. Patricia J. Fanning, *Influenza and Inequality: One Town's Tragic Response to the Great Epidemic of 1918* (Amherst: University of Massachusetts Press, 2010), 68.

21. Christopher M. MacNeil, interview with author, September 18, 2013, Grand Wayne Center, Fort Wayne, IN.

22. P. L. Kauble, letter to the editor, *Kokomo Tribune*, August 11, 1987. Trustee's "Notice to All Former Employees of Continental Steel Corporation," *ibid.*, March 11, 1988 (Classifieds section). "Multiple Factors Brought Mill's Downfall," *ibid.*, March 27, 1988.

23. Mary Ellen Podmolik, "Judge Divvies Up Part of Continental," *Kokomo Tribune*, April 6, 1988. Mary Ellen Podmolik, "All Parties Benefit with Settlement," *ibid.*, April 13, 1988.

24. *Ibid.*, April 13, 1988. Thomas Hamilton, letter to the editor, *ibid.*, September 23, 1988. Dave Phillips, "Continental Distribution Begins," *ibid.*, July 1, 1989. "Checks Mailed," *ibid.*, November 14, 1989.

25. Indiana Department of Environmental Management, *First Five-Year Review Report for Continental Steel Superfund Site, City of Kokomo, Howard County, Indiana* (July 2002), 10–12; http://www.epa.gov/region5/superfund/fiveyear/reviews_pdf/indiana/continental_steel.pdf, accessed March 21, 2013. *Health Effects of PCBs*, http://www.epa.gov/osw/hazard/tsd/pcbs/pubs/effects.htm, accessed February 2, 2014.

26. *First Five-Year Review Report* at 10–11.

27. Kate Conlon, "Lagoons May Get 'Superfund' Aid," *Kokomo Tribune*, June 22, 1988. "Status of Continental Site Itemized by Federal Agency," December 1,

1989; *First Five-Year Review Report* at 13; ND001213503, NPL Fact Sheet, Region 5 Superfund, U.S. EPA, *Continental Steel Corp.*, http://www.epa.gov/region5/superfund/npl/indiana/IND001213503.html, accessed February 7, 2013.

28. B. Haberfield, letter to the editor, *Kokomo Tribune*, July 7, 1988. Anne Schmitt, "New Zoning Could Spur Growth," *ibid.*, October 27, 1989. Maureen Groppe, "Group Concerned About Continental," *ibid.*, January 14, 1990. "EPA is Asking for Your Call," *ibid.*, March 7, 1990. Dave Phillips, "PSI Scraps Continental Steel Marketing Plans," *ibid.*, March 18, 1990. Amy Bell, "Wildcat's PCBs Plague Creek," *Logansport Pharos Tribune*, April 8, 1990.

29. Christopher M. MacNeil, interview with author, September 18, 2013, Grand Wayne Center, Fort Wayne, IN. Of Curie, Rich wrote: "She died a famous woman denying/her wounds/denying/her wounds came from the same source as her power." Adrienne Rich, "Power," in *The Dream of a Common Language: Poems 1974–1977* (New York: W. W. Norton, 1978, 2013), 3.

30. Trump family to Ryan White, 1987, Ryan White Collection, C—1986–1989 cards, letters, oversized envelopes, Uncatalogued, Children's Museum of Indianapolis, Indianapolis, Indiana. White and Dworkin, *Weeding Out the Tears: A Mother's Story of Love, Loss, and Renewal*, 115–116. Ryan White and Ann Marie Cunningham, *Ryan White: My Own Story* (New York: Signet, 1992), 159.

31. Judy Kessler, *Inside People: The Stories Behind the Stories* (New York: Villard Books, 1994), 180–182; *People*, August 3, 1987.

32. *People*, August 3, August 24, 1987.

33. *Ibid.*, August 24, 1987.

34. White and Cunningham, *Ryan White: My Own Story*, 171–173. John Norberg, "AIDS, School and Ryan White: People Friendlier in a New City," *USA Today*, August 28, 1987.

35. White and Cunningham, *Ryan White: My Own Story*, 167, 174–175. Beth L. Rosenberg, "Classmates Warmly Greet Ryan on 1st Day," *Indianapolis Star*, September 1, 1987. Associated Press, "White Reports to Class Monday," *Kokomo Tribune*, August 30, 1987. "News: Indiana," *USA Today*, August 31, 1987. "AIDS Boy Gets Welcome; School Went 'Really Great,'" *ibid.*, September 1, 1987. Associated Press,

"Indiana Teen-ager With AIDS Ready to Start School Today," *New York Times*, August 31, 1987. Associated Press, "A Warm Welcome in Indiana," *ibid.*, September 1, 1987.

36. White and Dworkin, *Weeding Out the Tears: A Mother's Story of Love, Loss, and Renewal*, 116. Kyle Niederpruem, "Orr Honors School for Accepting Ryan White," *Indianapolis Star*, December 19, 1987. Associated Press, "Governor to Honor Ryan and Jeanne White," *Kokomo Tribune*, December 17, 1987. Associated Press, "Governor Honors White, His Mother," *ibid.*, December 19, 1987. Cory SerVaas, "The Happier Days for Ryan White," *Saturday Evening Post* 260, no. 2 (Mar. 1988), 56.

37. *People*, May 30, June 20, 1988.

38. *People*, July 11, 1988. White and Cunningham, *Ryan White: My Own Story*, 195–212. Steve Hall, "Ryan White to Be in Film About His Life," *Indianapolis Star*, August 1, 1988. Michelle Cohen, "Ryan White Enjoys Filming Own Life," *ibid.*, September 14, 1988. Associated Press, "AIDS Victim Appears in Movie," *Kokomo Tribune*, August 22, 1988. Steve Marshall, "Ryan White to Play Part in Movie About Himself," *USA Today*, August 2, 1988.

39. Kate Conlon, "Ryan White Has Role in Movie," *Kokomo Tribune*, September 21, 1988. Matt Roush, "A Teen's Look at AIDS," *USA Today*, September 30, 1988. Don Shirley, "Teen's Story Puts Human Face on AIDS Education," Television Reviews, *Los Angeles Times*, October 29, 1988. Jeremy Gerard, "Teen-Ager With AIDS," TV Notes, *New York Times*, October 6, 1988. Advertisement, "I Have AIDS—A Teenager's Story," *ibid.*, October 7, 1988. John J. O'Connor, "Second Look at the Liberace Legend," *ibid.*, October 8, 1988. "Positive Attitude," For Children, *ibid.*, October 9, 1988.

40. Christopher Todd Cummings, "A Case Study of the Fan Letters of Ryan White: The Stigma of Disclosure" (PhD diss., Indiana State University, 2008), 58–60, 69–70, ISU Thesis Collection, RC606.55.A95 C86 2008. Ryan Atwell to Ryan White, September 1, 1988, Ryan White Collection, C, 1986–1989, Uncatalogued, Children's Museum of Indianapolis, Indianapolis, Indiana. "'Ryan White Story' to Appear on TV," *Kokomo Tribune*, December 19, 1988.

41. Paul Hendrie, "Ryan White Movie Depicts Hardships," *Kokomo Tribune*, January 8, 1989. *USA Weekend* magazine section, January 13–15, 1989.

42. Richard K. Shull, "Ryan White Revisited," *Indianapolis News*, January 14, 1989. BBC World Service, Witness Archive 2011, "Witness: Ryan White," podcast audio, December 1, 2011, http://downloads. bbc.co.uk/podcasts/worldservice/witness/witness_20111201-0900a.mp3. John J. O'Connor, "AIDS and Hemophilia," *New York Times*, January 16, 1989. Scott L. Miley, "Ryan White Film Flops in Kokomo," *Indianapolis Star*, January 18, 1989. Dave Wiethop, "Cop Movie Topples White Story," *Kokomo Tribune*, January 18, 1989. Garret Floyd, The Joe Campbells, Steve Alley, Susan Sandberg, Amy Royal, Stacy Miller, C. Main, and David and Robyn Schaetzel, letters to the editor, *ibid.*, January 20, 1989.

43. Dave Wiethop, "AIDS Movie Stirs Opposing Emotions," *Kokomo Tribune*, January 17, 1989.

44. Rosemary Curnutt to Ryan White, January 27, 1989; Gayle Schertenleib to city of Cicero, Indiana, undated; Gary Morgan to Ryan White, January 18, 1989, Ryan White Collection, D, 1989 cards and letters, Uncatalogued, Children's Museum of Indianapolis, Indianapolis, Indiana. Ken Ferries Collection, Box 33, MSC 336, Folder 1, Howard County Historical Society, Kokomo, Indiana.

45. Ken Ferries, interview by Allen Safianow, November 23, 2010, transcript, Ryan White Project, Howard County Historical Society, Kokomo, Indiana. Joan Shropshire to Robert Sargent, February 6, 1989, Ken Ferries Collection, Box 33, MSC 336, Folder 1, Howard County Historical Society, Kokomo, Indiana.

46. Alonzo and Reynolds, "Stigma, HIV and AIDS," 304.

47. John Wiles, Ken Ferries, interview by Judy Lausch, July 14, 2008, transcript, Ryan White Project, Howard County Historical Society, Kokomo, IN. David Whitman, "To a Poster Child, Dying Young," *U.S. News & World Report*, April 16, 1990, 8. Lee Edelman, *No Future: Queer Theory and the Death Drive* (Durham: Duke University Press, 2004), 19. Cathy J. Cohen, *The Boundaries of Blackness: AIDS and the Breakdown of Black Politics* (Chicago: University of Chicago Press, 1999), 172–173.

48. Alonzo and Reynolds, "Stigma, HIV, and AIDS," 304; Jeri Malone, interview by Judy Lausch, February 9, 2011,

Notes—Chapter 7 217

transcript, Ryan White Project, Howard County Historical Society, Kokomo, IN; Ken Ferries, interview transcript, Howard County Historical Society, Kokomo, IN.

49. White and Dworkin, *Weeding Out the Tears*, 125, 127, 131–133. White and Cunningham, *Ryan White: My Own Story*, 248, 255, 258–259. "AIDS TV Spot Features White," *Kokomo Tribune*, November 30, 1989. Associated Press, "Ryan Must Wait for Surgery," *ibid.*, December 1, 1989. Associated Press, "White Has Visit at Jackson Ranch," *ibid.*, January 3, 1990. Dave Wiethop, "Ryan's Doctor, Family Optimistic," *ibid.*, April 4, 1990. Associated Press, "TV Message by Ryan White Key in State AIDS Campaign," *Indianapolis Star*, December 3, 1989. Paul Clancy, "Teen Faces Surgery," *USA Today*, December 1, 1989. "News: Briefly," *ibid.*, December 7, 1989.

50. Linda Gillis, "Calls Pour in for Ryan White," *Indianapolis News*, April 4, 1990. George Stuteville, "Ryan's Fight for Life Garners Respect, Admiration of Many," *Indianapolis Star*, April 6, 1990. George Stuteville, "Celebrities Rally Around Ryan," *ibid.*, April 4, 1990. George Papajohn, "Ryan White's Old Town Fights 'Rap,'" *Chicago Tribune*, April 5, 1990. Judy Keen and Desda Moss, "Ryan Inspired Dignity for All AIDS Patients," *USA Today*, April 3, 1990. Steve Marshall and Richard Benedetto, "Ryan Continues Fight; Celebrities Honor Him," *ibid.*, April 4, 1990; Paul Leavitt, "News: Nationline," *ibid.*, April 5, 1990; Edna Gundersen and David Zimmerman, "Farm Aid IV Reaps $1.3 Million So Far," *ibid.*, April 9, 1990.

51. "Nation Grieves Ryan's Death," *Kokomo Tribune*, April 9, 1990. Associated Press, "Vigil Honors Ryan White," *ibid.*, April 10, 1990. Pamela Palmer and Patricia Bartlett, letters to the editor, *Kokomo Tribune*, April 10, 1990, Ken Ferries Collection, Box 33, MSC 336, Folder 1, Howard County Historical Society, Kokomo, IN.

52. Betty Mosteller to Western Middle School, April 10, 1990, correspondence, Western Middle School Library, Russiaville, IN.

53. Laura Cheng to Jeanne and Andrea White, April 10, 1990; Ryan White Collection, A, Condolence/sympathy cards, Uncatalogued; Michael E. Sharkey to Jeanne White, April 11, 1990, Ryan White Collection, E, Todd Cummings

Dissertation Sources, Children's Museum of Indianapolis, Indianapolis, Indiana. Ken Kusmer, "White Family Receives Friends at Mortuary," *Kokomo Tribune*, April 11, 1990. Dave Wiethop, "A Solemn Celebration for Ryan," *ibid.*, April 12, 1990.

Chapter 7

1. *People*, April 23, May 14, 1990.
2. *People*, May 14, 1990.
3. Debbie Howlett, "Mother Keeps Up Ryan's Fight," *USA Today*, April 27, 1990; Bob Minzesheimer, "Senate Nears Vote on AIDS Bill; Federal AIDS Funds," *ibid.*, May 16, 1990. Jeanne White and Susan Dworkin, *Weeding Out the Tears: A Mother's Story of Love, Loss, and Renewal* (New York: Avon Books, 1997), 16–19.
4. Susan F. Rasky, "How the Politics Shifted on AIDS Funds," *New York Times*, May 20, 1990; "Senate Approves Measures on Transit and AIDS," *ibid.*, August 6, 1990. Carol Memmott, "Activists: $882M in AIDS Help Falls Short," *USA Today*, August 20, 1990.
5. Elaine DePrince, *Cry Bloody Murder: A Tale of Tainted Blood* (New York: Random House, 1997), 15, 42–44, 173–176.
6. Holly Selby, "AIDS Virus Haunts a Generation of Hemophiliacs," *Baltimore Sun*, September 19, 1993. Heather M. Johnson, "Resolution of Mass Product Liability Litigation Within the Federal Rules: A Case for the Increased Use of Rule 23(b)(3) Class Actions," *Fordham Law Review* 64, no. 5 (1996), 2340; Lauren B. Leveton, Harold C. Sox, Jr., and Michael A. Stoto, eds., *HIV and the Blood Supply: An Analysis of Crisis Decisionmaking* (Washington, D.C.: National Academy Press, 1995), 22.
7. John Fairhall, "Miles Inc. Gets German Name of Parent-Company Bayer," *Baltimore Sun*, April 4, 1995; Johnson, "Resolution of Mass Product Liability Litigation Within the Federal Rules," 2341–2343; George W. Conk, "Is There a Design Defect in the *Restatement (Third) of Torts: Products Liability*?," *Yale Law Journal* 109 (1999–2000), 1113; *Wadleigh et al. v. Rhone-Poulenc Rorer et al.*, 157 F.R.D. 410 (N.D. Ill., 1994), at 414; Leveton, Sox, Jr., and Stoto, eds., *HIV and the Blood Supply: An Analysis of Crisis Decisionmaking*, 31.
8. *Ibid.*; Johnson, "Resolution of Mass Product Liability Litigation Within the

Federal Rules," 2343–2344; *In the Matter of: Rhone-Poulenc Rorer Incorporated, et al.*, 51 F.3d 1293 (7th Cir. 1995). United States Securities and Exchange Commission Form 10-Q, filed May 13, 1996, Rhone-Poulenc Rorer, Inc., http://www.sec.gov/Archives/edgar/containers/fix041/217028/0000217028-96-000014.txt., accessed March 30, 2014.

9. *JKB, Sr., and VB v. Armour Pharmaceutical Company, Cutter Laboratories, Division of Miles, Inc., Baxter Healthcare Corporation, and Alpha Therapeutics Corporation*, 660 N.E.2d 602 (Ind. Ct. App. 1996); Wailoo, *Pain: A Political History*, 7–8; David Ray Papke, "The American Legal Faith: Traditions, Contradictions and Possibilities," *Ind. L. Rev.* 30, no. 3 (1997), 646, 655.

10. Douglas Starr, *Blood: An Epic History of Medicine and Commerce* (New York: Alfred A. Knopf, 1998), 282; 303–315; 327–335. The French physicians' convictions were reversed after a law was passed in 2000 changing the degree of proof required in such cases. See Victoria A. Harden, *AIDS at 30: A History* (Washington, D.C.: Potomac Books, 2012), 91.

11. Leveton, Sox, Jr., and Stoto, eds., *HIV and the Blood Supply: An Analysis of Crisis Decisionmaking*, Chapter 8, "Conclusions and Recommendations," 207–235.

12. Starr, *Blood: An Epic History of Medicine and Commerce*, 341–342.

13. Robin Finn, "Arthur Ashe, Tennis Star, Is Dead at 49," *New York Times*, February 8, 1993. Katharine Q. Seelye, "Helms Puts the Brakes to a Bill Financing AIDS Treatment," *ibid.*, July 5, 1995. David W. Dunlap, "Different Faces of AIDS Are Conjured Up by Politicians," *ibid.*, July 8, 1995. Jim Smith, letter to the editor, *ibid.*, July 9, 1995.

14. Susan Resnik, *Blood Saga: Hemophilia, AIDS, and the Survival of a Community* (Berkeley: University of California Press, 1999), 184–185. Conk, "Is There a Design Defect in the *Restatement (Third) of Torts: Products Liability?*" at 1114. Harden, *AIDS at 30: A History*, 93.

15. DePrince, *Cry Bloody Murder*, 154, 170; Ind. Code 16–41–12–11, 2016 ed.

16. Associated Press, "Travel Ban Lifted," *Kokomo Tribune*, October 31, 2009. Harden, *AIDS at 30: A History*, 93.

17. Maureen Groppe, "Questions Raised About Safety of Mill Property," *Kokomo Tribune*, July 8, 1990.

18. Indiana Department of Environmental Management, *First Five-Year Review Report for Continental Steel Superfund Site, City of Kokomo, Howard County, Indiana* (July 2002), 13; Scott Smith, "Continental Steel Cleanup Timeline from 1989–2007," *Kokomo Tribune*, December 1, 2007; IND001213503, NPL Fact Sheet, Region 5 Superfund, U.S. EPA, *Continental Steel Corp.*, http://www.epa.gov/region5/superfund/npl/indiana/IND001213503.html, accessed February 7, 2013.

19. *Kokomo Perspective*, October 26, 2005, http://kokomoperspective.com/salute_to_labor/operating-engineers-are-big-boys-with-big-toys/article_4f9f0f9b-8588-56ef-9c48-9e38f599f945.html, accessed March 30, 2014.

20. Scott Smith, "Continental Steel Still a Part of Kokomo," *Kokomo Tribune*, October 21, 2009. Former Continental employees continue to stage reunions every two years. "Continental Steel Reunion," *Kokomo Tribune*, August 5, 2012.

21. Andrew Hurley traces the evolution of other former plant sites from abandoned campuses to garbage disposal centers in New Jersey, Missouri, and California in "From Factory Town to Metropolitan Junkyard: Postindustrial Transitions on the Urban Periphery," *Environmental History* 21 (2016): 3–29; Scott Smith, "Walk the Line: Industrial Heritage Trail Follows the Tracks," *Kokomo Tribune*, June 26, 2011; Scott Smith, "City to Announce Continental Plans," *ibid.*, October 25, 2011; Scott Smith, "Goal! City Backs 60-Acre Soccer Complex," *ibid.*, October 26, 2011; Scott Smith, "City Officials Leery of Taking Property," *ibid.*, October 30, 2011. "Walkpaths & Trails," City of Kokomo, http://www.cityofkokomo.org/departments/walkpaths_and_trails.php, accessed August 31, 2014; "Solar Farm Coming to Kokomo," *Kokomo Perspective*, http://kokomoperspective.com/kp/solar-farm-coming-to-kokomo/-article_f3b35b1e-9a9f-11e4-a451-f3a7453701d1.html, accessed February 22, 2015; Associated Press, "Kokomo Solar Park Set to Operate Next Month," *Indianapolis Star*, November 21, 2016, p. 2A.

22. Steve Marshall, "Ryan White's Legacy; Son's Crusade Now Mother's," *USA Today*, June 27, 1990.

23. "News: Briefly," *USA Today*, September 5, 1990; "Vandalism at Ryan White's Grave," *Indianapolis Star*, September 27,

1990; Associated Press, "Ryan White's Grave Found Damaged," *Kokomo Tribune*, September 27, 1990; "News: Briefly," *USA Today*, September 27, 1990; Dennis Hevesi, "Parents Vow to Protest AIDS Student," *New York Times*, September 16, 1990; "Ryan's Smile Shines in Video at Colts Game," *Indianapolis Star*, December 23, 1990; "News: Passages, 1990," *USA Today*, December 27, 1990; *People*, December 31, 1990; White and Dworkin, *Weeding Out the Tears: A Mother's Story of Love, Loss, and Renewal*, 188–190.

24. White and Dworkin, *Weeding Out the Tears*, 151; Associated Press, "Ryan's Memory Lives On," *Kokomo Tribune*, April 6, 1991; *People*, April 8, 1991; "Gannett Journalists Win 3 Pulitzer Prizes," *USA Today*, May 3, 1991; "Best Sellers," The New York Times Book Review, *New York Times*, May 5, 1991; "Book is White's Own Story of Life With AIDS," and Kris Kinkade, "Sales Mixed on Ryan White's Book," *Kokomo Tribune*, March 24, 1991; Rob Schneider, "Vandals Strike Ryan White's Grave," *Indianapolis Star*, July 9, 1991; Steve Marshall, "News: Ryan White's Tombstone Toppled," *USA Today*, July 8, 1991; Associated Press, "Grave of Boy Who Led Fight On AIDS Bias Is Vandalized," *New York Times*, July 10, 1991.

25. Associated Press, "White Honored as Champ for AIDS," *Kokomo Tribune*, August 30, 1995; *Indianapolis Monthly* 21, no. 1 (Sep. 1997) at 140, 144; Achy Obejas, "Ryan's Town Remembers," *Chicago Tribune*, October 28, 1998.

26. Obejas, "Ryan's Town Remembers," *Chicago Tribune*, October 28, 1998.

27. *People*, March 15, 1999; *Indianapolis Monthly* 23, no. 4 (Dec. 1999), at 133; Danielle Gates Rush, "How Far Have We Come?" *Kokomo Tribune*, April 8, 2000; *People*, May 15, 2000.

28. Scott Smith, "The Year the Media Came to Town," *Kokomo Tribune*, September 24, 2006; Scott Smith, "Ryan White Court Battle Captivated Nation," *ibid.*, March 25, 2007; Ken de la Bastide, "Indianapolis Exhibit Will Feature Model of Ryan White's Bedroom," September 13, 2007; Ken de la Bastide, "Exhibit Taking Shape," *ibid.*, November 2, 2007; Ken de la Bastide, "Power of Children," *ibid.*, November 11, 2007.

29. "The History," The Children's Museum of Indianapolis, https://thehistory. childrensmuseum.org, accessed February 29, 2020; "Quick Facts About the Museum," https://thehistory.childrensmuseum.org/about/about-the-museum, accessed February 29, 2020.

30. White and Dworkin, *Weeding Out the Tears*, 178, 182; Donna S. Mullinix, "After the Heartache, Ryan's Mom Finds Love," *Indianapolis Star*, July 3, 1992; Kevin Morgan, "Ryan's Mom Celebrates New Starts," *ibid.*, August 2, 1992. Jeanne White Ginder, interview with author, October 25, 2012, Children's Museum of Indianapolis, Indianapolis, IN; Andrea Hughes, e-mail messages to author, October 15 and 16, 2012.

31. Jennifer Pace-Robinson, conversation with author, October 29, 2012; Andrea Hughes, e-mail messages to author, October 15 and 16, 2012.

32. Jennifer Pace-Robinson, conversation with author, October 29, 2012.

33. Alex Patton, e-mail message to author, November 1, 2012; Domenica Bongiovanni, "The Children's Museum Will Build the First Permanent Exhibit of Education Activist Malala," *Indianapolis Star*, January 8, 2020, https://www.indystar.com/story/entertainment/arts/2020/01/08/-malala-yousafzais-story-coming-childrens-museum-indianapolis/2835181001/, accessed February 29, 2020.

34. Jeanne White Ginder, interview with author, October 25, 2012, Children's Museum of Indianapolis, Indianapolis, IN.

35. Wanda Bilodeau, interview by Allen Safianow, June 7, 2011, transcript, Ryan White Project, Howard County Historical Society, Kokomo, IN.

36. Edward T. Linenthal, *The Unfinished Bombing: Oklahoma City in American Memory* (New York: Oxford University Press, 2001): see Chapter 3, "Telling the Story: Three Narratives," at 41–80, for a discussion of the progressive, redemptive, and toxic narratives he encountered among residents.

37. Casy Smith, "State Marker to Honor White and His Activism about AIDS," *Indianapolis Star*, August 7, 2019.

38. Allen Safianow, "Ryan White and Kokomo, Indiana: A City Remembers," *Traces of Indiana and Midwestern History* 25, no. 1 (Winter 2013), 16, 25. Lauren Fitch, "Howard County Hall of Legends 2014 Inductees," *Kokomo Tribune*, July 1, 2014.

39. Sanford Levinson, *Written in Stone: Public Monuments in Changing Societies* (Durham: Duke University Press, 1993), 130.

Bibliography

Primary Sources

Serials

NEWSPAPERS

Baltimore Sun
Boston Globe
Chicago Tribune
Fort Wayne Journal Gazette
Fort Wayne News Sentinel
[Hamilton] Heights Herald
Indianapolis News
Indianapolis Star
Kokomo Perspective

Kokomo Tribune
Los Angeles Times
New York Times
Oklahoman
Philadelphia Inquirer
The Times [of London]
USA Today
Wall Street Journal
Washington Post

MAGAZINES

"AFRAIDS," *The New Republic* 193, October 14, 1985: 7.

"AIDS Epidemic: The Price of Promiscuity," *Human Events* 43, no. 25 (June 18, 1983): 5.

Barker, Susan. "Profiles in Courage," *Indianapolis Monthly* 21, no. 1 (September 1997): 140–144.

Bell, Steve. "Look Back in Anger," *Indianapolis Monthly* 9, no. 11 (July 1986): 54–58, 104.

Gelman, David, et al. "The Social Fallout from an Epidemic," *Newsweek*, August 12, 1985: 28–29.

Godwin, Ronald S. "AIDS: A Moral and Political Time Bomb," *Moral Majority Report*, July 1983: 2.

"Hoosier 50: A Chronicle of Indiana's Most Memorable Sons and Daughters," *Indianapolis Monthly* 23, no. 4 (December 1999): 133.

"Jerry's Castle," *Forbes*, June 15, 1976: 21–23.

Kotkin, Joel. "A Commitment Forged in Steel," INC., June 1983: 82–93.

Langone, John. "Special Report: AIDS," *Discover* 6, December 1985: 28–53.

Leishman, Katie. "San Francisco: A Crisis in Public Health," *The Atlantic* 256, no. 4 (October 1985): 18–41.

"The New Victims," *Life*, July 1985.

People, August 3, 1987; August 24, 1987; May 30, 1988; June 20, 1988; July 11, 1988; April 23, 1990; May 14, 1990; December 31, 1990; April 8, 1991; March 15, 1999; May 5, 2000.

"Protecting the Hemophiliacs," *Saturday Evening Post* 260, no. 2 (March 1988): 100–101.

"R. Alan Brubaker: Judge with a Secret," *Indianapolis Monthly* 18, no. 6 (January 1995): 68.

Safianow, Allen. "Ryan White and Kokomo, Indiana: A City Remembers," TRACES *of Indiana and Midwestern History* 25, no. 1 (Winter 2013): 14–25.

Stall, Sam. "Living with AIDS," *Indianapolis Monthly* 9, no. 5 (January 1986): 35–38.

Swenson, Robert M. "Plagues, History, and AIDS," *American Scholar* 57, no. 2 (Spring 1988): 183–200.

Wallis, Claudia, et al. "AIDS: A Growing Threat," *Time*, August 12, 1985: 40–47.

Whitman, David. "To A Poster Child, Dying Young," *U.S. News & World Report*, April 16, 1990: 8.

"WWKI Presents the Popular 'Mike' Show: 'Male Call for the Ladies,'" *Our Town* 2, no. 1 (Spring, 1980): 3–6.

JOURNALS

AIDS Policy & Law 1, 1986, BNA, Buraff Publications.

Barnes, Joseph W. "Rochester and the Automobile Industry," *Rochester History* 43, nos. 2 and 3 (April and July 1981): 1–39.

Eisenberg, Leon. "The Genesis of Fear: AIDS and the Public's Response to Science," *Law, Medicine & Health Care* 14, no. 5–6 (December 1986): 243–249.

Fauci, Anthony S. "The Acquired Immune Deficiency Syndrome: The Ever-Broadening Clinical Spectrum," *JAMA* 249, no. 17 (May 6, 1983): 2375–2376.

Francis, Donald P. "Commentary: Deadly AIDS Policy Failure by the Highest Levels of the US Government: A Personal Look Back 30 Years Later for Lessons to Respond Better to Future Epidemics," *Journal of Public Health Policy* 33, no. 3 (2012): 290–300.

Friedland, Gerald H., Brian R. Saltzman, Martha F. Rogers, Patricia A. Kahl, Martin L. Lesser, Marguerite M. Mayers, and Robert S. Klein. "Lack of Transmission of HTLV-III/LAV Infection to Household Contacts of Patients with AIDS or AIDS-Related Complex with Oral Candidiasis," *New England Journal of Medicine* 314, no. 6 (February 6, 1986): 344–349.

"The Global AIDS Situation: WHO Update, January, 1988," *American Journal of Public Health* 78, no. 4 (April, 1988): 410.

Goldsmith, Marsha F. "Hemophilia, Beaten on One Front, Is Beset on Others," *JAMA* 256, no. 23 (Dec. 19, 1986): 3200.

Howell, G. A. "Waste Pickle Liquor Disposal," *Sewage and Industrial Waste* 29, no. 11 (Nov. 1957): 1278–1281.

Johnson, Robert E., Dale N. Lawrence, Bruce L. Evatt, Dennis J. Bregman, Lawrence D. Zyla, James W. Curran, Louis M. Aledort, M. Elaine Eyster, Alan P. Brownstein, and Charles J. Carman, "Acquired Immune Deficiency Syndrome Among Patients Attending Hemophilia Treatment Centers and Mortality Experience of Hemophiliacs in the United States," *American Journal of Epidemiology* 121, no. 6 (June 1985): 797–810.

Kirp, David L. "Uncommon Decency: Pacific Bell Responds to AIDS," *Harvard Business Review* 67, no. 3 (May-June 1989): 140–151.

Lusher, Jeanne M. "Hemophilia: From Plasma to Recombinant Factors." American Society of Hematology. Accessed February 28, 2013. http://www.hematology.org/publications/50-years-in-hematology/4737.aspx.

Nelkin, Dorothy, and Stephen Hilgartner. "Disputed Dimensions of Risk: A Public School Controversy over AIDS," *The Milbank Quarterly* 64, Supplement 1. AIDS: The Public Context of an Epidemic (1986): 118–142.

Oleske, James, Anthony Minnefor, Roger Cooper, Kathleen Thomas, Antonio dela Cruz, Houman Abdieh, Isabel Guerrero, Vijay V. Joshi, and Franklin Desposito. "Immune Deficiency Syndrome in Children," *JAMA* 249, no. 17 (May 6, 1983): 2345–2349.

Pauling, Linus. "Reflections on the New Biology: Foreword," *UCLA Law Review* 15, no. 2 (1967–1968): 267–272.

Pierce, Glenn F., Jeanne M. Lusher, Alan P. Brownstein, Jonathan C. Goldsmith, and Craig M. Kessler. "The Use of Purified Clotting Factor Concentrates in Hemophilia: Influence of Viral Safety, Cost, and Supply on Therapy," *JAMA* 261, no. 23 (June 16, 1989): 3434–3438.

Ragni, Margaret V. "Medical Aspects of Hemophilia and AIDS," FOCUS: *A Guide to AIDS Research* 4, no. 5 (April 1989): 1–2.

Scheerhorn, Dirk. "Hemophilia in the Days of AIDS: Communicative Tensions Surrounding 'Associated Stigmas,'" *Communication Research* 17, no. 6 (Dec. 1990): 842–847.

Schwarz, Jr., Frederick A. O., and Frederick P. Schaffer. "AIDS in the Classroom," *Hofstra Law Review* 14, no. 1 (Fall 1985): 163–191.

Oral History Collections

Howard County Historical Society

Continental Steel Corporation: Steve Daily
Ryan White Project: Paula Adair, Alan Adler, Bev Ashcraft, Rita Bagby, Wanda Bilodeau, Daniel Carter, Ronald Colby, Ken Ferries, Donald Fields, Frances Sempsel Hardin, Mitzie Johnson, Chantel Kebrdle, Ruth Lawson, Jeri Malone, William Narwold, Ray (Bud) Probasco, Arletta Reith, David Rosselot, John Wiles, and Harold Williams

Government Documents

Constitutions

Indiana Constitution of 1851, Article 8

Cases & Statutes

Scott Bogart, b/n/f Daniel R. Bogart et al. v. Ryan White, b/n/f Jeanne White and Jeanne White, No. 49192 (Howard Cir. Ct., Ind. 1986)
Bogart, et al. v. Howard County Board of Health, No. 49192 (Howard Cir. Ct., Ind. 1986)
Bogart et al. v. White et al., No. 86–144 (Clinton Cir. Ct., Ind. 1986)
Bowers v. Hardwick, 478 U.S. 186 (1986)
District 27 Community School Board v. Board of Education, 130 Misc. 2d 398, 502 N.Y.S. 2d 325 (Sup. Ct. 1986)
In re Factor VIII or IX Concentrate Blood Products Litigation, 169 F.R.D. 632 (N.D. Ill. 1996)
In the Matter of: Rhone-Poulenc Rorer Incorporated, et al., 51 F. 3d 1293 (7th Cir. 1995) *JKB, Sr., and VB v. Armour Pharmaceutical Company, Cutter Laboratories, Division of Miles, Inc., Baxter Healthcare Corporation, and Alpha Therapeutics Corporation,* 660 N.E. 2d 602 (Ind. Ct. App. 1996)
Lawrence v. Texas, 539 U.S. 558 (2003)
Ryan White b/n/f/ Jeanne White v. Western School Corporation et al., IP 85–1192-C (S. D. Ind. 1985, 1986), U.S. Dist. Lexis 16540
State of Indiana v. R. Alan Brubaker, No. 06D019407CF-39 (Boone Sup. Ct. 1, Ind. 1994)
Wadleigh v. Rhone-Poulenc Rorer, Inc., Armour Pharmaceutical Company, Inc., Miles, Inc., Baxter Healthcare Corporation, Alpha Therapeutic Corporation, and National Hemophilia Foundation, 157 F.R.D. 410 (N.D. Ill. 1994)
Education for All Handicapped Children Act, Public Law 94–142
Ind. Code 16–1–9–7, -8, -9, 1985 ed.
Ind. Code 16–8–7–2, 1982 ed.
Ind. Code 16–41–12–11, 2016 ed.
Rehabilitation Act of 1973, Public Law 93–112

Centers for Disease Control and Prevention (CDC) Morbidity and Mortality Weekly Report (MMWR)

"A Cluster of Kaposi's Sarcoma and Pneumocystis carinii Pneumonia among Homosexual Male Residents of Los Angeles and Orange Counties, California," *MMWR* 31, no. 23 (June 18, 1982): 305–307.
Curran, James W., and Harold W. Jaffe. "AIDS: The Early Years and CDC's Response," *MMWR* 60, Supplement (October 7, 2011): 64–69.
"Current Trends Education and Foster Care of Children Infected with Human T-Lymphotropic Virus Type III/Lymphadenopathy-Associated Virus," *MMWR* 34, no. 34 (August 30, 1985): 517–521.

"Current Trends Prevention of Acquired Immune Deficiency Syndrome (AIDS): Report of Inter-Agency Recommendations," *MMWR* 32, no. 8 (March 4, 1983): 101–103.

"Current Trends Update on Acquired Immune Deficiency Syndrome (AIDS)—United States," *MMWR* 31, no. 37 (September 24, 1982): 507–508; 513–514.

"Current Trends Update: Acquired Immunodeficiency Syndrome (AIDS)—United States," *MMWR* 33, no. 47 (November 30, 1984): 661–664.

"Current Trends Update: Acquired Immunodeficiency Syndrome (AIDS)—United States," *MMWR* 35, no. 2 (January 17, 1986): 17–21.

"Epidemiologic Notes and Reports *Pneumocystis carinii* Pneumonia among Persons with Hemophilia A," *MMWR* 31, no. 27 (July 16, 1982), 365–367.

"Epidemiologic Notes and Reports Possible Transfusion-Associated Acquired Immune Deficiency Syndrome (AIDS)—California," *MMWR* 31, no. 48 (December 10, 1982): 652–654.

"Update: Acquired Immunodeficiency Syndrome (AIDS) in Persons with Hemophilia," *MMWR* 33, no. 42 (October 26, 1984): 589–591.

"Update on Acquired Immune Deficiency Syndrome (AIDS) among Patients with Hemophilia A," *MMWR* 31, no. 48 (December 10, 1982): 644–646; 652.

Indiana State Archives, Commission on Public Records

State Board of Health, Commissioners File, Commissioner's Correspondence
State Board of Health, Executive Board Minutes & Reports
State Board of Health, Woodrow Myers Correspondence, Commissioners Files

Indiana Department of Environmental Management

Indiana Department of Environmental Management. *First Five-Year Review Report for Continental Steel Superfund Site, City of Kokomo, Howard County, Indiana.* July 2002. Accessed March 21, 2013. http://www.epa.gov/region5/superfund/fiveyear/reviews_pdf/indiana/continental_steel.pdf.

National Archives and Records Administration

Ronald Reagan Presidential Library. Transcript of the President's News Conference, September 17, 1985. Accessed August 14, 2012. http://www.reagan.utexas.edu/archives/speeches/1985/91785c.htm.

United States Department of Commerce

Bureau of the Census. *1980 Census of Population and Housing, Census Tracts, Kokomo, Ind. Standard Metropolitan Statistical Area* (Washington, D.C.: U.S. Department of Commerce, Bureau of the Census, 1983): Tables P-2 and P-3.

United States Department of Health and Human Services

Health Resources and Services Administration. "Mom, I Want to Go to School," Transcript of audio recording of Jeanne White Ginder, The HIV/AIDS Program: Who Was Ryan White? Accessed October 26, 2014. http://hab.hrsa.gov/abouthab/ryanwhite.html.

U.S. National Library of Medicine, National Institutes of Health. "ELISA: MedlinePlus Medical Encyclopedia." Accessed February 6, 2013. http://www.nlm.nih.gov/medlineplus/ency/article/003332.htm.

_____. "ELISA/Western blot tests for HIV." Accessed July 13, 2014. http://www.nlm.nih.gov/medlineplus/ency/article/003538.htm.

United States Environmental Protection Agency

United States Environmental Protection Agency. "Health Effects of PCBs." Accessed February 2, 2014. http://www.epa.gov/osw/hazard/tsd/pcbs/pubs/effects.htm.

_____. *First Five-Year Review Report*, "NPL Fact Sheet, Region 5 Superfund, US EPA, *Continental Steel Corp.*" Accessed February 7, 2013. http://www.epa.gov/region5/superfund/npl/indiana/IND001213503.html.
_____. "NPL Site Narrative for Continental Steel Corp." Accessed February 13, 2013. http://www.epa.gov/superfund/sites/npl/nar1164.htm.
_____. Region 5 Cleanup Sites, "Continental Steel." Accessed February 4, 2013. http://www.epa.gov/region5/cleanup/continental/index.html.

UNITED STATES SECURITIES AND EXCHANGE COMMISSION
United States Securities and Exchange Commission Form 10-Q, filed May 13, 1996, Rhone-Poulenc Rorer, Inc. Accessed March 30, 2014. http://www.sec.gov/Archives/edgar/containers/fix041/217028/0000217028-96-00014.txt.

Manuscripts and Archival Materials

Boise, Glen R. *A Land Use Plan for the City of Kokomo, Indiana*. Kokomo: Kokomo-Howard County Plan Commission, 1976.
Continental Steel Corporation. *Getting Acquainted with Steel and Continental*. Kokomo, IN: Continental Steel Corporation, 1947.
Cummings, Christopher Todd. "A Case Study of the Fan Letters of Ryan White: The Stigma of Disclosure." PhD diss., Indiana State University, 2008. ISU Thesis Collection, RC606.55. A95 C86 2008.
Sparks, Charlie, ed. *Kokomo: City of Firsts*. Kokomo, IN: Kokomo Development Corp., 1982.

CHILDREN'S MUSEUM OF INDIANAPOLIS
Ryan White Collection

WESTERN MIDDLE SCHOOL, RUSSIAVILLE, INDIANA
Library Collection

HOWARD COUNTY HISTORICAL SOCIETY
Jeri Malone Collection
Ken Ferries Collection

HOWARD COUNTY PUBLIC LIBRARY
Howard County Memory Project Digital Collection

Books and Memoirs

Black, David. *The Plague Years: A Chronicle of AIDS, the Epidemic of Our Times*. London: Picador/Pan Books, 1985, 1986.
Decker, Shawn. "A Boy, a Virus, and the Education of a Community," *The Times Gone By*, January 15, 2014. Accessed January 20, 2014. http://www.waynesboroheritagefoundation.com/boy-virus-education-community.
_____. *My Pet Virus: The True Story of a Rebel Without a Cure*. New York: Penguin, 2006.
DePrince, Elaine. *Cry Bloody Murder: A Tale of Tainted Blood*. New York: Random House, 1997.
Griggs, John, ed. *AIDS: Public Policy Dimensions*. New York: United Hospital Fund of New York, 1987.
Hoyle, Jay. MARK: *How a Boy's Courage in Facing AIDS Inspired a Town and the Town's Compassion Lit Up a Nation*. South Bend, IN: Langford Books, 1988.
John, Elton. *Love Is the Cure: On Life, Loss, and the End of AIDS*. New York: Little, Brown, 2012.

Jones, Cleve, and Jeff Dawson. *Stitching a Revolution: The Making of an Activist.* New York: HarperCollins, 2000, 2001.

Kessler, Judy. *Inside People: The Stories Behind the Stories.* New York: Villard Books, 1994.

Kirp, David L., Steven Epstein, Marlene Strong Franks, Jonathan Simon, Douglas Conaway, and John Lewis. *Learning by Heart: AIDS and Schoolchildren in America's Communities.* New Brunswick, NJ: Rutgers University Press, 1989.

Koop, C. Everett. *Koop: The Memoirs of America's Family Doctor.* New York: Random House, 1991.

Scannell, Kate. *Death of the Good Doctor: Lessons from the Heart of the AIDS Epidemic.* San Francisco: Cleis Press, 1999.

Shilts, Randy. *And the Band Played On: Politics, People, and the AIDS Epidemic.* New York: St. Martin's, 1987, 2007.

Strub, Sean. *Body Counts: A Memoir of Politics, Sex, AIDS, and Survival.* New York: Scribner's, 2014.

Sullivan, Robert G. "*District 27 v. Board of Education,*" in John Griggs, ed., *AIDS: Public Policy Dimensions.* New York: United Hospital Fund of New York, 1987: 69–76.

Tarkington, Booth. *The Works of Booth Tarkington, vol. XXIII: The World Does Move.* Garden City, NY: Doubleday, Doran & Co., 1928, 1932.

White, Jeanne, and Susan Dworkin. *Weeding Out the Tears: A Mother's Story of Love, Loss, and Renewal.* New York: Avon Books, 1997.

White, Ryan, and Ann Marie Cunningham. *Ryan White: My Own Story.* New York: Signet, 1992.

Podcasts

BBC World Service, *Witness* Archive 2011, "Witness: Ryan White," podcast audio, December 1, 2011, interview with Wanda Bilodeau. http://downloads.bbc.co.uk/podcasts/worldservice/witness/witness_20111201-0900a.mp.3.

Websites

Academy of Motion Picture Arts and Sciences. "The 62nd Academy Awards—1990." Accessed February 21, 2015. http://www.oscars.org/oscars/ceremonies/1990.

Associated Press AP News Archive. "AIDS-Infected Boy to Be Taught at Home in Wake of Threats." September 10, 1987. Accessed February 21, 2015. http://www.apnewsarchive.com/1987/AIDS-Infected-Boy-To-Be-Taught-At-Home-In-Wake-of-Threats/id-2706dda8e5ae7d0d0bf657f4b10f630d.

_____. "Group That Fought AIDS Victim Ryan White Will Announce National Organization." September 5, 1986. Accessed May 21, 2013. http://www.apnewsarchive.com/1986/Group-That-Fought-AIDS-Victim-Ryan-White-Will-Announce-National-Organization/id-c0a3c751f6bac6968a89c1443b0e6d4a.

Baxter. "Company Profile: History." Accessed November 29, 2012. http://www.baxter.com/about_baxter/company_profile/history.html.

Bowling Green State University Journalism. "1990 Borgman Cartoons Reduced." Accessed September 11, 2016. http://bgsujournalism.com/pulitzer/jfoust/wordpress/wp-content/uploads/2016/01/1990-Borgman-Cartoons-reduced.pdf

The Children's Museum of Indianapolis. "Our History." Accessed February 29, 2020. https://thehistory.childrensmuseum.org/about/about-the-museum.

City of Kokomo. "Walkpaths & Trails." Accessed August 31, 2014. http://www.cityofkokomo.org/departments/walkpaths_and_trails.php.

Forbes. "Woodrow Myers Profile." Accessed February 20, 2013. http://www.forbes.com/profile/woodrow-myers/ (profile no longer available).

General Motors Heritage Center. "Generations of GM." Accessed January 15, 2013. https://history.gmheritagecenter.com/wiki/index.php/1936-1996_Delco_Electronics_60th_Anniversary_Video.

Haynes International. "Haynes Heritage—80 Years Plus of Innovative Metallurgy." Accessed December 19, 2012. www.haynesintl.com/Heritage.htm.

Howard County Memory Project. "Ryan White: Howard County Board of Health, 1986–02–13." Accessed April 17, 2012. http://www.howardcountymemory.net/item. aspx?details=23446.

_____. "Ryan White: Kokomo Tribune 1986–02–26 page 1c." Accessed July 12, 2012. http:// www.howardcountymemory.net/item.aspx?details=23719.

Kokomo Perspective. "Nothin' Like 1950s Lunch Counters." November 2, 2005. Accessed February 22, 2015. http://kokomoperspective.com/generations/nothin-like-s-lunch-counters/-article_49bee847-eb0d-52ba-b29d-f251e4573eb5.html.

_____. "Salute to Labor." October 26, 2005. Accessed March 30, 2014. http:// kokomoperspective.com/salute_to_labor/operating-engineers-are-big-boys-with-big-toys/article_4f9f0f9b-8588-56ef-9c48-9e38f599f945.html.

_____. "Solar Farm Coming to Kokomo." January 13, 2015. Accessed February 22, 2015. http://kokomoperspective.com/kp/solar-farm-coming-to-kokomo/article_f3b35b1e-9a9f-11e4-a451-f3a7453701d1.html.

The Living Room Candidate. "The Living Room Candidate-Commercials-1984-Prouder, Stronger, Better." Accessed August 25, 2016. www.livingroomcandidate.org/ commercials/1984/prouder-stronger-better.

National Hemophilia Foundation. "History of Bleeding Disorders." Accessed August 28, 2012. https://www.hemophilia.org/Bleeding-Disorders/History-of-Bleeding-Disorders.

National Institutes of Health. "The NIH Almanac: Chronology of Events." Accessed February 21, 2015. http://nih.gov/abouthttp://nih.gov/about/almanac/historical/chronology_of_ events.htm#nineteenthirty.

The Oklahoman/NewsOK. "Sheffield Buys Joliet." Accessed February 12, 2013. http://newsok. com/article/2158296, Archive ID: 279964.

People Online Archives. "Breaking America's Heart: Aug. 3, 1987." Accessed March 4, 2012. http://www.people.com/people/archive/issue/0,,7566870803,00.html.

_____. "Candle in the Wind: Apr. 23, 1990." Accessed March 4, 2012. http://www.people.com/ people/archive/issue/0,,7566900423,00.html.

The Recording Academy. "Winners—Dionne Warwick." Accessed May 23, 2013. http://www. grammy.com/nominees/search?artist=dionne+warwick&field_nominee_work_value=%2 2That%27s+What+Friends+Are+For%22&year=1986&genre=All.

Swansea Schools. "Mark G. Hoyle Elementary." Accessed May 23, 2013. http://hoyle. swanseaschools.org.

United Steelworkers Local 12–369. "Past/Current International Presidents." Accessed February 4, 2013. http://www.uswl2-369.org/?ID=22.

Worcester Polytechnic Institute. "Profiles in Innovation: Stainless Steel, Invented by Elwood Haynes, Class of 1881." Accessed January 8, 2013. http://www.wpi.edu/about/history/steel. html.

WWKI-WE CARE. "History." Accessed October 1, 2012. http://www.wecareonline.com/files/ history.html.

Secondary Sources

Aamidor, Abe, and Ted Evanoff. *At the Crossroads: Middle America and the Battle to Save the Car Industry.* Toronto: ECW Press, 2010.

Abraham, Julie. *Metropolitan Lovers: The Homosexuality of Cities.* Minneapolis: University of Minnesota Press, 2009.

Alonzo, Angelo A., and Nancy R. Reynolds. "Stigma, HIV and AIDS: An Exploration and Elaboration of a Stigma Trajectory," *Social Science & Medicine* 41, no. 3 (1995): 303–315.

Babson, Steve. *The Unfinished Struggle: Turning Points in American Labor, 1877-Present.* Critical Issues in History Series. Lanham, MD: Rowman & Littlefield, 1999.

Baldwin, Peter. "Beyond Weak and Strong: Rethinking the State in Comparative Policy History," *Journal of Policy History* 17, no. 1 (2005): 12–33.

Beauregard, Robert A. *Voices of Decline: The Postwar Fate of U. S. Cities,* second ed. New York: Routledge, 2003.

Bellah, Robert N., Richard Madsen, William M. Sullivan, Ann Swidler, and Steven M. Tipton. *Habits of the Heart: Individualism and Commitment in American Life*. Berkeley: University of California Press, 1985, 1996, 2008.

Bender, Thomas M. *Community and Social Change in America*. Baltimore: Johns Hopkins University Press, 1978.

Bluestone, Barry, and Bennett Harrison. *The Deindustrialization of America: Plant Closings, Community Abandonment, and the Dismantling of Basic Industry*. New York: Basic Books, 1982.

Brandt, Allan M. *No Magic Bullet: A Social History of Venereal Disease in the United States Since 1880*. New York: Oxford University Press, 1987.

Brier, Jennifer. *Infectious Ideas: U. S. Political Responses to the AIDS Crisis*. Chapel Hill: University of North Carolina Press, 2009.

———. "'Save Our Kids, Keep AIDS Out': Anti-AIDS Activism and the Legacy of Community Control in Queens, New York," *Journal of Social History* 39, no. 4 (Summer 2006): 965–987.

Brown, Michael P. *RePlacing Citizenship: AIDS Activism and Radical Democracy*. Mappings: Society/Theory/Space Series. New York: Guilford Press, 1997.

Castells, Manuel. *The City and the Grassroots: A Cross-Cultural Theory of Urban Social Movements*. Berkeley: University of California Press, 1983.

Chase, Sophia. "The Bloody Truth: Examining America's Blood Industry and Its Tort Liability Through the Arkansas Prison Plasma Scandal," *William & Mary Business Law Review* 3, no. 2 (2012): 597–644.

Cohen, Cathy J. *The Boundaries of Blackness: AIDS and the Breakdown of Black Politics*. Chicago: University of Chicago Press, 1999.

Conk, George W. "Is There a Design Defect in the *Restatement (Third) of Torts: Products Liability*?" *Yale Law Journal* 109 (1999–2000): 1087–1133.

Cowie, Jefferson. *Capital Moves: RCA's Seventy-Year Quest for Cheap Labor*. New York: The New Press, 1999, 2001.

Cowie, Jefferson, and Joseph Heathcott, eds. *Beyond the Ruins: The Meanings of Deindustrialization*. Ithaca, NY: ILR Press, 2003.

Curran, James W. and Harold W. Jaffe. "AIDS: The Early Years and CDC's Response," *MMWR* 60, Supple,ment (October 7, 2011): 64–69.

Dandaneau, Steven P. *A Town Abandoned: Flint, Michigan, Confronts Deindustrialization*. SUNY Series in Popular Culture and Political Change. Albany: State University of New York Press, 1996.

De Santis, Vincent P. *The Shaping of Modern America: 1877–1920*, Third ed. Wheeling, IL: Harlan Davidson, 2000.

Douglas, Mary. *Purity and Danger: An Analysis of Concept of Pollution and Taboo*. London: Routledge, 1966, 2002.

Edelman, Lee. *No Future: Queer Theory and the Death Drive*. Durham: Duke University Press, 2004.

Epstein, Steven. *Impure Science: AIDS, Activism, and the Politics of Knowledge*. Medicine and Society Series. Berkeley: University of California Press, 1996.

Fanning, Patricia J. *Influenza and Inequality: One Town's Tragic Response to the Great Epidemic of 1918*. Amherst: University of Massachusetts Press, 2010.

Fee, Elizabeth, and Daniel M. Fox, eds. *AIDS: The Burdens of History*. Berkeley: University of California Press, 1988.

———, and ———, eds. *AIDS: The Making of a Chronic Disease*. Berkeley: University of California Press, 1992.

Feldman, Douglas A., ed. *Culture and AIDS*. New York: Praeger, 1990.

Feldman, Eric A., and Ronald Bayer, eds. *Blood Feuds: AIDS, Blood, and the Politics of Medical Disaster*. New York: Oxford University Press, 1999.

Franchini, Massimo. "Plasma-derived versus recombinant Factor VIII concentrates for the treatment of haemophilia A: recombinant is better," *Blood Transfusion* 8, no. 4 (2010): 292–296.

Franklin, Marc A. "Tort Liability for Hepatitis: An Analysis and a Proposal," *Stanford Law Review* 24 (1971–1972): 439–480.

Glass, James A. "The Gas Boom in East Central Indiana," *Indiana Magazine of History* 96, no. 4 (Dec. 2000): 313–335.

Goffman, Erving. *Stigma: Notes on the Management of Spoiled Identity*. New York: Simon & Schuster, 1963, 1986.

Gould, Deborah B. *Moving Politics: Emotion and ACTUP's Fight Against AIDS*. Chicago: University of Chicago Press, 2009.

Grmek, Mirko D. *History of AIDS: Emergence and Origin of a Modern Pandemic*. Translated by Russell C. Maulitz and Jacalyn Duffin. Princeton, NJ: Princeton University Press, 1990.

Harden, Victoria A. *AIDS at 30: A History*. Washington, D.C.: Potomac Books, 2012.

Harvey, David. *A Brief History of Neoliberalism*. Oxford: Oxford University Press, 2005.

Hensler, Deborah R., Nicholas M. Pace, Bonnie Dombey-Moore, Elizabeth Giddens, Jennifer Gross, and Erik Moller. *Class Action Dilemmas: Pursuing Public Goals for Private Gain*. Santa Monica, CA: RAND, 2000.

High, Steven. *Industrial Sunset: The Making of North America's Rust Belt, 1969–1984*. Toronto: University of Toronto Press, 2003.

High, Steven, and David W. Lewis. *Corporate Wasteland: The Landscape and Memory of Deindustrialization*. Ithaca, NY: ILR Press, 2007.

Hoerr, John P. *And the Wolf Finally Came: The Decline of the American Steel Industry*. Pittsburgh: University of Pittsburgh Press, 1988.

Hurley, Andrew. "From Factory Town to Metropolitan Junkyard: Postindustrial Transitions on the Urban Periphery," *Environmental History* 21 (2016): 3–29.

Ingram, G.I.C. "The History of Haemophilia," *Journal of Clinical Pathology* 29 (1976): 469–479.

Johnson, Heather M. "Resolution of Mass Product Liability Litigation Within the Federal Rules: A Case for the Increased Use of Rule 23(b)(3) Class Actions," *Fordham Law Review* 64, no. 5 (1996): 2329–2379.

Leveton, Lauren B., Harold C. Sox, Jr., and Michael A. Stoto, eds. *HIV and the Blood Supply: An Analysis of Crisis Decisionmaking*. Washington, D.C.: National Academy Press, 1995.

Levinson, Sanford. *Written in Stone: Public Monuments in Changing Societies*. Public Planet Books. Durham: Duke University Press, 1998.

Lichtenstein, Nelson. *State of the Union: A Century of American Labor*, rev. ed. Princeton: Princeton University Press, 2013.

Linenthal, Edward T. *The Unfinished Bombing: Oklahoma City in American Memory*. New York: Oxford University Press, 2001.

Linkon, Sherry Lee, and John Russo. *Steeltown U.S.A.: Work and Memory in Youngstown*. Lawrence: University Press of Kansas, 2002.

Lipset, Seymour Martin, and William Schneider. *The Confidence Gap: Business, Labor, and Government in the Public Mind*, rev. ed. Baltimore: Johns Hopkins University Press, 1987.

Longworth, Richard C. *Caught in the Middle: America's Heartland in the Age of Globalism*. New York: Bloomsbury, 2008, 2009.

Lynd, Robert S., and Helen Merrell Lynd. *Middletown: A Study in Modern American Culture*. New York: Harcourt, Brace, 1929, 1956.

Madison, James H. *Indiana Through Tradition and Change: A History of the Hoosier State and Its People, 1920–1945*. The History of Indiana Series, Vol. 5. Indianapolis: Indiana Historical Society, 1982.

Maharidge, Dale, and Michael S. Williamson. *Journey to Nowhere: The Saga of the New Underclass*. New York: Hyperion, 1985, 1996.

_____, and _____. *Someplace Like America: Tales from the New Great Depression*. Berkeley: University of California Press, 2011.

Mannucci, Pier Mannuccio. "Plasma-derived versus recombinant factor VIII concentrates for the treatment of haemophilia A: plasma-derived is better," *Blood Transfusion* 8, no. 4 (2010): 288–291.

Martin, Bradford. *The Other Eighties: A Secret History of America in the Age of Reagan*. New York: Hill and Wang, 2011.

McKay, Richard A. *Patient Zero and the Making of the AIDS Epidemic*. Chicago: University of Chicago Press, 2017.

Milkman, Ruth. *Farewell to the Factory: Auto Workers in the Late Twentieth Century.* Berkeley: University of California Press, 1997.

Miller, Michael J. "Strict Liability, Negligence and the Standard of Care for Transfusion-Transmitted Disease," *Arizona Law Review* 36 (1994): 473–513.

Palfrey, Judith S., Terence Fenton, Alison T. Lavin, Stephanie M Porter, Deirdre M. Shaw, Kenneth S. Weill, and Allen C. Crocker. "Schoolchildren with HIV Infection: A Survey of the Nation's Largest School Districts," *Journal of School Health* 64, no. 1 (Jan. 1994): 22–26.

Papke, David Ray. "The American Legal Faith: Traditions, Contradictions and Possibilities," *Ind. L. Rev.* 30, no. 3 (1997): 645–657.

Parmet, Wendy E. and Daniel J. Jackson. "No Longer Disabled: The Legal Impact of the New Social Construction of HIV," *American Journal of Law and Medicine* 23, no. 1 (1997): 7–43.

Patton, Cindy. *Inventing AIDS.* New York: Routledge, 1990.

Pemberton, Stephen. *The Bleeding Disease: Hemophilia and the Unintended Consequences of Medical Progress.* Baltimore: Johns Hopkins University Press, 2011.

Pepin, Jacques. *The Origins of AIDS.* Cambridge: Cambridge University Press, 2011.

Quam, Michael D. "The Sick Role, Stigma, and Pollution: The Case of AIDS," in Douglas A. Feldman, ed. *Culture and AIDS.* New York: Praeger, 1990: 29–44.

Resnik, Susan. *Blood Saga: Hemophilia, AIDS, and the Survival of a Community.* Berkeley: University of California Press, 1999.

Rich, Adrienne. "Power," in *The Dream of a Common Language: Poems 1974–1977.* New York: W.W. Norton, 1978, 2013.

Rosenberg, Charles E. "What is an Epidemic? AIDS in Historical Perspective," in *Explaining Epidemics and Other Studies in the History of Medicine.* New York: Cambridge University Press, 1992: 278–292.

Rueda, Andres. "Rethinking Blood Shield Statutes in View of the Hepatitis C Pandemic and Other Emerging Threats to the Blood Supply," *Journal of Health Law* 34, no. 3 (Summer, 2001): 419–458.

Scheuerman, William. *The Steel Crisis: The Economics and Politics of a Declining Industry.* New York: Praeger, 1986.

Scott, James C. *Domination and the Arts of Resistance: Hidden Transcripts.* New Haven: Yale University Press, 1990.

Sennett, Richard. *Flesh and Stone: The Body and the City in Western Civilization.* New York: W.W. Norton, 1994, 1996.

Shah, Nayan. *Contagious Divides: Epidemics and Race in San Francisco's Chinatown.* Berkeley: University of California Press, 2001.

Starr, Douglas. *Blood: An Epic History of Medicine and Commerce.* New York: Alfred A. Knopf, 1998.

Sugrue, Thomas J. *The Origins of the Urban Crisis: Race and Inequality in Postwar Detroit.* Princeton Studies in American Politics. Princeton: Princeton University Press, 1996, 2005.

Teaford, Jon C. *Cities of the Heartland: The Rise and Fall of the Industrial Midwest.* Midwestern History and Culture Series. Bloomington: Indiana University Press, 1993, 1994.

Tiemeyer, Phil. *Plane Queer: Labor, Sexuality, and AIDS in the History of Male Flight Attendants.* Berkeley: University of California Press, 2013.

Titmuss, Richard M. *The Gift Relationship: From Human Blood to Social Policy.* New York: Pantheon Books, 1971.

Wailoo, Keith. *Dying in the City of the Blues: Sickle Cell Anemia and the Politics of Race and Health.* Studies in Social Medicine Series. Chapel Hill: University of North Carolina Press, 2001.

_____. *Pain: A Political History.* Baltimore: Johns Hopkins University Press, 2014.

_____. "Stigma, Race, and Disease in 20th Century America," *The Lancet* 367 (February 11, 2006): 531–533.

Waldby, Catherine. *AIDS and the Body Politic: Biomedicine and Sexual Difference.* Writing Corporealities Series. London: Routledge, 1996.

Index